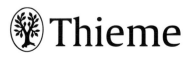

Chinese Herbal Medicine

The Formulas of Dr. John H.F. Shen

Leon I. Hammer, MD

Founder
Dragon Rises College of Oriental Medicine
Gainesville, Florida
USA

Hamilton Rotte, MSTCM, AP

Dragon Rises College of Oriental Medicine
Gainesville, Florida
USA

With contributions by
Ray Rubio, DAOM, LAc, FABORM

24 illustrations

Thieme
Stuttgart · New York

Library of Congress Cataloging-in-Publication Data is available from the publisher.

Illustrator: Laisha Canner, AP, MAOM, Gainesville, Florida, USA

© 2013 Georg Thieme Verlag KG,
Rüdigerstrasse 14, 70469 Stuttgart, Germany
http://www.thieme.de
Thieme Medical Publishers, Inc., 333 Seventh Avenue,
New York, NY 10001, USA
http://www.thieme.com

Cover design: Thieme Publishing Group
Typesetting by SOMMER media GmbH & Co. KG,
Feuchtwangen, Germany
Printed in Germany by Grafisches Centrum Cuno, Calbe

ISBN 978-3-13-150071-7
eISBN 978-3-13-169721-9

Foreword

Numerous schools of thought and various methods are found within the vast historical tradition of Chinese medicine…
It sustains itself in part by adjusting to changing conditions and will continue to develop differently in each country and era in
relation to the social demands and belief systems that prevail there.

(Beinfield H, Korngold, E. Between Heaven and Earth: A Guide to Chinese Medicine. New York: Ballantine; 1991:xiv)

Chinese medicine was just beginning to join the greater social, cultural, and medical landscape of US health care in the 1980s. Only a few acupuncture colleges were established by this time in the coastal cities in which the largest Chinese immigrant communities had settled a century earlier.

Doctors from China began immigrating to the United States in the mid-1970s to become licensed acupuncture practitioners. They brought with them practical experience and systematic training in both conventional Western medicine and what is now known as Traditional Chinese Medicine or TCM. Formulated in the 1950s, TCM was the product of a government initiative to reexamine, reframe, homogenize, and standardize traditional medical knowledge in accord with the principles of modern scientific medicine and the prevailing political ideology of China. TCM is a 20th-century reinvention.

In the last 20 years, US students, teachers, practitioners, and researchers have been gaining a greater appreciation of the enormously diverse historical currents in Chinese traditional health care—thanks primarily to the work of Western scholars who have published the results of their anthropological, historical, and linguistic investigations. As a result, we are beginning to fathom, value, and gain access to knowledge transmitted over generations by families and communities outside of and in parallel with officially approved Chinese medical curricula.

Dr. John Shen was initiated into a 17th-century medical tradition known as the Menghe lineage. In 1971 he brought this knowledge tradition with him to the United States. Not only was he a transporter of the Menghe current, he was himself an ingenious innovator who readily tailored what he knew to the conditions and the people he encountered here. I believe that he saw in Leon Hammer an enlightened physician devoted to seeking the comprehension and skill that would enable him to be ever more efficacious in his medical mission.

No doubt it was Dr. Hammer's ardent pursuit of Chinese medicine teachings that led him, as if by chance, to an encounter with Dr. John Shen in the early 1970s. The result of this fortuitous meeting between men with entirely different cultural and medical backgrounds is that we are offered an entrée into the Menghe current. The opportunity to explore, incorporate, and shape this tradition of knowledge and practice to the context of our lives is ours to choose. In accepting this offer, are we not called upon to develop our own current and our own tradition? I believe this is what Drs. Shen and Hammer had in mind.

Because of his diligence, perseverance, fertile imagination, and critical intelligence, Leon Hammer recognized the authenticity of John Shen's insight and the depth of his skill. He was determined to acquire and absorb as much as he could and then pass it on to the rest of us. Along with his students—and I am proud to be one—and the teachers he has trained, he has made Dr. Shen's method of pulse diagnosis comprehensible *and* teachable—no small feat!

With this book, Leon Hammer and Hamilton Rotte generously share the bounty of Dr. Shen's herbal prescriptions. Rotte's adept analysis of their contents, indications, and conceptual foundation makes this an eminently practical clinical guide. These formulas are now available for us as inspiration, to study and to put to good use.

Efrem Korngold, OMD, LAc

Preface

The Herbal Heritage of Dr. John H. F. Shen

This book has been organized and written by Hamilton Rotte, MSTCM, AP, and Leon I. Hammer, MD. Hamilton Rotte is a graduate of the American College of Oriental Medicine in San Francisco, a member of the faculty and previously Clinical Director at Dragon Rises College of Oriental Medicine (DRCOM, www.dragonrises.edu), and an herbalist and teacher. Analysis of the formulas, a larger part of this book, is written by Hamilton Rotte. There are denoted by a gray sidebar and the appellation "Hamilton Rotte." Many of the etiologic, diagnostic comments and references to Dr. Shen's concepts are by Dr. Hammer. The latter are denoted by a red sidebar and the appellation "Leon Hammer" and are repeated for each formula for which they are appropriate. The illustrations were provided by Laisha Canner, AP, a faculty member at Dragon Rises College of Oriental Medicine.

The principal purpose of this book is to share with the world the clinical perspective of a Chinese practitioner trained prior to the Traditional Chinese Medicine (TCM) system, and who is widely recognized throughout the world as one of the great diagnosticians and herbalists of the 20th century by many of our well-regarded colleagues. He is frequently referred to by Giovanni Maciocia in his books, who stated that "Dr. Shen was the most influential teacher in my professional development" (Maciocia, 2001). You will find Dr. Shen listed in Volume I of *A Commemorative Book of Challenge and Courage* as one of the American Association of Acupuncture and Oriental Medicine's (AAAOM) top ten "Pioneers & Leaders." Dr. Shen was a clinician with 70 years of experience whose views often differed from convention and from the classics. One of his most common comments when presented with the difference was "Book wrong." We found this assertion commonly to be true.

Sources for this Book

One source for this book is a collection of herbal formulas given directly to Dr. Hammer by Dr. Shen during the 8 years of weekly association and 19 years of looser contact. Many are for Chinese medical conditions that were unique to Dr. Shen such as "nervous system tense" or "heart closed," which are fully expounded in the text and translated into formal Chinese medical terminology. These formulas have been clinically tested by Dr. Hammer for the past 36 years and by practitioners associated with him, especially at the DRCOM clinic, including Hamilton Rotte for the past 10 years.

A second source for this book began as a 3-day meeting between Dr. Shen and Dr. Hammer in the 1990s, which was recorded as a video when Dr. Hammer formulated questions for him as the stimulus for some of the material in this book. Dr. Hammer wrote the first three versions from a stream of consciousness recorded on a computer at the time by a student. Others, especially Ray Rubio, LAc, a graduate of Emperor's College, California, Dr. Shen's last student (in Shanghai), made significant contributions to this book. However, in the intervening period between Dr. Hammer's first edits and Ray Rubio's contribution, Dr. Shen employed Chinese translators whose English was sometimes arcane and who introduced language and ideas that were clearly their own and would have been foreign to Dr. Shen. An attempt has been made to return the text to something more faithful to Dr. Shen's, and to good English.

The third source is from transcripts of Dr. Shen's lectures. Those formulas prescribed for his unique conditions sometimes vary from the ones that he gave Dr. Hammer years before. Formulas contributed by individuals from all over the world are the fourth and final source.

Structure of this Book

The book is divided into two parts based on the experience of the authors. In the first part, "Dr. Shen's Formulas in Systems," are those formulas with which they have the greatest clinical familiarity and are most closely correlated with Dr. Shen's conditions and concepts of the medicine. For these formulas personal comments were added about the conditions for which they were created in terms of etiology, symptoms, pathogenesis, and signs based on conversations with Dr. Shen and from the authors' own experience. The first part includes those formulas that are significantly different from those already extant in the field. The formulas are organized, in alphabetical order, by standard systems ranging from cardiovascular to respiratory.

The second part of the book, "Dr. Shen's Life-cycle Formulas," includes Dr. Shen's comments about his formulas, expressed in language meant for the layperson about many Chinese medical conditions. This part essentially covers many of the significant events of people's lives, beginning with conception, that are appropriate for the medical problems of that developmental era, with the emphasis on lifestyle.

Appendix 1 contains material that was composed by Dr. Shen in a later version of his writings that resulted in the second part of this book. With regard to the formulas that are difficult to explain, Dr. Shen referred to many of these as "experience" formulas, meaning that while they are ancient and effective they cannot always be explained by recent concepts about herbs such as pharmacology and channels. However, herbalists may recognize familiar formulas changed by Dr. Shen for his unique understanding of the condition and individual he was treating.

The diagnostic system on which these formulas are based is Dr. Shen's pulse system, as described in *Chinese Pulse Diagnosis: A Contemporary Approach* (Hammer, 2001), and chinese tongue diagnosis, primarily from personal contact with Dr. Shen. This book and Chapter 14 of *Dragon Rises Red Bird Flies* (Hammer, 2005) reflect his diagnostic life's work. A few detailed references to the pulse have been included, since the system, unique to Dr. Shen and his lineage and developed by Dr. Hammer, may be familiar to the some of the readers. Others can refer to *Chinese Pulse Diagnosis: A Contemporary Approach* and to seminars listed on the dragonrises.org website.

The authors anticipate that readers are trained Chinese medical practitioners and do not require detailed descriptions of all of the symptoms associated with solid-hollow (*zang-fu*) patterns that either they know or can find in the many well-known books on that subject. They also hope that each of these formulas will be altered according the needs of the individual patient, no two of whom are exactly the same.

Acknowledgments

The authors are particularly grateful to Angelika Findgott for her support in initiating this work and her extraordinary patience in seeing it through. Brian La Forgia, LAc, was exceedingly generous with his editing and, as mentioned above, Ray Rubio, LAc, shared Dr. Shen's herbal information in his possession. Dr. Terry Tang provided material from the Chinese literature describing the founder of the Shanghai Technical College Ding Gan Ren's use of herbs and made his impressive knowledge of herbal medicine available to the authors. The authors are thankful to Stacey Liu, AP, for helping to translate Ding Gan Ren's material on herbal medicine (from the book *Collection of Ding Gan Ren's Medical Cases*, edited by Shen Zhong Li). Giovanni Maciocia generously shared information gleaned from the time he spent with Dr. Shen. Damien Bell provided a wealth of information from Dr. Shen's various teaching engagements. Ross Rosen, LAc, provided many insightful comments about the text.

The authors hope that this work will satisfy those interested in the herbal and diagnostic perspective of one of the great herbalists of recent times, offering a pragmatic window into the mind and practice of a Chinese physician who comes from a much, much older tradition than TCM. The authors also hope that this volume will contribute to a different outlook on the clinical use of herbs in the practice of Chinese medicine.

Leon I. Hammer
Hamilton Rotte

Caution

Leon Hammer   The action of a substance depends upon its dose and upon the terrain upon which it acts. At one dose a substance might enhance physiology and at another compromise it. The safest procedure whenever administering herbs is to begin with a low dose and build to tolerance over about nine days, especially in highly vulnerable individuals.

Using aconite (*fu zi*) as an example: the recommended dosage for most people, between 0.12 g and 9 g, restores devastated *yang*. In toxic doses it may cause suffocation, loss of consciousness, precipitated atrial fibrillation, atrial tachycardia, or other symptoms.

Dr. Shen's Biography

The following history was told to me by Dr. Shen over the period of our 27-year association, especially during the increasingly intimate first 8 years. This was edited by his son Paul, with whom I have maintained a continuous friendship.

Dr. Shen was born in Shanghai in 1914 into one of the wealthiest families in China, as the eighth of nine children. The first and fourth died when young, possibly before Dr. Shen was born, which is why Dr. Shen always referred to being the sixth of seven. At the fall of the Imperial Qing dynasty in 1911, Dr. Shen's paternal grandfather, formerly an officer in that dynasty, founded and was president of the first private bank in China's long history.

Dr. Shen described his backyard as being the size of Central Park in New York City. Dr. Shen's mother, whom he worshipped all his life, was a very religious Catholic. On her death bed she made him promise to attend Catholic church every Sunday, which he did faithfully during all the time that I worked with him.

Some of Dr. Shen's siblings were sent abroad to study. I met all six of his living siblings. His only sister attended the Paris Conservatory of Music, where she became an accomplished pianist. One son became an accomplished engineer in Germany, another a linguist proficient in 12 languages. According to Dr. Shen, some had advanced degrees from prestigious European universities.

Not so for Dr. Shen. He did not have the opportunity to study abroad. From birth his mother, performing the duty of all Chinese mothers, assessed his lung qi to be very weak. He was therefore educated at home and never allowed to dress himself until he was around 15 years of age. His mother continued to be the center of his existence throughout his life. When he was 17 his mother, again fearing his propensity to become like his less than responsible father, insisted that he become a doctor, choosing either Western or Chinese medicine. He thumbed through books on both and discovered that he would have to work too hard to learn Western medicine. Chinese medicine seemed familiar to him already and easy for him to learn, so he chose that option.

After graduating in 1935 from the Shanghai Technical College operated by the famous Ding family of Chinese physicians, he opened a very low-cost clinic for poor people, seeing as many as 200 patients a day and affording him a great deal of clinical experience.

In 1935 his principal teacher Ding Ji Wan, the grandson of the founder of the Shanghai Technical College, Ding Gan Ren, began to teach the ancient pulse secrets handed down only within the clan from father to son since at least the 15th century. Ding Ji Wan taught this to only a few of the most wealthy students, who were required to pay large amounts of money, of whom Dr. Shen was one. This continued in Hong Kong to where he and Ding Ji Wan fled during the Japanese invasion of Shanghai in 1937.

He followed the master Ding Ji Wan whom he could question only during their daily "nap," at which time they lay on separate cots in a room, sharing an opium pipe, and during which time he could ask questions and get answers. Smoking opium was common practice among the upper classes in China at that time. His responsibilities to the Ding family included baby-sitting and other domestic duties. Shen married the widow of Ding Ji Wan's elder son, who died in a car accident.

He remained addicted to opium until 1941 when the Japanese invaded Hong Kong. Walking down the street with two fellow addicts, he in the middle, the other two, one on either side, were killed by Japanese snipers in the hills. He took this as a divine sign (perhaps from his mother) and at that point decided to withdraw from opium. It was at that point that he began to meditate, which he continued until his death 66 years later from lung cancer (the cause of death for all his siblings). His photographic memory and mental lucidity he attributed to his meditation.

With the invasion of Hong Kong by the Japanese in 1941, Dr. Shen was forced to flee again, running after the last train to Chongqing and hanging onto the outside for a long time until a passenger pulled him in. He spent the war in that city treating many people and learned from patients the importance of their psychological condition to their recovery. He spoke of one young lady with tuberculosis with whom he spent hours every day listening and talking to her.

After the war he returned to Shanghai where he owned a factory, from where he sold rice to Chiang Kai-shek. In 1949 this made him highly unpopular with the victorious communists, who came to arrest him. However, he managed to trick and evade them, claiming that he had to swim to a boat in the river to escape to Taiwan.

His personal life at that time is not entirely clear. When he was on Mainland China he had three children, whom he left. In Taiwan he married the widow of Ding Ji Wan's eldest son, and had several children. Much to the dissatisfaction of his wife at that time, he had difficulty supporting them. With relatively few patients, he said that he found time to spend hours with each of them, and in the 12 years he lived there he perfected the pulse system.

He also said that for him Chinese medicine was an avocation, not a vocation, and that other men of his social station who had other kinds of work had similar avocations associated with Chinese medical and related traditions. They would meet every afternoon to play *mahjong*, drink tea, and share their knowledge. It was here that he learned face reading, at which he was remarkably accomplished. In fact, he earned his living by it when he first went to the United States in 1971. This became a seamless part of his diagnostic acumen along with his other remarkable observational skills, especially the pulse.

Dr. Shen stated that in 1965 he was invited to many countries in Southeast Asia to practice his form of medicine. He would arrive in a city, be visited by the local police whom he had to bribe, and would stay for several days prescribing to over 100 patients a day. He did this for several years, marrying a Vietnamese woman of Chinese extraction, a Cantonese. In 1971 Dr. Shen and his wife were brought to the United States by his older sister and by one of his original three children, who were already living there.

We met in the office of another physician in my hometown of East Hampton, New York, who brought Dr. Shen there twice a week to treat his patients. I saw a Chinese man sitting at a desk taking another man's pulse, after which he took me and the physician to one side and said, "In 1943 this man killed a man and contracted venereal disease." The physi-

cian spoke privately with this patient (who was blind). The patient said that he had been a part of General de Gaulle's Free French forces in North Africa in 1943 after the Americans invaded and that in fighting against the Vichy French had killed a man, and had also developed venereal disease that year. At that point I knew I had to learn more about this seemingly magical skill; thus began a 27-year odyssey. The other "physician" lost interest.

At the beginning of my 8-year intensive apprenticeship (2 or 3 days a week), Dr. Shen told me that "you may not learn anything but you eat well" and he was true to his word. He also said "you Western doctor; now forget everything you learned." He was willing to teach me if I helped him open a clinic in Boston, for which he needed a medical doctor as director. Ultimately this led to many complications, but again he was true to his word and very reluctantly shared some of his knowledge, which required great persistence and insistence on my part. In particular, I learned the pulse and some of his face-reading skills. He was a diagnostician par excellence and his herbal formulas were very successful.

These 8 years were spent with him in a humble apartment in Chinatown, New York, before he developed his socially elite clientele in the 1980s. At this point in his career and forever after he became increasingly famous in the United States and Europe for his extraordinary diagnostic and herbal skills, the latter being the subject of this book. His fame spread with the help of several students who arranged workshops for him in the United States, Europe, and Australia.

Our more intimate relationship ended when I moved 6 hours from New York City; that trip in the winter from the mountains was more than I could handle as I was 58 years old. He was 10 years older than me and throughout our relationship until his death we addressed each other as "doctor." I spoke with him during the last 3 weeks before his death when he could barely speak and he insisted that his only problem was low *qi,* though we all knew that he was dying from lung cancer that he developed after a lifetime of heavy cigarette smoking.

The following story is related by his son Paul. "In his last days, he chose to go back to Shanghai where he was born and raised. My father stayed in a hospital mainly treating patients with Chinese medicine, using Western medicine only as an auxiliary tool. The doctors prescribed many Chinese medicine formulas to my father. My father refused them all after reviewing their formula and called them rubbish. The night before his death, he spoke with Auntie Mary and told her that he would be gone that night and asked her and Uncle Peter to take care of themselves. He then asked one of his domestic helpers to go out to buy some Chinese cough medicine as he felt itchy in his throat. I remember this vividly as I was thinking then that till the last moment he still preferred Chinese to Western medicine. He passed away at 4 a.m. that night with a clear mind till almost the very last minute (one of my aunts kept asking him questions such as "Do you feel peaceful?" etc. and although he could not speak he nodded and shook his head to answer)."

Dr. Shen was a unique person and master of Chinese medicine. As I have said before, "There are few like him, and his kind shall not pass this way again. I am grateful for the sometimes trying gift of having known him so well. He taught me the many faces of reality."

Leon I. Hammer

Contents

Dr. Shen's Formulas in Systems

Leon Hammer The following herbal formulas were chosen from among the many for their relative uniqueness from the extant current Chinese medical herbal formulae.

The term 'systems' by which this was organized, refers to the biomedical organization of medical conditions that we conceived as both familiar and convenient.

Cardiovascular Conditions

Blue-green Color around the Mouth in Children

FROM DR. SHEN: Symptoms: crying a lot, insomnia, possible constipation. Do not use if there is fever. Give throughout night. Children 6 months to 3 years old easily develop this problem, for example, from being frightened after falling down.

Formula for the newborn:

Pin Yin	Latin	English	Dosage
Shi chang pu	Acori Tatarinowii Rhizoma	Grass-leaved sweetflag rhizome, acorus	2.4–3 g
Chuan xiong	Chuanxiong Rhizoma	Chuanxiong root, Szechuan lovage root, cnidium	3–4.5 g
Chao jing jie	Schizonepetae Herba	Dry-fried schizonepeta	3–4.5 g
Zhu fu shen	Poria Cocos Pararadicis Sclerotium	Dried Poria fungus	9 g
Yuan zhi	Polygalae Radix	Chinese senega root, polygala root	3 g
Suan zao ren	Ziziphi Spinosae Semen	Spiny zizyphus seeds, sour jujube seeds, zizyphus	9 g
Long chi	Fossilia Dentis Mastodi	Dragon teeth, fossilized teeth	18 g
Ci shi	Magnetitum	Magnetite	24 g
Chao huang qin	Scutellariae Baicalensis Radix	Fried baical skullcap root, scutellaria, scute	3 g
Chao gu ya	Oryzae Germinatus Fructus	Fried rice sprout	9 g
Chao mai ya	Hordei Germinatus Fructus	Fried barley sprout	9 g
Zhu deng xin cao (with zhu sha[a])	Medulla Junci Effusi (with Cinnabaris)	Dried rush pith, juncus (with cinnabar)	3 pieces

[a] Unavailable due to supposed toxicity.

FROM DR. SHEN: For a fever, around 40°C, low in morning, which in the afternoon goes up, still playing, open mouth and eyes.

Administer previous formula and add:

Pin Yin	Latin	English	Dosage
Dan dou chi	Sojae Preparatum Semen	Prepared soybean	9 g
Bo he	Menthae Haplocalycis Herba	Field mint, mentha, peppermint leaves	2.4 g
Hei shan zhi zi	Gardeniae Jasminoidis Fructus	Charred cape jasmine fruit, gardenia fruit	9 g
Lian qiao	Forsythiae Suspensae Fructus	Forsythia fruit	9 g

Hamilton Rotte   The blue-green color around the mouth is an indication that a shock occurred at birth. Trauma impairs *qi* and blood circulation in the heart and is accompanied by disturbances of the spirit (insomnia, anxiety, and fear). Shock also depletes heart *qi* and *yin*.

This formula contains the following herbs to calm the spirit: *shi chang pu, fu shen, yuan zhi, suan zao ren, long chi*, and *ci shi*. It is a mixture of herbs that resolve "phlegm misting the orifices" (*shi chang pu, fu shen, yuan zhi*, and *chuan xiong* [according to Ding Gan Ren]), and nourish the heart *yin* (*suan zao ren*) and heavy mineral substances that settle the spirit (*long chi* and *ci shi*). According to Ding Gan Ren, *ci shi* is especially indicated for fear from kidney deficiency, a common outcome of an early trauma. The emphasis is on resolving phlegm and settling the spirit. Experi-

ence has shown that "phlegm misting the orifices" is the pathogenic process that is central in mental-emotional disturbances.

We also find herbs in this formula to clear heat, including *huang qin* and *deng xin cao*. Ding Gan Ren indicated that "in order to clear the heart one must use *deng xing cao*." These may address the heat that develops from stagnation in trauma.

Mai ya and *gu ya* address food stagnation. It is well documented in the literature that children easily develop food stagnation. This could easily be exacerbated by the heavy minerals contained in this formula. According to Ding Gan Ren, *mai ya* activates and unblocks the *san jiao*, addressing stagnation that results from trauma.

If a fever is present then *dan dou chi, bo he, zhi zi*, and *lian qiao* are included to clear heat.

Blue-green Color around the Mouth in Adults

FROM DR. SHEN: Very frightened.

Use base formula and add:

Pin Yin	Latin	English	Dosage
Chuan lian zi	Meliae Toosendan Fructus	Szechuan pagoda tree fruit, Szechuan chinaberry, melia	1.5 g
Chen xiang	Aquilariae Lignum	Aloeswood, aquilaria	1.8 g
Yu jin	Curcumae Radix	Curcuma tuber	9 g

Hamilton Rotte   The focus of the formula for the blue-green color around the mouth in children is to open the orifices and calm the spirit. This modification of the formula for adults contains ingredients to regulate the *qi*, especially of the liver. The etiology of

qi stagnation in the liver is repression of emotions. An individual who suffered a trauma early in life will have mental-emotional difficulties that make functioning more difficult. One of the most common maladaptive coping mechanisms is repression.

Example of Modification of Blue-green Color around the Mouth from Dr. Hammer's Records

Hyperactive patient aged 5 years:

Pin Yin	Latin	English	Dosage
Shi chang pu	Acori Tatarinowii Rhizoma	Grass-leaved sweetflag rhizome, acorus	3 g
Chuan xiong	Chuanxiong Rhizoma	Chuanxiong root, Szechuan lovage root, cnidium	3 g
Chao jing jie	Schizonepetae Herba	Dry-fried schizonepeta	5 g
Hei fang feng	Saposhnikoviae Radix	Charred ledebouriella root, saposhnikoviae root, siler	5 g
Mu xiang	Saussureae Lappae Radix or Aucklandia Lappae Radix	Costus root, saussurea, aucklandia	3 g
Zhu fu shen	Poria Cocos Pararadicis Sclerotium	Dried Poria fungus	10 g
Chao suan zao ren	Ziziphi Spinosae Semen	Fried spiny zizyphus seeds, sour jujube seeds, zizyphus	12 g
Long chi	Fossilia Dentis Mastodi	Dragon teeth, fossilized teeth	25 g
Ci shi	Magnetitum	Magnetite	25 g
Huang qin	Scutellariae Baicalensis Radix	Baical skullcap root, scutellaria, scute	3 g
Chao gu ya	Oryzae Germinatus Fructus	Fried rice sprout	12 g
Chao mai ya	Hordei Germinatus Fructus	Fried barley sprout, fried malt	12 g
Zhu deng xin cao (with zhu sha[a])	Medulla Junci Effusi (with Cinnabaris)	Dried rush pith, juncus (with cinnabar[a])	3 pieces

[a] Unavailable due to supposed toxicity.

Leon Hammer When the entire face is blue, the shock was either extraordinary at any age or occurred at a very early point in development, most likely in-utero, and less likely at birth or shortly after. The other possible scenario is the combination of a shock during a later stage of life superimposed on an early shock. Usually this person is fearful their entire life. This is often associated with heart blood stagnation when the pulse's left distal position is very flat or deep, feeble and the rate either normal, slightly rapid, or slightly slow.

When the blue color occurs only around the chin, the problem is either due to genetics or a defect due to an interference with the normal development in-utero. When the blue color appears around the mouth, the etiology is trauma during the birth process. When this color appears on the nose the shock occurred during a later stage of development. When the color is only on the temples and around and between the eyes and forehead, the problem is probably one or the other or both. The addition of a blue color on the temples to color around the chin or mouth means that the condition is more serious. When blue veins are found at the temples the person is often very frightened much of the time for no apparent reason.

Circulatory System, Original Formula

FROM DR. SHEN: Symptoms include tiring easily, cold hands, migrating joint problems, anxiety, easily angered, swollen joints.

Pin Yin	Latin	English	Dosage
Qiang huo	Notopterygii Rhizoma et Radix	Notopterygium root and rhizome, chiang-huo	6 g
Si gua luo	Fasciculus Vascularis Luffae	Dried skeleton of vegetable sponge	6 g
Dan shen	Salviae Miltiorrhiziae Radix	Salvia root	6 g
Sang ji sheng	Taxilli Herba	Mulberry mistletoe stems, loranthus, taxillus, mistletoe	12 g
Yuan zhi	Polygalae Radix	Chinese senega root, polygala root	6 g
Da zao	Zizyphi Jujubae Fructus	Chinese date, jujube	10 g
Dang gui	Angelicae Sinensis Radix	Chinese angelica root, tang-kuei	6 g
Mu gua	Chaenomelis Fructus	Chinese quince fruit, chaenomeles	12 g
Fang feng	Saposhnikoviae Radix	Ledebouriella root, saposhnikoviae root, siler	6 g

Hamilton Rotte   Dr. Shen indicated that circulatory system problems were caused by physical and emotional trauma. The effects manifest in the channels (migrating joint problems, swelling joints), in poor circulation in general (cold hands), and in changes in the mental-emotional state (anxiety, easily angered). Even though there are some apparent signs of deficiency (fatigue, cold hands), the focus of this formula is to unblock stagnation in the channels and the chest in order to restore heart function. In this case, the stagnation is what is causing poor heart function, not heart weakness itself.

The following herbs open the channels in this formula: qiang huo, si gua luo, sang ji sheng, mu gua, and fang feng.

This formula contains ingredients that move the qi and especially target the chest. These include yuan zhi and si gua luo. It also contains blood-invigorating ingredients, including dan shen, dang gui, and to a lesser degree si gua luo.

The moistening nature of da zao and dang gui offset the drying tendencies of some of the moving ingredients such as qiang huo and yuan zhi.

Dan shen, da zao, and yuan zhi are included to calm the spirit, as spirit disturbances present as part of pathology of the circulatory system.

Circulatory System, Additional Formula

Formula from February 2000:

Pin Yin	Latin	English	Dosage
Qiang huo	Notopterygii Rhizoma et Radix	Notopterygium root and rhizome, chiang-huo	6 g
Jiu chao dang gui	Angelicae Sinensis Radix	Wine-fried Chinese angelica root, tang-kuei	6 g
Fang feng	Saposhnikoviae Radix	Ledebouriella root, saposhnikoviae root, siler	4.5 g
Sang ji sheng	Taxilli Herba	Mulberry mistletoe stems, loranthus, taxillus, mistletoe	9 g
Mu gua	Chaenomelis Fructus	Chinese quince fruit, chaenomeles	9 g
Ji xue teng	Jixueteng Radix et Caulis	Spatholobus or milettia root and vine	9 g
Mu xiang	Saussureae Lappae Radix or Aucklandia Lappae Radix	Costus root, saussurea, aucklandia	4.5 g
Sang zhi	Ramulus Mori Albae	Mulberry twig, morus twig	12 g

Leon Hammer There is no clear equivalent to the "circulatory system" in TCM. Conditions of the circulatory system involve the entire organism, the entire pulse is also involved, and the system cannot be delineated in terms of a single organ disharmony except the heart, which controls circulation.

Circulation, in Chinese medicine, is either of the *qi*, that is, the moving force of the body, or of the nourishing blood, a Chinese medicine concept that is not exactly the same as the Western concept of blood but refers to a heavier, more dense form of energy. Traditionally, it is said that the *qi* moves the blood and that the blood nourishes the *qi*. They are, in this sense, interdependent. With both there is either deficiency or excess (stagnation). Generally speaking, the less serious the problem, the more likely it is to be just a *qi* disease; the more serious the problem, the more likely it is that there will also be a blood disease.

There are two general categories: one where the circulatory problem is secondary to an energy problem, and one where the circulatory problem creates the energy problem. With the first a person has either overworked or over-exercised, creating deficient heart *qi* and a deficient body condition, "terrain." This in turn affects circulation because heart *qi* moves the blood, and the *qi* is the moving part of the energy. The pulse is generally slow and feeble, though in the extremes there may be "circulation out of control" (arrhythmias).

The second category, in which the circulation has secondarily affected the energy (heart *qi*), is caused by some kind of relatively strong and sudden experience, such as physical or mental trauma (emotional shock), or very severe weather conditions. In this case we find rough vibration on the entire pulse. The vessels respond by constricting peripheral blood vessels and diminishing blood flow, especially to the sur-

face, to protect vital organs and call upon the heart to work harder to maintain flow.

In this situation, the pulse may at first be initially very slow due to the sudden diminishment of circulation and later more rapid as the heart has to work harder to restore circulation. Later, as the heart *qi* is depleted, the pulse will be somewhat slower than when circulation is affected by the body condition or energy.

Both over-exercise (beyond a person's energy) over an extended period of time ("yielding hollow full-overflowing and slow"), and the sudden cessation of heavy, prolonged exercise ("yielding hollow full-overflowing and rapid"), may cause a separation of *yin* and *yang* in the vessels, resulting in "circulation out of control," and in turn chaos in the *qi* ("*qi* wild"), since the blood nourishes the *qi*. Milder manifestations are fluctuating symptoms of being easily fatigued, cold hands and feet, migrating joint problems, and being easily angered. More serious manifestations are severe anxiety, depersonalization, and major personality decompensation, frequently and tragically confused with serious mental illness (Hammer, 2011a).

The effects described below are related to a "nervous system tense" disorder. The cause may be constitutional or based on life experience. With the former, the person is tense only under stress; with the latter, the person is always tense. Due to the increasing demands of modern living we have become hyperactive supermen and women. It is the nervous system that is most often the culprit that adversely affects all of the other systems.

Pulse:

When the nervous system is affecting the circulatory system, the rate is normal, the "*qi* depth" is tight and thin, the middle "blood depth" separates on pressure (partially hollow), and the "organ depth" is tense or tight.

Heart Blood Deficiency ("Heart Weak")

FROM DR. SHEN: Heart problems can be caused by:
- Congenital deficiency
- Working too hard
- A weak heart and heavy lifting
- Emotions, sudden anger when tired
- Suddenly frightened, affects heart
- High fever in children causing valve problems
- Very angry: heart large, size the same but inside the pressure is great

Pin Yin	Latin	English	Dosage
Dang gui	Angelicae Sinensis Radix	Chinese angelica root, tang-kuei	6 g
Chuan xiong	Chuanxiong Rhizoma	Chuanxiong root, Szechuan lovage root, cnidium	4.5 g
Shu di huang	Rehmanniae Preparata Radix	Prepared Chinese foxglove root (cooked in red wine), rehmannia rhizome	9 g
Yuan zhi	Polygalae Radix	Chinese senega root, polygala root	4.5 g
Wu wei zi	Schisandrae Chinensis Fructus	Schisandra fruit	3 g
Dan shen	Salviae Miltiorrhiziae Radix	Salvia root	4.5 g
Sha ren	Amomi Fructus	Cardamom	2.4 g
Mai men dong	Ophiopogonis Radix	Ophiopogon tuber/root	9 g
Fo shou	Fructus Citri Sarcodactylis	Finger citron fruit, Buddha's hand	4.5 g

Hamilton Rotte All major formulas for heart blood deficiency in the standard formula repertoire (such as *Gui Pi Tang* [Restore the Spleen Decoction] and *Yang Xin Tang* [Nourish the Heart Decoction]) contain ingredients to nourish liver blood and those that calm the spirit and treat the heart more directly. Liver blood provides the foundation for heart blood. This formula follows this principle with the inclusion of the liver blood tonics *dang gui* and *shu di huang*. *Chuan xiong* is included to move blood, essential in a blood tonic formula (such as in *Si Wu Tang* [Four Substance Decoction]).

The ingredients that target the heart more directly include *yuan zhi*, *wu wei zi*, *dan shen*, and *mai men dong*. *Yuan zhi* and *wu wei zi* are a two-herb combination that is commonly utilized in heart tonic formulas. The two together harmonize heart and kidneys, calm the spirit, and create a dynamic tension in that *wu wei zi* is sour, moistening, and stabilizing and *yuan zhi* is drying, acrid, and moving. It is included in *Tian Wang Bu Xin Dan* (Emperor of Heaven's Special Pill to Tonify the Heart), *Yang Xin Tang* (Nourish the Heart

Decoction) and *Ren Shen Yang Rong Tang* (Ginseng Decoction to Nourish Luxuriance). They act somewhat as guide herbs for the heart in that they direct other herbs to the heart.

Dan shen is included as a mild heart blood tonic that also moves blood in the heart. As previously mentioned, including blood-moving herbs among tonic herbs is essential in blood tonic formulas.

Spirit-calming ingredients in this formula include *dan shen*, *yuan zhi*, and *wu wei zi*. *Mai men dong*, a favorite of Dr. Shen's in the treatment of heart conditions, is also described by Ding Gan Ren when treating disturbances of the heart marked by agitation and becoming easily startled or shocked. Deficiency of heart blood and heart *yin* frequently overlap, explaining the inclusion of the heart *yin* tonics *dan shen*, *wu wei zi*, and *mai men dong*.

Sha ren and *fo shou* are *qi*-regulating herbs that prevent damp excess and *qi* stagnation that can result from blood tonic herbs. *Sha ren* in particular aids in the digestion of *shu di huang*, a very greasy substance. *Qi*-moving herbs are recommended in any tonic formula, especially *yin*-blood tonics.

Leon Hammer
Pulse:
- First impressions (FI) of entire pulse:
  - "Rate on exertion" exceeds the "rate at rest" by more than 20 beats
  - Blood depth slightly–moderately hollow
- Heart blood deficiency:
  - Left distal position (LDP): thin (3–5)
  - Change of rate on exertion: pulse rises more than 20 beats/minute from resting rate

This condition is one in which the heart blood is deficient, with some attendant heart *qi* deficiency, both of which cause a deficit in heart function. The pulse shows a large change in rate on exertion, more than 20 beats per minute if the heart is very blood deficient, and a lesser change (12–20 beats) if the heart is only slightly blood deficient. The rate may be a little rapid, normal, or slow, depending upon the chronicity of the condition: the longer the duration of the condition, the slower the pulse. The left distal position is often thin when the blood deficiency is more severe, sometimes accompanied by reduced substance if the heart *qi* is also mild to moderately deficient.

While constitutional heart *qi* deficiency is sometimes a predisposing factor, heart blood deficiency is most often due to prolonged and severe heart *qi* agitation ("heart nervous"). However, heart blood deficiency can be due to one or any combination of the following: kidney essence deficiency, spleen *qi* deficiency, and gradual blood loss over time. When any of these three is the cause, the entire pulse is thin and a little feeble and the vessels inside the lower eyelid are pale.

The patient may experience palpitations throughout the day, especially with activity, because there is not enough blood in the heart. There is also a general feeling of weakness and depression, with poor concentration and memory. The sleep pattern is one of waking up after 5 hours of solid sleep, after which sleep returns, sometimes lightly, and sometimes deeply. One will be tired in the morning, though less so than with heart *qi* deficiency. A very prolonged "heart weak" pattern can lead to serious "heart large" and "heart disease," with manifestations such as congestive heart failure.

Hamilton Rotte **General comments about Dr. Shen's heart formulas:**

These apply to "Heart Closed," Heart Large," "Heart Full," "Heart Small," "Heart Tight," "Heart Vibration" and "Heart Weak."

Because of their low dosage, *shi chang pu, chuan xiong, mu xiang, yuan zhi, huang lian, chen xiang, ding xiang,* and *huang qin* primarily have an effect on *qi* circulation. The drying effects of these herbs is reduced by their light dosage and offset by the moistening *suan zao ren* and *bai shao.*

Commonly used ingredients that calm the spirit include *shi chang pu, fu shen,* and *yuan zhi.* Commonly used orifice-opening ingredients include *shi chang*

pu, fu shen, yu jin, and, according to Ding Gan Ren, *chuan xiong.*

As a means of treating stagnation in the upper burner, most of the herbs are descending, including *mu xiang* (as described by Ding Gan Ren), *fu shen, yuan zhi, yu jin, suan zao ren, huang lian, chen xiang, ding xiang, huang qin, chen pi, gua lou pi,* and *deng xin cao. Shi chang pu* and *chuan xiong* are ascending, as utilizing herbs together that move in opposite directions is very beneficial in moving *qi.*

Dr. Shen indicated that *wu wei zi, mu li,* and *mai men dong* are indicated for enlargement of the heart and used them frequently for this purpose.

Heart Closed

Pin Yin	Latin	English	Dosage
Shi chang pu	Acori Tatarinowii Rhizoma	Grass-leaved sweetflag rhizome, acorus	2.4 g
Chuan xiong	Chuanxiong Rhizoma	Chuanxiong root, Szechuan lovage root, cnidium	4.5 g
Mu xiang	Saussureae Lappae Radix or Aucklandia Lappae Radix	Costus root, saussurea, aucklandia	4.5 g
Fu shen	Poria Cocos Pararadicis Sclerotium	Poria fungus	9 g
Yuan zhi	Polygalae Radix	Chinese senega root, polygala root	4.5 g
Suan zao ren	Ziziphi Spinosae Semen	Spiny zizyphus seeds, sour jujube seeds, zizyphus	9 g
Yu jin	Curcumae Radix	Curcuma tuber	9 g
Huang lian	Coptidis Rhizoma	Coptis rhizome	1.8 g
Chen xiang	Aquilariae Lignum	Aloeswood, aquilaria	2.1 g

Leon Hammer In terms of Traditional Chinese Medicine (TCM), the closest equivalent term to the "heart closed" pattern would be heart *qi* stagnation. This is a pattern where a moderately flat pulse quality at the left distal position is a sign that circulation of *qi* has been partially blocked from entering the heart, usually due to a shock. This ultimately leads to heart *qi* deficiency and diminished peripheral blood circulation. With "heart nervous" the shock affects the nervous innervations of the heart. With "heart closed" the substance of the heart (parenchyma) is slightly affected, though much less so than in the case of either "heart small" or "heart full" (see below).

The shock is most often an emotional one experienced during childhood while the body's *qi* is still immature, and usually involves the loss of someone very close, such as a parent. A common shock to the heart also occurs at birth with the cord around the neck. However, the "heart closed" condition can occur later in life due to a major emotional shock, such as sudden bad news or the sudden break-up of a romance when the person withdraws their "heart" feelings. With adult onset and a stronger more mature heart *qi*, the "heart closed" condition is more reversible and easily overcome. Other causes include heart *qi* agitation ("heart nervous") over a long period of time, or even a mild physical shock to the chest when heart *qi* is deficient.

This type of person seems to be in some kind of constant emotional difficulty. According to Dr. Shen, a "heart closed" person tends to be vengeful and spiteful. The "spirit" of the eyes can be somewhat narrow and withdrawn, the pupils wide, and color dark. The person may experience some chest pain in connection with the closing of *qi* circulation, especially under stress.

Heart Enlarged

FROM DR. SHEN: Can cause thyroid problems.

Formula from February 2000:

Pin Yin	Latin	English	Dosage
Shi chang pu	Acori Tatarinowii Rhizoma	Grass-leaved sweetflag rhizome, acorus	2.4 g[a]
Chen xiang	Aquilariae Lignum	Aloeswood, aquilaria	2.1 g
Chao huang lian	Coptidis Rhizoma	Dry-fried coptis rhizome	2.1 g
Chao bai shao	Paeoniae Alba Radix	Dry-fried white peony root	6 g
Fu shen	Poria Cocos Pararadicis Sclerotium	Poria fungus	9 g
Yuan zhi	Polygalae Radix	Chinese senega root, polygala root	4.5 g
Wu wei zi	Schisandrae Chinensis Fructus	Schisandra fruit	4.5 g
Duan mu li	Ostreae Concha	Calcined oyster shell	12 g
Mai men dong	Ophiopogonis Radix	Ophiopogon tuber/root	9 g

[a] A small amount makes the heart relax.

Heart Full, Original Formula

Pin Yin	Latin	English	Dosage
Shi chang pu	Acori Tatarinowii Rhizoma	Grass-leaved sweetflag rhizome, acorus	2.4 g
Chuan xiong	Chuanxiong Rhizoma	Chuanxiong root, Szechuan lovage root, cnidium	4.5 g

Pin Yin	Latin	English	Dosage
Mu xiang	Saussureae Lappae Radix or Aucklandia Lappae Radix	Costus root, saussurea, aucklandia	4.5 g
Fu shen	Poria Cocos Pararadicis Sclerotium	Poria fungus	9 g
Yuan zhi	Polygalae Radix	Chinese senega root, polygala root	4.5 g
Suan zao ren	Ziziphi Spinosae Semen	Spiny ziziphus seeds, sour jujube seeds, zizyphus	9 g
Yu jin	Curcumae Radix	Curcuma tuber	9 g
Huang lian	Coptidis Rhizoma	Coptis rhizome	2.4 g
Chen xiang	Aquilariae Lignum	Aloeswood, aquilaria	2.1 g
Wu wei zi	Schisandrae Chinensis Fructus	Schisandra fruit	4.5 g
Mu li	Ostreae Concha	Oyster shell	15 g
Mai men dong	Ophiopogonis Radix	Ophiopogon tuber/root	9 g

Heart Full, Formula from the late 1990s

FROM DR. SHEN: Heart is too large due to anger—has relation to liver. Size is the same, but inside the pressure is great.

Pin Yin	Latin	English	Dosage
Shi chang pu	Acori Tatarinowii Rhizoma	Grass-leaved sweetflag rhizome, acorus	2.4 g
Huang lian	Coptidis Rhizoma	Coptis rhizome	2.1 g
Chen xiang[a]	Aquilariae Lignum	Aloeswood, aquilaria	2.1 g
Chuan xiong	Chuanxiong Rhizoma	Chuanxiong root, Szechuan lovage root, cnidium	4.5 g
Fu ling[b]	Poria Cocos Sclerotium	Sclerotium of tuckahoe, poria, China root, hoelen, Indian bread	4.5 g
Yuan zhi	Polygalae Radix	Chinese senega root, polygala root	4.5 g
Yu jin	Curcumae Radix	Curcuma tuber	6 g
Huang qin	Scutellariae Baicalensis Radix	Baical skullcap root, scutellaria, scute	4.5 g
Bai shao	Paeoniae Radix Alba	White peony root	4.5 g

[a] For heart nerves.
[b] Fu ling and fu shen are different but related herbs; both counter damp conditions (diuretics), but fu shen (as the shen part of the term indicates) calms the spirit as well.

If bleeding, add:

Pin Yin	Latin	English	Dosage
Tan ou jie	Nelumbinis Nodus Rhizomatis	Charred node of lotus rhizome, lotus root node	12 g
Tan di yu	Sanguisorbae Radix	Charred sanguisorba, burnet-bloodwort root	12 g
Chuan bei mu	Fritillariae Cirrhosae Bulbus	Szechuan fritillaria bulb, tendrilled fritillary bulb, fritillaria	9 g

FROM DR. SHEN: If "heart full" condition is due to lifting, and there is great anger when fatigued then this takes the *qi* out of the heart (this only affects the heart, not the liver). Add these:

Pin Yin	Latin	English	Dosage
Wu wei zi	Schisandrae Chinensis Fructus	Schisandra fruit	4.5 g
Mai men dong	Ophiopogonis Radix	Ophiopogon tuber/root	9 g
Mu li	Ostreae Concha	Oyster shell	12 g

Leon Hammer   This is a condition in which the *qi* is unable to exit the heart that I call "trapped *qi* in the heart." There is no known equivalent in TCM, but in quasi-biomedical terms, it would be a very slight energetic enlargement of the heart undetected by x-ray, and might also be accompanied by incipient mild hypertension.

This condition manifests on the pulse as a yielding or tense inflated quality at the left distal position with the rate normal or a little rapid. According to Dr. Shen, but outside my own experience, when the condition is more serious the left distal position is deep, thin, and tight, and the entire pulse rate is rapid.

A minor cause is sudden and very profound repressed anger at a time when a person is extremely active. A more serious etiology is a very prolonged birth with the head inside (breech delivery). Other causes are trauma to the chest, prolonged grief, or following an episode of sudden extreme lifting beyond one's energy. Uncorrected, "heart full" can develop into either an energetically or even biomedically enlarged heart (see "Enlarged Heart" above) or hypertension, or both.

Such individuals will feel tired their entire lives, have little energy, and may be rather depressed. They are frequently very quick to anger. The entire body may be uncomfortable. There is more difficulty breathing out than in, and some discomfort when lying down on the left side. In a more advanced stage there may be coughing up of blood, because frequently the lungs become secondarily stagnant due to insufficient cardiopulmonary circulation from diminished heart function.

FROM DR. SHEN: Heart large versus heart small:
• Heart large—must sleep on right side, cannot lie on back or left
• Heart small affects heart nerves, not heart organ condition; chest pain same place—small like needle

Heart Large

Pin Yin	Latin	English	Dosage
Ge jie	Gekko Gecko Linnaeus	Gecko	1 pair
Chuan bei mu	Fritillariae Cirrhosae Bulbus	Szechuan fritillaria bulb, tendrilled fritillary bulb, fritillaria	6 g
Wu wei zi	Schisandrae Chinensis Fructus	Schisandra fruit	3 g
Xi yang shen	Panacis Quinquefolii Radix	American ginseng root	4.5 g

Hamilton Rotte   This formula, gleaned from Dr. Shen's records of treating patients, represents an approach to treat his "heart large" condition, described in detail below.

A severe heart *qi*-deficient condition usually involves underlying deficiency of kidney *yang*. *Ge jie* is included for this purpose. *Xi yang shen* tonifies heart *qi*. The enlargement of the heart from deficiency is addressed by the astringent qualities of *wu wei zi*. *Chuan bei mu* is included because it treats stagnation in the chest, as described by Ding Gan Ren.

Leon Hammer This is the equivalent of severe heart *qi* deficiency in TCM. Some of the qualities at the left distal positions associated with this condition are deep, feeble-absent, change in intensity or qualities and rough vibration, with a labile rate often in excess of 100 beats per minute. If the distal end of the diaphragm position (between the left distal and left middle positions), is more inflated and/or rough than the proximal end, this is a sign of an enlarged heart (energetically and/or by x-ray).

A tense hollow full-overflowing quality at the left distal position, with a rate exceeding 100 beats per minute, is another combination associated with the "heart large" condition. An interrupted or intermittent rhythm, and a slippery quality at the mitral valve position (MV prolapse), can also be found. The rate will precipitously and temporally increase with movement and stress, and one will find widely different rates at different times during a pulse examination.

Dr. Shen associates these signs with prolonged overwork in a person with constitutionally deficient heart *qi*. The underlying causes are constitutional heart *qi* deficiency, any of the other heart conditions, especially trapped *qi* in the heart ("heart full") and heart blood stagnation ("heart small") with coronary occlusion over a long period of time, and rheumatic heart disease. All of these etiologies may be exacerbated by chronic, repressed, and profound anger that occurs especially while active.

Also, more common before the advent of child labor laws, but still prevalent in the underdeveloped world, is child labor with excessive physical work at an early age, together with malnutrition. With this etiology there is usually an interrupted or intermittent rhythm, and the pulse is yielding hollow.

Symptoms include excessive and easy fatigue, severe shortness of breath especially on exertion, difficulty breathing if lying flat on the back or on the left side, and chronic chest discomfort. Sleep cycle involves frequent waking and retuning to sleep without agitation and fatigue in the morning. Hypertension due to heart *qi* deficiency is sometimes present.

Heart Small, Original Formula

Pin Yin	Latin	English	Dosage
Shi chang pu	Acori Tatarinowii Rhizoma	Grass-leaved sweetflag rhizome, acorus	2.4 g
Chuan xiong	Chuanxiong Rhizoma	Chuanxiong root, Szechuan lovage root, cnidium	4.5 g
Mu xiang	Saussureae Lappae Radix or Aucklandia Lappae Radix	Costus root, saussurea, aucklandia	4.5 g
Fu shen[a]	Poria Cocos Pararadicis Sclerotium	Poria fungus	9 g
Yuan zhi	Polygalae Radix	Chinese senega root, polygala root	4.5 g
Suan zao ren	Ziziphi Spinosae Semen	Spiny zizyphus seeds, sour jujube seeds, zizyphus	9 g
Yu jin	Curcumae Radix	Curcuma tuber	9 g
Gua lou pi	Trichosanthis Pericarpium	Peel of trichosanthes fruit	9 g
Chen pi	Citri Reticulatae Pericarpium	Tangerine peel	6 g
Ding xiang	Caryophilli Flos	Clove flower bud	2.4 g

[a] *Fu ling* and *fu shen* are different but related herbs; both counter damp conditions (diuretics), but *fu shen* (as the *shen* part of the term indicates) calms the spirit as well.

Heart Small, Formula from the late 1990s

Pin Yin	Latin	English	Dosage
Shi chang pu	Acori Tatarinowii Rhizoma	Grass-leaved sweetflag rhizome, acorus	4.5 g
Xiang fu	Cyperi Rotundi Rhizoma	Nut grass rhizoma, cyperus	4.5 g
Chuan xiong	Chuanxiong Rhizoma	Chuanxiong root, Szechuan lovage root, cnidium	4.5 g
Fu ling	Poria Cocos Sclerotium	Sclerotium of tuckahoe, poria, China root, hoelen, Indian bread	9 g
Yuan zhi	Polygalae Radix	Chinese senega root, polygala root	4.5 g
Yu jin	Curcumae Radix	Curcuma tuber	4 g
Huang qin	Scutellariae Baicalensis Radix	Baical skullcap root, scutellaria, scute	4.5 g
Bai shao	Paeoniae Alba Radix	White peony root	9 g
Ding xiang	Caryophilli Flos	Clove flower bud	4.5 g

Leon Hammer   In terms of TCM, the closest equivalent term to "heart small" would be heart blood stagnation, and in biomedicine, the closest equivalent condition would be coronary artery spasm and angina. There are mild and temporary, and serious and enduring, varieties.

The spasm pattern is usually the result of a sudden shock during which time the coronary arteries constrict, depriving the heart of *qi* and blood. This spasm leads to an insufficient oxygen supply to the coronary muscles. In Dr. Shen's terms, the heart is "suffocating." The left distal position of the pulse can become extremely flat.

The etiology of the more serious "heart small" disorder is a profound shock at birth when there is prolonged labor and the head has already reached the outside of the birth canal, but is being held back by something like the suffocating cord around the neck of the infant. With the more serious chronic form the pulse at the left distal position becomes at first extremely flat and later very deep, thin, and feeble. The rate is normal, slightly rapid, or slightly slow. A choppy quality has been observed with this condition, indicating blood stagnation in the coronary arteries.

Prolonged fear and unexpressed anger may also lead to this condition, though these emotions may also be the consequence, since one finds in people with the "heart small" condition a lifelong, unexpressed, and unexplained fear, as well as some anger and tension. Night terrors and being easily startled are common complaints. There is shortness of breath, in that it is easy to expel air and difficult to take it in. There may be chest pain, usually of a needlelike or stabbing quality in one spot, or stabbing pain in the left shoulder and/or down the left arm. Other symptoms are palpitations and cold extremities.

"Heart small" is permanent unless treated, and is equated by Dr. Shen with what he calls "true heart disease," by which he means coronary artery disease.

Heart Tight

Pin Yin	Latin	English	Dosage
Shi chang pu	Acori Tatarinowii Rhizoma	Grass-leaved sweetflag rhizome, acorus	2.4 g
Chuan xiong	Chuanxiong Rhizoma	Chuanxiong root, Szechuan lovage root, cnidium	4.5 g
Mu xiang	Saussureae Lappae Radix or Aucklandia Lappae Radix	Costus root, saussurea, aucklandia	4.5 g

Pin Yin	Latin	English	Dosage
Fu shen	Poria Cocos Pararadicis Sclerotium	Poria fungus	9 g
Yuan zhi	Polygalae Radix	Chinese senega root, polygala root	4.5 g
Suan zao ren	Ziziphi Spinosae Semen	Spiny zizyphus seeds, sour jujube seeds, zizyphus	9 g
Yu jin	Curcumae Radix	Curcuma tuber	9 g
Gua lou pi	Trichosanthis Pericarpium	Peel of trichosanthes fruit	9 g
Chen pi	Citri Reticulatae Pericarpium	Tangerine peel	6 g

Leon Hammer "Heart tight" is equivalent to moderate heart *qi* agitation due to heart *yin* deficiency. An early sign of heart *yin* deficiency is the hesitant wave on the entire pulse associated with obsession and the obsessive-compulsive personality. Later, tightness is felt over the entire left distal position. If the condition has existed for a short period of time owing to an emotional shock, immediately afterward the pulse is usually relatively rapid, between 84 and 90 beats per minute. Over a much longer period of time, the pulse rate will be slower, as this condition weakens heart *qi* and affects overall circulation.

Heart *yin* deficiency accompanies heart shock. Other etiologies include a prolonged condition of excess heat of the heart (heart fire flaring up as in mania and Graves disease), and consequent depletion of heart *yin*. With excess heat the pulse's left distal position will at first feel tight in the pericardium position, as if a strong, sharp point is pressing the middle of the finger with each beat. If the heat becomes overwhelming, the entire position can feel tense with robust pounding. This heat usually has its origins in the liver, gallbladder, and stomach.

Occasionally, there will be some discomfort in the left side of the chest over a relatively large area. This discomfort is an early form of mild angina that is due to excess heat from the liver, gallbladder, or stomach, causing a mild spasm of the coronary arteries, or stagnant liver *qi* migrating to the pericardium with the same result (the liver controls the autonomic nervous system). There may also be some shortness of breath during these episodes with palpitations and anxiety.

The "heart tight" (heart *yin*-deficient) condition is characterized by more restless sleep marked by constant awakening throughout the night, and tossing and turning. There is mild to moderate anxiety and irritability, and often complaints of constant worry, a "racing mind." (Symptoms associated with excess heat are marked by tension, severe irritability, outbursts of anger, and difficulty getting to sleep. This heat, now fire, is found in the manic phases of bipolar disease and with substances such as cocaine or *ma huang* [ephedra stem] in the early phases and less often with Graves [acute hyperthyroid] disease.)

An alternative to Dr. Shen's formula is *Tian Wang Bu Xin Dan* (Emperor of Heaven's Special Pill to Tonify the Heart).

Heart Vibration

Pin Yin	Latin	English	Dosage
Shi chang pu	Acori Tatarinowii Rhizoma	Grass-leaved sweetflag rhizome, acorus	2.4 g
Chuan xiong	Chuanxiong Rhizoma	Chuanxiong root, Szechuan lovage root, cnidium	4.5 g
Mu xiang	Saussureae Lappae Radix or Aucklandia Lappae Radix	Costus root, saussurea, aucklandia	4.5 g
Fu shen	Poria Cocos Pararadicis Sclerotium	Poria fungus	9 g
Yuan zhi	Polygalae Radix	Chinese senega root, polygala root	4.5 g

Pin Yin	Latin	English	Dosage
Suan zao ren	Ziziphi Spinosae Semen	Spiny zizyphus seeds, sour jujube seeds, zizyphus	9 g
Yu jin	Curcumae Radix	Curcuma tuber	9 g
Gua lou pi	Trichosanthis Pericarpium	Peel of trichosanthes fruit	9 g
Chen pi	Citri Reticulatae Pericarpium	Tangerine peel	6 g
Zhu deng xin cao	Medulla Junci Effusi	Dried rush pith, juncus	1.5–4.5 g

Leon Hammer   The vibration quality over the entire pulse or at individual positions is defined by whether it is transient or consistent, superficial or deep, and rough or smooth. Transient, superficial, and smooth vibration at the left distal position or even over the entire pulse indicates a relatively innocuous process involving passing worries or a tendency to worry, which I define as mild heart *qi* agitation. This sometimes begins with a very mild emotional shock (very mild heart *yin* deficiency), and often there is a background of vulnerability due to a very mild heart *qi* deficiency.

Consistent smooth vibration over the entire pulse is a sign that one is highly susceptible to worry, and will find something to worry about even when there is no reason. Here there may be vulnerability due to a background of "nervous system weak" as well as heart *qi*-blood deficiency. The hesitant wave is a sign of obsession and over a period of time of an obsessive-compulsive personality. Consistent vibration that is rougher and deeper over the entire pulse is a sign of more severe shock, guilt, or fear, and at individual positions indicates parenchymal damage.

Heart Weakness

FROM DR. SHEN: Lifting, chest area problem, chest pain, *qi* doesn't move. *Cun* position pulses weak or tight: weak in a long-term problem, tight in a short-term problem.

Pin Yin	Latin	English	Dosage
Xie bai	Albi Bulbus	Bulb of Chinese chive, macrostem onion, bakeri	6 g
Gua lou pi	Trichosanthis Pericarpium	Peel of trichosanthes fruit	9 g
Xiang fu	Cyperi Rotundi Rhizoma	Nut grass rhizoma, cyperus	4.5 g
Chuan xiong	Chuanxiong Rhizoma	Chuanxiong root, Szechuan lovage root, cnidium	4.5 g
Fu ling	Poria Cocos Sclerotium	Sclerotium of tuckahoe, poria, China root, hoelen, Indian bread	9 g
Yuan zhi	Polygalae Radix	Chinese senega root, polygala root	1.5 g
Yu jin	Curcumae Radix	Curcuma tuber	6 g
Huang qin	Scutellariae Baicalensis Radix	Baical skullcap root, scutellaria, scute	4.5 g
Bai shao	Paeoniae Alba Radix	White peony root	4.5 g

Leon Hammer   For heart *qi* deficiency Dr. Shen recommended the following formula, which we gave several affectionate names such as "Dr. Shen's Rock-et Fuel" and "Kick-a-Poo Joy Juice" to acknowledge its powerful ability to provide at least short-term stamina.

Formula for heart *qi* deficiency:

Pin Yin	Latin	English	Dosage
Ren shen	Ginseng Radix	Ginseng root	4.5 g
Gao li shen	Ginseng Coreensis Radix	Korean ginseng root[a]	4.5 g
Zi he che or tai pan	Placenta Hominis	Human placenta, placenta	2 g
Fu zi	Aconiti Lateralis Praeparata Radix	Aconite	0.25 g

[a] The Korean ginseng was soaked in aconite.

Hypertension

Leon Hammer   According to Dr. Shen there are two kinds of hypertension: one is the "true hypertension," when the pressure remains steadily elevated, and the other a pseudo-hypertension in which the elevation is variable associated with anxiety and stress.

True hypertension:

"True hypertension" in my own Chinese medical experience is usually associated with excess heat in the blood. One would assume from other comments by Dr. Shen that he would attribute this excess heat to the organ involved working beyond its capacity over a long period of time. Overwork can involve a normal workload by a deficient organ or a normal organ that is confronted with an excessive load.

The organ that is overworked the most in our culture is the gastrointestinal system due to poor food quality, too much food, eating too fast, and eating irregularly. Metabolic heat is required for work. Like any engine that overworks more heat accumulates than the organism can eliminate through ordinary mechanisms—the bowels, the urine, the skin—and becomes a retained pathogen in the blood.

Excess heat in the blood will eventually affect the intima of the vessel walls by draining the yin (fluid) of the walls to balance the heat. This inflammatory process makes the vessel walls less flexible and forces the heart to work harder, which is manifested as an increase in blood pressure (hypertension).

The body sends fluid to the blood vessels to balance the heat, increasing the volume and creating the thicker phlegm that adds more material to the blood, requiring more pressure from the heart to move it. This excess material clings to the inflamed walls (arteriosclerosis), requiring even more pressure.

Overwork of other organs, the liver and heart in particular, will likewise create excess heat that will eventually go to the blood, re-enacting the scenario described above. Since the liver stores the blood its excess heat will more readily go directly into the blood. The formula presented here for pseudo-hypertension contains herbs that are more appropriately useful in "true hypertension."

Pseudo-hypertension:

Dr. Shen stated that stress and states of ongoing tension could elevate blood pressure temporarily, which he stated was "pseudo-hypertension" ("white coat hypertension"). In this context, Dr. Shen did not explain the physiological mechanisms accounting for the relationship between the functions of the organs or the role of emotions in the elevation of blood pressure.

There are several physiological scenarios in Chinese medicine that can explain how the heart is forced to work harder and raise the blood pressure temporarily. We know that anxiety is the principal cause of blood pressure that is elevated in circumstances involving an examination in a doctor's office. We also know that the kidney yin will balance excesses in the heart, and kidney yang will balance deficiencies in the heart, and will always be a factor in all of the following.

The heart is the organ that increases blood pressure when it is forced to work harder. Anxiety, fear in this instance, of a particular situation is mediated through kidney yang (adrenal medulla—epinephrine; adrenal cortex—cortisol) that stimulates the heart. In Chinese medical terms I call this "heart qi agitation" in which the heart is stimulated to increase rate and force without a normal physiological signal.

Other sources of temporary stimulation to the heart include liver qi or yang, and/or excess heat, escaping from a qi-stagnant liver to a vulnerable heart. Stress requires the liver to repress emotion and contain more qi and heat. If the demand exceeds the ability of the liver (liver qi deficiency) to contain the ensuing excess qi and heat, they will escape and disrupt function in a vulnerable organ. The "rising *yang*" is associated with the more serious liver condition, "separation of *yin* and *yang*" in which the *yang* is out of control and will also go to the most vulnerable organ, in this case the heart where it will interfere with function.

Another pathway for the above is through the liver's control of the autonomic nervous system causing constriction of peripheral arteries and increased pressure since the heart has to work harder to move the circulation. Excess heat in the liver might excite the sympathetic nerves and cause vasoconstriction of the blood vessels.

Again, anything that causes the heart to pump harder temporarily will increase blood pressure temporarily. If the lungs are vulnerable, temporary escaping liver *qi* or heat causes constriction of the blood vessels in the lungs and requires more work by the heart to maintain this function.

We see from examining the above that the several etiologies of pseudo-hypertension would each require a separate herbal approach not addressed by Dr. Shen's herbal formulas available to the authors.

Formula for pseudo-hypertension:

Pin Yin	Latin	English	Dosage
Tian ma	Gastrodiae Rhizoma	Gastrodia rhizome	9 g
Chuan xiong	Chuanxiong Rhizoma	Chuanxiong root, Szechuan lovage root, cnidium	4.5 g
Chao jing jie	Schizonepetae Herba	Dry-fried schizonepeta	4.5 g
Bai ji li	Tribuli Terrestris Fructus	Caltrop fruit, puncture-vine fruit, tribulus	9 g
Fu ling	Poria Cocos Sclerotium	Sclerotium of tuckahoe, poria, China root, hoelen, Indian bread	9 g
Yuan zhi	Polygalae Radix	Chinese senega root, polygala root	4.5 g
Long chi	Fossilia Dentis Mastodi	Dragon teeth, fossilized teeth	18 g
Ci shi	Magnetitum	Magnetite	18 g
Chuan lian zi	Meliae Toosendan Fructus	Szechuan pagoda fruit, Szechuan chinaberry fruit, melia	9 g
Huai niu xi or niu xi	Achyranthis Bidentatae Radix	Ox-knee root, achyranthes root from Huai	9 g

FROM DR. SHEN: First boil the *long chi* (fossil teeth) and *ci shi* (magnetite) for 20 minutes, then add other medicines and boil into tea. Continue until the blood pressure returns to normal. The patient has to refrain from consuming alcohol and spicy food and must remain relaxed and rested.

Hamilton Rotte In the literature, hypertension is attributed to liver *yin* deficiency and *yang* rising (often causing wind), liver fire, liver *qi* stagnation, phlegm-heat, damp-heat in the middle burner, *qi* and *yin* deficiency and blood stagnation. Most commonly the literature cites liver *yin* deficiency and *yang* rising.

This formula addresses the following conditions: liver *yin* deficiency and *yang* rising, liver *qi* stagnation, liver heat, and dampness in the middle burner. The following herbs nourish liver *yin*: *tian ma* and *huai niu xi*.

The following herbs descend the liver *yang*: *tian ma*, *ci shi*, *huai niu xi*, and *long gu*, *bai ji li*, and *chuan lian zi*. The following herbs regulate liver *qi*: *chuan lian zi* and *bai ji li*. *Chuan lian zi* is also included to clear liver heat. *Chuan xiong* addresses blood stagnation and it is likely that it is also included along with *jing jie* to reduce nervous tension. *Chuan xiong* and *jing jie* are included in Dr. Shen's "Nervous System Tense" formula. *Chuan xiong* and *jing jie* are used by Dr. Shen in a way that is not described by the standard texts.

Leon Hammer Personal experience suggests that the use of *fu shen* rather than *fu ling* calms the heart and relaxes the nervous system.

Formula for hypertension:

Pin Yin	Latin	English	Dosage
Yu jin	Curcumae Radix	Curcuma tuber	12 g
Du zhong	Eucommiae Cortex	Eucommia bark	12 g

Hamilton Rotte This formula, gleaned from Dr. Shen's records, contains two herbs that are descending in nature. It is indicated for a hypertensive individual that presents with liver *qi* stagnation (addressed by *yu jin*) and kidney *yang* deficiency (addressed by *du zhong*).

Insomnia

FROM DR. SHEN: Insomnia may happen as a result of long-term overwork, over deliberation and worry. As a matter of fact people never rest their heads on a sleepless pillow when they are perfectly exhausted. So the first course of treatment is to compose the troubled mind. A patient with a recent case of insomnia should never feel nervous about his sleeplessness. He must try to relax himself and go into dreamland without taking sleeping pills. He should avoid eating too much food in the evening as a heavy stomach will contribute to his insomnia.

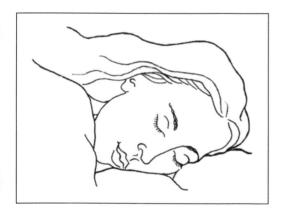

Fig. 1 Sleeping woman.

Leon Hammer The following information was imparted to me during my apprenticeship to Dr. Shen. According to Chinese medicine, sleep occurs when a significant amount of circulating blood is stored in the liver and removed from the heart circulation (**Fig. 1**).

All heart conditions affect sleep in different, often predictable, ways. These conditions are almost always in combination with other deficiencies or excesses of *qi*, *yin*, *yang*, and blood. With most heart conditions affecting sleep the person wakes up tired, especially with heart *qi* and *yang* deficiency, and to a lesser extent with heart blood stagnation ("heart small") and trapped *qi* in the heart ("heart closed").

Difficulty getting to sleep occurs with all the following heart patterns but especially with liver and heart fire (frequent dreams and nightmares):

• "Heart *qi* agitation" with worry ("heart nervous") in which with this heart activity blood cannot return to the liver. The "heart nervous" person can also have difficulty getting to sleep if they have overworked or have been under great stress during the prior day.

- "Heart tight," excess heat type brought on by worry similar to heart *qi* agitation. The mind is racing, worried, and the person restless, uptight, and in Dr. Shen's terms "the nerves are tight."

Difficulty falling asleep can occur with eating before sleep, especially food difficult to digest, though this problem usually manifests later (see below). Some people cannot sleep at all some nights, obsessing about presumed insults and vengeance, which is associated with heart *qi* stagnation ("heart closed").

Sleep reversal can be a "normal" cycle in some people. In others it is a sign of "*qi* wild," a condition in which the *yin* and *yang* of many of the solid organs have separated. This is always associated with some profound deficiency of one or more of the substances, blood, *qi*, *yin*, and *yang*. We see this in large cities like New York when a different population emerges when the day people retire. Very often the "*qi* wild" people are severely emotionally and mentally disturbed (a "*Qi* Wild" herbal formula is discussed below).

People who awake frequently fall into two general categories. First are those who are extremely restless, tossing and turning, generally associated with heart *yin* deficiency (with profuse dreaming) or "heart *qi* agitation" who are very sensitive to sound, up and down all night but not restless, tossing and turning. Second, there are the heart *qi*-deficient people who wake up frequently and are not restless, with few dreams and fall back asleep easily.

Then there are those who, due to stomach food and *qi* stagnation, awake after a few (often just 2) hours of sleep and have difficulty returning to sleep. Eating lightly in the evening is advised.

There is another group of people who wake after about 5 hours of sleep. Those who fall back to sleep in less than an hour are considered heart blood deficient ("heart weak"), and those who cannot are considered heart blood stagnant ("heart small").

The heart blood-deficient condition is paradoxical since the heart rests best when there is less blood. However, there must be enough to maintain life throughout the night and when what is used for that purpose depletes the blood to maintain heart muscle function, the liver that stores the blood urgently releases it to the heart and causes temporary wakening until homeostasis is restored.

Insomnia due to difficulty breathing occurs due to severe heart *qi* and *yang* deficiency ("heart large"; "heart disease") with difficulty breathing when they lie on their back and they wake up to find a more comfortable position. With "trapped *qi* in the heart" ("heart full") there is difficulty lying especially on the left side and they wake up to find more comfortable position.

Excessive dreaming is associated with liver-heart fire (difficulty getting to sleep), heart *yin* deficiency and "phlegm misting the orifices."

Gallbladder damp-heat combined with heart *qi* deficiency and possibly "phlegm misting the orifices" is marked by a fear of sleeping alone, waking frightened, being easily startled and paranoid, with profuse phlegm. The gallbladder is implicated in the sleep disorder, related also to liver blood not supporting the "ethereal soul," though this relationship is obscure.

We can also consider sleep patterns in terms of kidney–heart disharmony. The heart "controls" the mind and kidney essence nourishes the brain. If the water of the kidney cannot control the fire of the heart the mind will become restless. If the fire of the heart cannot warm the water of the kidney it cannot rise and nourish the brain and normal patterns will be disrupted (Hammer, 2011b).

Formula I for insomnia:

Pin Yin	Latin	English	Dosage
Chao huang lian	Coptidis Rhizoma	Dry-fried coptis rhizome	1.5 g
Rou gui	Cinnamomi Cassiae Cortex	Inner bark of Saigon cinnamon	0.3 g
Suan zao ren	Ziziphi Spinosae Semen	Spiny zizyphus seeds, sour jujube seeds, zizyphus	15 g

FROM DR. SHEN: Boil the wild jujube seeds for 30 minutes, then add other medicines to be boiled for another 10 minutes; drink the tea 1 hour before sleep. If the dose proves to be ineffective, the second insomnia formula is indicated.

Hamilton Rotte This formula is a modification of *Jiao Tai Wan* (Grand Communication Pill). *Jiao Tai Wan* is descending in nature and is indicated for heat-above and cold-below patterns, though normally the dosages of the ingredients (*huang lian* and *rou gui*) are usually much higher. His dosages are generally lower—the herbs in his time were stronger. The heat in the upper part of the body can be viewed as the kidney *yang*, which is out of place and floating upward, giving rise to agitation and insomnia. This condition is underappreciated in Chinese medicine and can give rise to a variety of mental-emotional conditions. The condition of the kidney *yang* being "out of the box" is described by Heiner Fruehauf in his discussion of the Szechuan fire school of herbal medicine (Fruehauf, 2009).

In this formula we also find *suan zao ren*, which is an especially potent herb for the treatment of insomnia. It treats heart *yin* and blood patterns and has a distinct sedating effect, which is why it is commonly utilized in standard formulas as well as prepared medicines in the treatment of insomnia. Its sour property draws the spirit inward, which enables the spirit to be nourished and calmed by heart blood and *yin*.

It is also possible that the dosages were kept lower in order not to be harmful to laypeople.

Formula II for insomnia:

Pin Yin	Latin	English	Dosage
Chao huang lian	Coptidis Rhizoma	Dry-fried coptis rhizome	1.5 g
Rou gui	Cinnamomi Cassiae Cortex	Inner bark of Saigon cinnamon	0.3 g
Suan zao ren	Ziziphi Spinosae Semen	Spiny zizyphus seeds, sour jujube seeds, zizyphus	12 g
Fu shen	Poria Cocos Pararadicis Sclerotium	Poria fungus	9 g
Long chi	Fossilia Dentis Mastodi	Dragon teeth, fossilized teeth	15 g
Ci shi	Magnetitum	Magnetite	15 g
Zhi yuan zhi	Polygalae Radix	Prepared Chinese senega root, polygala root	6 g
Yu jin	Curcumae Radix	Curcuma tuber	9 g
Bai shao	Paeoniae Alba Radix	White peony root	6 g
Zhu deng xin cao	Medulla Junci Effusi	Dried rush pith, juncus	3 bundles

FROM DR. SHEN: Boil the medicines into tea and drink 1 hour before going to bed. One dosage of medicine may be saved and boiled again.

Hamilton Rotte This formula is stronger than Dr. Shen's first formula for insomnia. It contains the ingredients of the first formula in addition to other spirit-calming ingredients. Here we find heavy minerals, notably *long chi* and *ci shi*. These two ingredients, along with *zhen zhu* (pearl) are the strongest spirit-sedating substances still readily available (some stronger substances such as *zhu sha* [cinnabar] are unavailable due to supposed toxicity). Heavy minerals are the strongest substances among the materia medica for intractable cases of insomnia.

Yuan zhi, apparently one of Dr. Shen's favorite herbs, calms the spirit, resolves phlegm, and moves *qi* in the chest. *Yu jin* is included to move blood, resolve phlegm, and clear heat. *Bai shao* nourishes liver blood, thereby indirectly supporting the heart. *Zhu deng xin cao* clears excess heat from the heart, a favorite of both Dr. Shen and Ding Gan Ren.

Leon Hammer Resolving "phlegm misting the orifices" is in my experience a critical step in dealing with the emotional component of any condition (Hammer, 2007). The question about the location of the orifices, external (nose, mouth, eyes, and ears) or internal, the "orifices of the heart organ" is controversial and the subject of investigation by me and a collaborator, Stephen Higgins, LAc.

Move *Qi* in the Chest

Pin Yin	Latin	English	Dosage
Dang shen	Codonopsis Pilosulae Radix	Codonopsis root	4.5 g
Xie bai	Albi Bulbus	Bulb of Chinese chive, macrostem onion, bakeri	4.5 g
Gua lou pi	Trichosanthis Pericarpium	Peel of trichosanthes fruit	9 g
Chuan xiong	Chuanxiong Rhizoma	Chuanxiong root, Szechuan lovage root, cnidium	4.5 g
Sang ji sheng	Taxilli Herba	Mulberry mistletoe stems, loranthus, taxillus, mistletoe	9 g
Zhi shi	Aurantii Immaturus Fructus	Immature bitter orange, unripe bitter orange, *chih-shih*	4.5 g
Yuan zhi	Polygalae Radix	Chinese senega root, polygala root	4.5 g
Wu wei zi	Schisandrae Chinensis Fructus	Schisandra fruit	4.5 g
Yu jin	Curcumae Radix	Curcuma tuber	9 g
Xiang fu	Cyperi Rotundi Rhizoma	Nut grass rhizoma, cyperus	4.5 g
Lu lu tong	Liquidambaris Fructus	Sweetgum fruit, liquidambar fruit	12 g

For flat pulse remove:

Pin Yin	Latin	English	Dosage
Wu wei zi	Schisandrae Chinensis Fructus	Schisandra fruit	4.5 g

And add:

Pin Yin	Latin	English	Dosage
Chen xiang	Aquilariae Lignum	Aloeswood, aquilaria	1.5 g
Ding xiang	Caryophilli Flos	Clove flower bud	3 g
Xie bai	Albi Bulbus	Bulb of Chinese chive, macrostem onion, bakeri	3 g

For a deficient person (usually with flat quality), add:

Pin Yin	Latin	English	Dosage
Xi yang shen	Panacis Quinquefolii Radix	American ginseng root	4.5 g
Gao li shen	Ginseng Coreensis Radix	Korean ginseng root	4.5 g
Zi he che or tai pan	Placenta Hominis	Human placenta, placenta	4.5 g

Hamilton Rotte This formula utilizes pungent, moving substances that address *qi* stagnation in the upper burner. Most of the *qi* regulators are described in the TCM literature as entering the spleen and stomach or liver, and here we see an expanded view of some of the moving substances commonly used in TCM.

The combination of *gua lou pi* and *xie bai* to address *qi* stagnation is based on the classical combination of *quan gua lou* and *xie bai*, which addresses chest "*bi* syndrome," where cold and damp pathogens lodge in the chest and obstruct circulation. In this case *gua lou pi* is selected because its ability to move *qi* is stronger than *quan gua lou*.

Chuan xiong is considered both *qi* and blood moving, and its effect on the upper body is well known.

Zhi shi has a marked effect on the chest. According to Bensky, it is indicated for "focal distention and fullness in the chest" (Bensky, 2004, p. 517).

Yuan zhi and *wu wei zi* are a two-herb combination, with *yuan zhi* drying and moving and *wu wei zi* moistening and consolidating. We find that formulas that are moving to *qi* or blood contain ingredients that move in opposite directions (as in the *chai hu*/*bai shao* and *tao ren*/*hong hua* combinations).

Yu jin is a *qi* and blood mover that is known to enter the heart, and *xiang fu* enters the triple burner, which enables it to treat stagnation in the chest. Furthermore, *xiang fu*'s ability to treat mental-emotional conditions demonstrates its ability to affect the upper burner.

Dang shen and *sang ji shen* are probably included as tonics to balance the moving nature of the other ingredients in the formula.

Descending herbs, widely used by Dr. Shen for stagnation in the upper burner, include *gua lou pi*, *sang ji sheng*, *zhi shi*, *yuan zhi*, *yu jin*, and *xiang fu*.

When the pulse is flat, *wu wei zi* is omitted because it has a consolidating effect on the *qi*. Also when the flat pulse is present, the addition of other *qi* regulators *chen xiang*, *ding xiang*, and *xie bai* are used.

Leon Hammer I have found this formula particularly effective with *qi* stagnation in the heart, lungs, and diaphragm. It should be kept in mind that *qi* stagnation can come from deficiency as well as excess and is usually milder with the latter since there is less *qi* to stagnate.

Symptoms:
- Heart
  - Depression—usually due to a sudden shock
  - Tightness and oppressed feeling, especially in middle of chest
  - Tendency to vengefulness and spite
  - Constant interpersonal strife
  - Insomnia
  - Ruminating about revenge
  - Palpitations with movement (less than heart *qi* and blood deficiency)
  - Circulatory problems
  - Difficulty healing
  - Migratory joint pains
- Lungs
  - Shortness of breath
  - Fullness and oppression of the chest
  - Other symptoms depend on cause.
    Example: Lung *qi* deficiency: shortness of breath (asthma), sitting still and on exertion; weak cough; weak voice; hoarse voice (phlegm may also be involved); fatigue; thin, watery sputum; daytime sweating
- Diaphragm
  - Lump in throat
  - Breathing difficulty—rapid, labored
  - Cannot get a full breath, worse when lying down
  - Cannot lie on chest
  - Discomfort in chest: pressure—fullness; pain—angina in any location in the chest; "gas" pains in chest—felt as heart; coughing—unproductive

Etiology:
- Heart
  - Repressed heart feelings due to loss of love
  - Feelings of revenge
  - Shock due to sudden loss (e.g., money in stock market)
- Lungs
  - Repressed grief
  - Physical trauma causing person to hold breath
  - Poor posture
  - Exterior pathogenic factor—retained cold turned to heat
- Diaphragm
  - Separation with repression of tender feeling replaced by anger
  - Lifting beyond capacity of "terrain" (body condition)

Hamilton Rotte The separation of *yin* and *yang* involves a functional alienation between *yin* and *yang* where *yin* no longer is able to hold *yang* and *yang* moves up and out. This process involves *yin* deficiency or *yang* deficiency. In addition to tonifying the substances it is necessary to restore contact between *yin* and *yang*.

This formula contains astringent, stabilizing herbs that bring the *yang* back to the *yin*. These include *wu wei zi*, *long gu*, and *mu li*. In addition, there are substances that calm the spirit, which address the men-tal-emotional aspects of a "*qi* wild" condition (anxiety, depersonalization): *yuan zhi*, *wu wei zi*, *long gu*, and *mu li*.

This formula contains tonic herbs for *qi* (*dang shen* and *huang qi*) and *yin* (*wu wei zi* and *mai men dong*).

Yuan zhi and *wu wei zi* are a two-herb combination. Both calm the spirit, while *yuan zhi* is moving and *wu wei zi* is stabilizing.

Si gua luo and *sang ji sheng* are moving for the channels and collaterals.

Leon Hammer This is a condition of extreme functional deficit in that, for one reason or another, the *yin* and *yang* have lost operative contact and are unable to support each other over a large part of the organism. The underlying condition is an extreme deficiency of either *yin* or *yang* or both in many individual organs where it is known as "separation of *yin* and *yang*."

The *yin*, that is, the material energy of the universe, can be thought of as a gravitational force that holds the more effervescent *yang* energies in check, and when drained can no longer serve that function. Under these circumstances, without the organizing force of the *yin*, the lighter *yang* energies wander aimlessly to all parts of the organism, especially organs or areas that are vulnerable, disturbing function and resulting in physiological disarray.

Thus, "*qi* wild" is a condition characterized by chaos and represents a very serious physiological disorganization and disruption. A person suffering from this condition is highly vulnerable to serious and fast-spreading, even life-threatening, disease within a very short time, including cancer, other autoimmune diseases, and degenerative central nervous system disease. Mental illness is another form of this chaos if the "nervous system" is vulnerable.

While this formula is an important first step to reunite the *yin* and *yang* and settle the associated physiological chaos it is important to remember that the "*qi* wild separation of *yin* and *yang*" is usually the result of a profound deficiency of some substance, *yin*, *yang*, blood, *qi* or of an equally profound shock to the heart and circulation.

The pulse qualities associated with the "*qi* wild" condition are on the entire pulse and include empty; leather; empty and thread-like; scattered; minute; and change in qualities: yielding hollow interrupted-intermittent; yielding hollow full-overflowing (rapid or slow) (Hammer, 1998).

The tongue will have areas that have no color, will appear milky-white, or lose its shape

Stopping Exercise Suddenly

FROM DR. SHEN: The following formula is for those persons who lose their concentration or suddenly stop exercising, which causes poor blood circulation.

Pin Yin	Latin	English	Dosage
Huang qi	Astragali Radix	Milk vetch root, astragalus root	9 g
Dang gui	Angelicae Sinensis Radix	Chinese angelica root, *tang-kuei*	6 g
Chuan xiong	Chuanxiong Rhizoma	Chuanxiong root, Szechuan lovage root, cnidium	4.5 g
Shan yao	Dioscoreae Oppositae Rhizoma	Chinese yam root, dioscorea rhizome	9 g
Fu ling	Poria Cocos Sclerotium	Sclerotium of tuckahoe, poria, China root, hoelen, Indian bread	9 g

Pin Yin	Latin	English	Dosage
Suan zao ren	Ziziphi Spinosae Semen	Spiny zizyphus seeds, sour jujube seeds, zizyphus	12 g
Wu wei zi	Schisandrae Chinensis Fructus	Schisandra fruit	4.5 g
Long gu	Fossilia Ossis Mastodi	Dragon bone, fossilized vertebrae and bones of the extremities (usually of mammals)	15 g
Mu li	Ostreae Concha	Oyster shell	15 g
Sang ji sheng	Taxilli Herba	Mulberry mistletoe stems, loranthus, taxillus, mistletoe	12 g
Mai men dong	Ophiopogonis Radix	Ophiopogon tuber/root	9 g
Mai ya	Hordei Germinatus Fructus	Barley sprout, malt	12 g
Gu ya	Oryzae Germinatus Fructus	Rice sprout	12 g
Sang zhi	Ramulus Mori Albae	Mulberry twig, morus twig	12 g

Hamilton Rotte   This formula is indicated for an individual who stops exercise suddenly, an event that has profound and devastating effects on physiology. Sudden cessation of exercise induces a separation of yin and yang as blood volume reduces more quickly than blood vessels can accommodate.

This formula contains stabilizing ingredients that bring floating yang back into contact with yin. Sour and astringent ingredients include suan zao ren, wu wei zi, long gu, and mu li.

This formula also includes many qi- and blood tonic ingredients, suggesting that this condition also includes a significant element of deficiency. Qi tonics include huang qi, shan yao, and fu ling. Blood tonics include dang gui, suan zao ren, and sang ji sheng. Mai men dong, a fluid tonic, increases blood volume as well. Blood tonics have a particular significance in this formula, as the decrease in blood volume is largely responsible for the separation of yin and yang.

This formula also contains moving ingredients to the blood and channels. Dang gui and chuan xiong move the blood. Sang ji sheng and sang zhi open the channels.

Mai ya and gu ya may be included to aid in the digestion of the tonic herbs.

Leon Hammer   This formula was developed by Dr. Shen to resolve a problem that he recognized from his experience that in our time has become an international epidemic. The reason is the overall increased pressure on children to perform athletically, mentioned under the discussion of scoliosis.

Colleges are eager to give athletic scholarships for large numbers of entering freshmen in the hope that a few of them will qualify for varsity teams. In fact only a tiny percentage of these athletic scholarship students succeed and the rest are discarded from the athletic programs.

These are students who have spent their entire childhoods preparing for this moment in their life when they would enter the limelight and even go on with professional careers. The unending physical work they have performed during their formative years is phenomenal.

When they are rebuffed, usually that rigorous training ends abruptly, partially because there is no program to follow, trainers to assist, and even more often because the rejection and sense of failure is accompanied by severe depression. For all these reasons they stop exercising abruptly.

Having been a psychiatrist in a college clinic for 7 years I saw what has now become a flood of calls for help at college health clinics with the presenting symptoms of depression and, especially, severe anxiety and bizarre emotional and physical experiences.

I have also found this syndrome in adults who cease long-term exercise suddenly. This includes another large group of people especially of the baby-boomer and long-term effect is difficulty with healing and the onset of migrating joint pain, both associated with decreased circulation. Another important consequence is structural defect, often manifested as pain and discomfort in other parts of the body. While we often treat the pain, which is often local, we usually ignore the long-term effects since the patient is long gone from our practice and often shows up years later in the office of a rheumatologist or orthopedic surgeon. Other later manifestations of the effect on circulation and the heart are sleep and "shen" disturbances, chronic fatigue, and fibromyalgia.

Signs:

Signs are most important because often trauma and shock are forgotten or never known.

Pulse:

The immediate effect of trauma and shock is a significant increase in rate and a very tight quality on the entire pulse if the trauma is great, or in positions associated with a particular area with a localized injury. Over the years the rate becomes very slow, further decreasing circulation and the tight quality persists with the presence of pain.

The flat quality is associated with a cord around the neck at birth, the loss of a loved one in childhood or physical trauma to the chest early in life. The inflated quality is associated with a breech birth, trauma to the chest, and/or emotional shock after the age of maturity.

When the problem begins during parturition or at birth, frequently the proximal positions are deep or feeble-absent indicating a kidney *yang-jing* deficiency. This is one dependable sign of an early physiological insult with failure to mature in one of a variety of ways and severity (unable to keep up with peers, cerebral palsy to autism, mental dysfunction or retardation).

Tongue:

With physical trauma there can be a long-lasting ecchymosis or purple blister on the same side of the body as the trauma (**Fig. 3**). A purple color can eventually pervade the entire tongue. With birth trauma or inherited heart *qi* deficiency there can be a thin, vertical line going to the tip that will get deeper over time if the heart condition is not resolved.

Eyes:

Under the lower eyelid on the side of the physical trauma at the base of the red vertical lines there will be a red horizontal line (**Fig. 4a, b**).

Structural:

Long leg syndrome is a condition in which one leg is longer than the other, indicating that the pelvis is out of balance. This is often the result of physical trauma. Frequently there are vertebral problems alluded to in chiropractics as fixations and subluxations. This can be the result of trauma any time from birth. The result is pain, often of the lower back and of the legs (sciatica, meralgia), knees, and ankles. (For more information please consult Hammer, 2006).

Asking:

A detailed probing history of the patient's parturition and birth and subsequent trauma during life is a very important part of the asking diagnosis, often overlooked.

Face and hands:

With birth trauma there is a pronounced blue-green color around the mouth. When there has been significant oxygen deprivation as a form of birth trauma the entire face may be blue. These colors last the entire life. When the face is more red than the hands the heart is affecting circulation (heart shock). When the hands are red and the face pale, the circulation is affecting the heart (physical trauma).

EMOTIONAL SHOCK

Physiology:

While daily stress tends to affect the liver, shock affects the heart. Emotional shock evokes protective measures by the pericardium to keep the heart functioning. That involves vasoconstriction of the peripheral circulation and an emptying of the heart in its attempt to maintain the circulation in the other vital organs.

The traditional use of the herbal formula *Sheng Mai San* (Generate the Pulse Powder) (see below) for the treatment of shock to the heart implies that with shock the heart empties itself of *yin*. Each of the three herbs protects or provides *yin*.

It is my opinion supported by pulse findings described below, that unless the *qi* of the heart and the organism is strong enough to restore the *yin*, or without healing intervention, the *yin* and *yang* of the heart will separate ("separation of *yin* and *yang*") and circulatory chaos will ensue. When *yin* and *yang* separate the *yin* loses control of the *yang*; substance (*yin*) loses control over function (*yang*). When function is out of control, physiological anarchy is the consequence.

Since the heart "controls" the mind the chaos is expressed by a chaotic lifestyle and mental instability. In terms of the *shen–hun–po*, the *shen* and *hun* become separated from the *po*, the spirit from its ground, and the former is fragmented and dissociated, the organism a "ship without a captain" ("*hun* flies and *po* scatters"). The *Su Wen* refers to "shock scatters the *qi*" under "Simple Questions," Chapter 39 (Maciocia 1989, p.132). A lesser psychological consequence of depletion of heart *yin* is a tendency toward obsessional thinking

My own experience is that likewise this is later accompanied by heart *qi* and blood stagnation (coronary artery) if not treated promptly. With failure to overcome stagnation of *qi* and blood, excess heat will accumulate, later a compensatory accumulation of damp leading to "phlegm misting the orifices" associated with severe mental and emotional conditions (neurosis and psychosis).

The failure of the heart to move *qi*, according to Dr. Shen, is intractable preoccupation with vengeance. Heart blood stagnation is associated by Dr. Shen with lifelong fear.

Complicating the above, if the *yin* and blood supply to the nervous innervation of the heart is permanently reduced, types of fibrillation (sinoatrial node) will ensue and remain throughout life until some form of therapy intervenes.

A vicious cycle begins with diminished heart function, in turn leading to decreased peripheral circulation. The physiological effect is the same as with trauma in reverse order, the heart affecting circulation rather than circulation affecting the heart. As with physical trauma, every cell in the body is affected by a decrease in the nutrients and increase in waste products.

Etiology:

Conception involves the ages of the parents, the abuse of substances (legal or otherwise), physical condition and illness, including venereal disease, past births, miscarriages and abortions, and the length of time since the last birth.

Emotional shock to the mother during pregnancy affects the fetus in-utero through the change in cortisol and epinephrine levels as well as the corticosteroids of the mother transmitted through the placenta. Other shocks to the fetus include physical trauma, placenta previa, mother's drug abuse, and prolonged vomiting and profound physical illness (toxemia), prematurity, cesarean section, high forceps delivery, cord around the neck, and abnormal presentation (breech). With early shock the kidney essence will be depleted, negatively affecting kidney–heart harmony.

The loss of a caretaker or loved one through death or separation, especially in childhood, profoundly affects the heart, which as a protective device withdraws and stagnates *qi* and blood. Translated in behavioral terms, the person withdraws their heart feelings so as not to be hurt, which when it occurs in childhood leaves a permanent challenge for interpersonal relations throughout life. More often than not shocks that occur during early life are often repressed and forgotten, including those by people who are physically abused and raped.

Accurate data about pregnancy, delivery, and early childhood are often obscured by a mother's need to put the painful past to rest, and require focused investigation by the patient, from which the information is almost always forthcoming through relatives and family friends. Information about shock in adulthood such as a break-up of a marriage or loss of a loved one or a severe auto accident are more clearly recalled.

Signs:
Pulse:

With emotional shock to the heart the rate can stay elevated for many years until the *qi* of the heart diminishes significantly to slow the rate. The pulse will also be very tight, commensurate with emotional pain. The long-term most dependable pulse sign is a rough vibration (4–5) (Hammer, 2001, p.370), felt as a first impression upon taking the entire radial pulse with both hands especially if the general *qi* is deficient. Changes in rate at rest including interrupted and intermittent pulses will be found when the effects of the shock on the heart are not relieved by some sort of healing intervention.

With some patients where the shock occurred at birth, or as a severe loss early in life up to the age of approximately 14, the effect is a flat quality at the left distal position. At the left distal position the quality is inflated if the emotional shock occurs after maturity. And according to Dr. Shen, with unusual presentations the two sides of the pulse can be seriously imbalanced, including possibly the rate.

(The inflated quality is also associated with a breech birth and trauma to the chest, and/or emotional shock after the age of maturity and the flat quality also with birth with the cord around the neck.)

Tongue:

With emotional trauma affecting the heart the tip might have raised red spots and be contracted.

Face and hands:

With fear the entire face has a green color and constricted pupils. With shock the face has a blue tinge if severe, especially between the eyes (*yin tang*) and temples (*tai yang*) later in life, and with guilt no change in color.

With mild to moderate shock in-utero a bluish tinge will occur around the mouth and chin and with shock

Ingredient	Action	Dosage	Reference
Bai niu dan, 25 mg	A substitute for xiong dan (bear gallbladder) that clears heat from the heart and liver and stops spasms (for convulsions, epilepsy, etc.), clears heat and resolves toxicity (for skin problems, sore throat, etc., topical application is especially effective for relieving pain), clears liver heat and benefits the eyes, may be similar to niu huang (cow gallbladder stones): cools heat, dredges phlegm, clears the consciousness (opens the orifices and awakes the spirit), clears the liver, resolves toxicity, extinguishes wind, cools the blood	n. a.	Bensky, 2004 (p. 1064)
Bing pian, 7.5 mg	Acrid-dispersing, aromatically mobilizing and piercing, opens the orifices and disperses fire constraint	0.01–0.3 g	Bensky, 2004 (p. 953)

When modifying the trauma and shock treatment, it is advisable to treat co-existing conditions that affect the heart. Here are common modifications utilized by Dr. Hammer for this purpose:

Formula for heart phlegm (very common and important addition), promotes awareness:

Pin Yin	Latin	English	Dosage
Shi chang pu	Acori Tatarinowii Rhizoma	Grass-leaved sweetflag rhizome, acorus	3 g
Yuan zhi	Polygalae Radix	Chinese senega root, polygala root	3 g

For birth trauma, problems that start early:

Pin Yin	Latin	English	Dosage
Zi he che or tai pan	Placenta Hominis	Human placenta, placenta	2–3 g

For heart blood deficiency:

Pin Yin	Latin	English	Dosage
Bai zi ren	Platycladi Semen	Biota seed	3–9 g
Suan zao ren	Ziziphi Spinosae Semen	Spiny zizyphus seeds, sour jujube seeds, zizyphus	9–15 g
Long yan rou	Longan Arillus	Longan aril	9–15 g
Ye jiao teng	Polygoni Multiflori Caulis	Polygonum vine, fleece flower vine	15–30 g

For heart yang deficiency:

Pin Yin	Latin	English	Dosage
Rou gui	Cinnamomi Cassiae Cortex	Inner bark of Saigon cinnamon	1 g
Fu zi	Aconiti Lateralis Praeparata Radix	Aconite	0.25 g

For greater heart qi deficiency:

Pin Yin	Latin	English	Dosage
Ren shen	Ginseng Radix	Ginseng root	6 g

For liver and kidney deficiency:

Pin Yin	Latin	English	Dosage
He shou wu	Polygoni Multiflori Radix	Fleece-flower root, polygonum hosuwu	9 g

For blood stagnation, also to move blood (a good idea when tonifying):

Pin Yin	Latin	English	Dosage
Yu ji	Curcumae Radix	Curcuma tuber	6–12 g

For agitation, depression:

Pin Yin	Latin	English	Dosage
He huan pi	Albiziae Cortex	Silk tree bark	6–15 g

For great lability:

Pin Yin	Latin	English	Dosage
Long chi	Fossilia Dentis Mastodi	Dragon teeth, fossilized teeth	15–30 g

For anxiety, constant worry, weak nervous system (flight rather than fight). *Gan Mai Da Zao Tang* (Licorice, Wheat, and Jujube Decoction):

Pin Yin	Latin	English	Dosage
Gan cao	Glycyrrhizae Radix	Licorice root	9 g
Fu xiao mai or xiao mai	Tritici Levis Fructus	Light wheat grain	9–15 g
Da zao	Zizyphi Jujubae Fructus	Chinese date, jujube	10–30 g

Other additions: *dan shen, chuan xiong, gan jiang, hu po.*

Trauma to Heart, Phlegm, Heart Nervous

Pin Yin	Latin	English	Dosage
Shi chang pu	Acori Tatarinowii Rhizoma	Grass-leaved sweetflag rhizome, acorus	1.8 g
Chuan xiong	Chuanxiong Rhizoma	Chuanxiong root, Szechuan lovage root, cnidium	1.8 g
Chuan bei mu	Fritillariae Cirrhosae Bulbus	Szechuan fritillaria bulb, tendrilled fritillary bulb, fritillaria	9 g
Zhe bei mu	Fritillariae Thunbergii Bulbus	Zhejiang fritillaria, Thunberg fritillaria bulb, fritillaria	9 g
Ju hong	Pars Rubra Epicarpii Citri Erythrocarpae	Red part of tangerine peel	3 g
Fu shen	Poria Cocos Pararadicis Sclerotium	Poria fungus	6 g
Zhi yuan zhi	Polygalae Radix	Honey-fried Chinese senega root, polygala root	2.4 g

Hamilton Rotte   This formula, which is related to "Move *Qi* in the Chest," is somewhat stronger and contains more blood-invigorating ingredients. The *qi*-moving ingredients are very similar to "Move *Qi* in the Chest" (with the addition of *chai hu* and *chen pi* in this formula), though the following blood-moving ingredients are included as well: *hu po, yan hu suo,* and *shan zha tan* (charred *shan zha* has more of an affinity for the blood level).

"Yielding Hollow Full-overflowing"

Hamilton Rotte   Here is a formula that is closely related to the "Stopping Exercise Suddenly" formula that Dr. Shen indicated for the yielding hollow full-overflowing pulse quality, associated with the sudden cessation of exercise. This formula is also closely related to the "*Qi* Wild" formula. The "*qi* wild" condition is commonly caused by the sudden cessation of exercise.

Pin Yin	Latin	English	Dosage
Dang shen	Codonopsis Pilosulae Radix	Codonopsis root	9 g
Chuan xiong	Chuanxiong Rhizoma	Chuanxiong root, Szechuan lovage root, cnidium	4.5 g
Qiang huo	Notopterygii Rhizoma et Radix	Notopterygium root and rhizome, chiang-huo	4.5 g
Sang ji sheng	Taxilli Herba	Mulberry mistletoe stems, loranthus, taxillus, mistletoe	12 g
Yuan zhi	Polygalae Radix	Chinese senega root, polygala root	4.5 g
Wu wei zi	Schisandrae Chinensis Fructus	Schisandra fruit	4.5 g
Long gu	Fossilia Ossis Mastodi	Dragon bone, fossilized vertebrae and bones of the extremities (usually of mammals)	12 g
Mu li	Ostreae Concha	Oyster shell	12 g
Xiang fu	Cyperi Rotundi Rhizoma	Nut grass rhizoma, cyperus	4.5 g

Dental Conditions

Dental Work

Pin Yin	Latin	English	Dosage
Chuan xiong	Chuanxiong Rhizoma	Chuanxiong root, Szechuan lovage root, cnidium	4.5 g
Bai zhi	Angelicae Dahuricae Radix	Angelica root	4.5 g
Jing jie	Schizonepetae Herba	Schizonepeta	4.5 g
Gan cao	Glycyrrhizae Radix	Licorice root	3 g
Ge gen	Puerariae Radix	Kudzu root, pueraria	3 g
Xiang fu	Cyperi Rotundi Rhizoma	Nut grass rhizoma, cyperus	4.5 g
Qiang huo	Notopterygii Rhizoma et Radix	Notopterygium root and rhizome, chiang-huo	4.5 g

Hamilton Rotte   This formula is indicated for painful conditions that develop from dental work procedures. Dental work always involves a trauma to the mouth and pain can be persistent afterward. This formula includes many herbs that target the head. These include *chuan xiong*, *bai zhi*, *ge gen*, and *qiang huo*. *Jing jie*, as a surface-releasing ingredient, may be included here as a guide to the upper body, as surface-releasing herbs tend to go upward. The very low dosages of the ingredients also give it the tendency to affect the head; it is a general principle that lighter dosages of herbs tend to direct them to the upper part of the body.

In this formula we also find *qi*- and blood-moving and pain-relieving ingredients. These include *chuan xiong*, *bai zhi*, *xiang fu*, and *qiang huo*. *Ge gen* is also considered by some sources to have a blood-moving effect as well.

This formula targets many different channels in the head, including *tai yang* (*qiang huo* and *ge gen*), *yang ming* (*bai zhi* and *ge gen*), *shao yang* (*xiang fu*). In particular, addressing the *yang ming* channel is especially relevant if pain involves the teeth and gums.

Dermatological Conditions

Acne

FROM DR. SHEN: Acne is small papules with little blackheads, appearing commonly on the faces of boys and girls in puberty. They mostly arise from indigestion together with the overheating of blood. Poor dietary habits, sweet, spicy, and pungent foods together with a defective digestive system will cause acne. Sometimes nervous tension or maladjustment in the nervous system will also lead to acne. Improving the diet by avoiding hot and pungent foods, sweets, and alcohol will help to clear acne. Patients are advised to keep their mood as relaxed as possible.

Formula for acne:

Pin Yin	Latin	English	Dosage
Chao hei jing jie	Schizonepetae Herba	Fried, charred schizonepeta	4.5 g
Chao hei fang feng	Saposhnikoviae Radix	Fried, charred ledebouriella root, saposhnikoviae root, siler	4.5 g
Di fu zi	Kochiae Fructus	Broom cypress, kochia fruit	9 g
Xia ku cao	Prunellae Spica Vulgaris	Self-heal spike, prunella	6 g
Gan cao	Glycyrrhizae Radix	Licorice root	4.5 g
Luo han guo	Momordicae Fructus	Grosvenor momordica fruit	9 g
Mu dan pi	Moutan Radicis Cortex	Tree peony root bark, moutan root bark	6 g
Jin yin hua	Lonicerae Flos	Honeysuckle flower	9 g
Sheng yi yi ren	Coicis Semen	Fresh seeds of Job's tears, coix seeds	12 g
Sheng di huang	Rehmannia Radix	Fresh Chinese foxglove root, rehmannia root	12 g
Chao chi shao	Paeoniae Rubra Radix	Fried red peony root	6 g
Lu gen	Phragmitis Communis Rhizoma	Reed rhizome	9 g

Boil the medicine into tea and drink twice a day for 1 to 2 months until the acne disappears.

Hamilton Rotte The literature attributes this common skin condition to wind-heat, heat in the lungs, blood heat, damp-heat in the intestines, blood stasis, spleen deficiency, and dampness and yin-deficient heat. Most commonly, it is caused by excess heat, especially if lesions are slightly raised with pronounced redness.

This formula addresses the most common causes of acne, namely wind-heat, lung heat, blood heat, and dampness of the spleen. The herbs that address wind-heat include jing jie, fang feng, jin yin hua, and di fu zi.

The herbs that cool the lungs include luo han guo and lu gen.

The herbs that clear blood heat or liver heat include xia ku cao, mu dan pi, sheng di huang, and chi shao. Xia ku cao is also included because of its ability to treat nodules.

Yi yi ren strengthens the spleen and resolves dampness, another prominent cause of acne.

FROM DR. SHEN: There are four main reasons for the many different types of skin problems: fecal matter that is not adequately expelled from babies before they first eat, eating hot foods such as seafood, sugar, and alcohol, nervous tension impairing circulation and accumulation of chemicals in the blood.
If the skin feels hot when you first touch it, then stops being hot, the heat is from *qi*. If the skin feels hot when you first touch it then gets hotter this indicates blood heat.

Leon Hammer Dr. Shen attributed these skin problems in children to the failure to pass meconium prior to their first feeding, which we discuss below under

the formula "*San Huang Tang* (Three Yellow Decoction) for discharging the meconium."

Adulthood Skin Problems

Pin Yin	Latin	English	Dosage
Jing jie	Schizonepetae Herba	Schizonepeta	4.5 g
Di fu zi	Kochiae Fructus	Broom cypress, kochia fruit	12 g
Yuan zhi	Polygalae Radix	Chinese senega root, polygala root	4.5 g
Huang qin	Scutellariae Baicalensis Radix	Baical skullcap root, scutellaria, scute	4.5 g
Fang feng	Saposhnikoviae Radix	Ledebouriella root, saposhnikoviae root, siler	4.5 g
Gan cao	Glycyrrhizae Radix	Licorice root	4.5 g
Long chi	Fossilia Dentis Mastodi	Dragon teeth, fossilized teeth	9 g
Chuan xiong	Chuanxiong Rhizoma	Chuanxiong root, Szechuan lovage root, cnidium	4.5 g
Mu dan pi	Moutan Radicis Cortex	Tree peony root bark, moutan root bark	6 g
Hei shan zhi zi	Gardeniae Jasminoidis Fructus	Charred cape jasmine fruit, gardenia fruit	9 g

Hamilton Rotte This is a broad-spectrum formula for early stages of various skin conditions. The most common chronic skin conditions, including eczema, psoriasis, and urticaria, usually begin as wind-heat and excess heat in the blood. Over time the effects of the exterior wind- and blood heat consume blood and body fluids and develop into what is described in dermatology as "blood dryness." Skin conditions due to excess heat are more acute and have a bright red color. Skin conditions due to blood dryness are pale, very dry, and may have fissures.

This formula is indicated for excess heat and wind-heat and would not be suitable for *yin* or blood deficiency. The herbs that release the exterior include *jing jie, di fu zi, fang feng*, and *chuan xiong*. Herbs that clear blood heat include *mu dan pi, huang qin*, and *zhi zi*.
Chuan xiong moves blood. Because the skin is the largest organ in the body, blood-invigorating ingredients aid in delivering herbs to the skin.
Long chi and *yuan zhi* are included because itching often causes severe irritability and emotional distress. Ding Gan Ren also noted that *yuan zhi* is indicated for heat affecting the skin.

Childhood Skin Problems

Pin Yin	Latin	English	Dosage
Da huang	Rhei Rhizoma et Radix	Rhubarb root and rhizome	3 g
Gan cao	Glycyrrhizae Radix	Licorice root	4.5 g
Ji nei jin	Corneum Gigeriae Galli Endothelium	Chicken gizzard's inner lining	12 g
Di fu zi	Kochiae Fructus	Broom cypress, kochia fruit	9 g
Xia ku cao	Prunellae Spica Vulgaris	Self-heal spike, prunella	6 g
Shen qu	Massa Medicata Fermentata	Medicated leaven (dough)	9 g
Chan tui	Periostracum Cicadae	Cicada moultings	9 g
Chuan bei mu	Fritillariae Cirrhosae Bulbus	Szechuan fritillaria bulb, tendrilled fritillary bulb, fritillaria	6 g
Zhi shi	Aurantii Immaturus Fructus	Immature bitter orange, unripe bitter orange, chih-shih	4.5 g
Sheng jiang	Zingiberis Officinalis Recens Rhizoma	Fresh ginger rhizome	2 pieces

Hamilton Rotte Dr. Shen emphasized that skin problems from childhood were usually due to feeding infants before they discharge the meconium. He advocated the use of San Huang Tang (Three Yellow Decoction) first to discharge the meconium before feeding them.

The formula above contains ingredients that are cleansing to the digestive system. Da huang is purgative and clears damp-heat from the intestines. It may aid in eliminating any remaining waste products that are related to feeding an infant too early. Ding Gan Ren indicated that da huang is able to clean up the stomach and intestines when there is old and chronic stagnation, thus improving digestive function. This differs substantially from a more conventional use of da huang for acute problems involving heat in the intestines.

Ji nei jin and shen qu resolve food stagnation. It is widely understood in pediatrics that children easily develop food stagnation and that this can lead to many of the problems that they experience. Zhi shi resolves dampness and regulates qi, further cleaning up the digestive system. It is also widely understood that respiratory problems are a major contributor to problems in pediatrics, explaining the presence of chuan bei mu that clears heat from the lungs.

Di fu zi and chan tui release the exterior, and are especially indicated for itching.

Hives (Red Hot Rash)

Pin Yin	Latin	English	Dosage
Jing jie	Schizonepetae Herba	Schizonepeta	4.5 g
Chuan xiong	Chuanxiong Rhizoma	Chuanxiong root, Szechuan lovage root, cnidium	4.5 g
Mu dan pi	Moutan Radicis Cortex	Tree peony root bark, moutan root bark	6 g
Man jing zi	Viticis Fructus	Vitex fruit	6 g
Lu lu tong	Liquidambaris Fructus	Sweetgum fruit, liquidambar fruit	3 g
Fang feng	Saposhnikoviae Radix	Ledebouriella root, saposhnikoviae root, siler	4.5 g
Gan cao	Glycyrrhizae Radix	Licorice root	4.5 g

Pin Yin	Latin	English	Dosage
Han lian cao	Ecliptae Prostratae Herba	Eclipta	6 g
Chan tui	Periostracum Cicadae	Cicada moultings	4.5 g
Chi shao	Paeoniae Rubra Radix	Red peony root	9 g
Huang qin	Scutellariae Baicalensis Radix	Baical skullcap root, scutellaria, scute	4.5 g

Hamilton Rotte   The TCM literature attributes hives (urticaria) to wind-heat, wind-cold, heat in the heart, heat toxins in the *ying* level, disharmony of the spleen and stomach, deficiency of *qi*, and blood and blood stasis.

This formula is indicated for wind-heat and blood heat causing hives. The lesions in this case will be bright red, acute, and itchy. Chronic conditions, which constitute a certain percentage of hives cases, tend to manifest in individuals who are more deficient. The herbs that relieve the exterior and/or stop itching include *jing jie, fang feng, lu lu tong, chan tui,* and *niu bang zi*. Herbs that cool the blood include *mu dan pi, han lian cao, chi shao,* and *huang qin*.

Chuan xiong may be included in order to aid in releasing the exterior, or it may address blood stasis that sometimes exists in hives. *Gan cao* is used to detoxify and also harmonize other ingredients in the formula.

Psoriasis

Pin Yin	Latin	English	Dosage
Di fu zi	Kochiae Fructus	Broom cypress, kochia fruit	12 g
Gan cao	Glycyrrhizae Radix	Licorice root	6 g
Huang bai	Phellodendri Cortex	Amur corktree bark, phellodendron bark	9 g
Bai xian pi	Dictamni Dasycarpi Radicis Cortex	Cortex of Chinese dittany root, dictamnus root bark	12 g
Bi xie	Discoreae Hypoglaucae Rhizoma	Fish poison yam rhizome, tokoro	6 g
Xia ku cao	Prunellae Spica Vulgaris	Self-heal spike, prunella	6 g
Fang feng	Saposhnikoviae Radix	Ledebouriella root, saposhnikoviae root, siler	6 g
Zhi shi	Aurantii Immaturus Fructus	Immature bitter orange, unripe bitter orange, *chih-shih*	4.5 g
Chi shao	Paeoniae Rubra Radix	Red peony root	9 g

Hamilton Rotte   In the TCM literature, psoriasis is attributed to wind-heat, wind-cold, blood heat, blood stasis, blood deficiency, damp-heat, wind-dampness, spleen deficiency or *ying*-level heat.

This formula addresses wind-heat, damp-heat, and blood heat. The lesions would present without any extreme dryness (this is associated with blood deficiency), and would be significantly itchy. Itchiness in skin problems indicates the use of surface-releasing herbs.

The herbs that release the exterior and stop itching include *di fu zi, bai xian pi,* and *fang feng*. Herbs that treat dampness include *huang bai* and *bai xian pi*. *Chi shao* is used to cool and move the blood. *Xia ku cao* is included because it cools the liver, and it also softens hardness, addressing the thickening and hardening of the skin present in psoriasis. *Gan cao* is used to gently moisten (offsetting the drying tendencies of other herbs in the formula) and clear heat and toxicity.

Spider Bites

Poultice in about 350 g sesame oil, use for 2 to 3 days:

Pin Yin	Latin	English	Dosage
Huang bai	Phellodendri Cortex	Amur corktree bark, phellodendron bark	3–12 g
Gan cao	Glycyrrhizae Radix	Licorice root	1.5–9 g
Jin yin hua	Lonicerae Flos	Honeysuckle flower, lonicera	6–20 g
Mu dan pi	Moutan Radicis Cortex	Tree peony root bark, moutan root bark	6–12 g
Dan shen	Salviae Miltiorrhiziae Radix	Salvia root	6–15 g

Hamilton Rotte   Poisonous insect and snake bites result in a heat toxicity condition in the local area where the bite occurred. At the site where the bite occurs there is redness, swelling, pain, and itching, all indicators of heat toxicity (also called "*yang* sores" in Chinese medicine). The herbs that clear heat and toxicity in this formula include *huang bai*, *gan cao*, *jin yin hua*, and *mu dan pi*. In addition to treating heat toxicity, this formula moves blood. *Mu dan pi* and *dan shen* are the blood-moving ingredients. Herbs that clear heat and toxicity are more effective when they are combined with blood-invigorating ingredients. This is because the herbs are better able to reach the site of the heat toxicity and the waste products from the heat toxin lesion are better eliminated by the body if blood circulation is restored.

Ear, Nose, and Throat Conditions

Sore Throat, Acute with Fever

FROM DR. SHEN: This is similar in cause to the "Sore Throat, Sudden Laryngitis" (see p. 45). It is slightly more severe due to lifestyle or body condition.

Pin Yin	Latin	English	Dosage
Chan tui	Periostracum Cicadae	Cicada moultings	4.5 g
Sang bai pi	Mori Cortex	Mulberry root bark, morus bark	6 g
Bo he ye	Menthae Haplocalycis Herba	Dried field mint leaf, mentha, peppermint leaves	4.5 g
Huang qin	Scutellariae Baicalensis Radix	Baical skullcap root, scutellaria, scute	4.5 g
Jing jie	Schizonepetae Herba	Schizonepeta	4.5 g
Ma bo	Fructificatio Lasiosphaera seu Calvatia	Fruiting body of puff-ball	4.5 g
Gan cao	Glycyrrhizae Radix	Licorice root	4.5 g
Mu dan pi	Moutan Radicis Cortex	Tree peony root bark, moutan root bark	6 g
Fang feng	Saposhnikoviae Radix	Ledebouriella root, saposhnikoviae root, siler	4.5 g
Sang ye	Folium Mori	White mulberry leaf	6 g
Lu gen	Phragmitis Communis Rhizoma	Reed rhizome	6 g
Hei shan zhi zi	Gardeniae Jasminoidis Fructus	Charred cape jasmine fruit, gardenia fruit	9 g

Hamilton Rotte This formula contains ingredients that clear lung heat, target the throat, and clear internal heat (especially from the liver). Surface-releasing herbs may be included in order to aid the lung in discharging the internally generated heat.

The herbs that clear heat and target the lungs and throat include *sang bai pi*, *bo he*, *huang qin*, *ma bo*, and *sang ye*. Of these, *bo he* and *ma bo* are especially effective in treating a sore throat.

Herbs that cool the liver include *huang qin*, *mu dan pi*, and *zhi zi*.

Surface-releasing herbs include *bo he*, *jing jie*, *fang feng*, and *sang ye*. *Lu gen* aids in releasing the exterior by generating fluids.

Leon Hammer
Pulse:
- See p. 46 under "Sore Throat, Sudden Laryngitis" for a fuller pulse description
- Add to the body of the pulse a robust pounding (3–5) and perhaps flooding excess

Sore Throat, Chronic Laryngitis

FROM DR. SHEN: In this condition, a person gradually loses their voice. This is a very serious situation in which the lungs can become damaged as in TB. A medical doctor must always be consulted about this condition. The following formula may help if taken over a long time. During the course of treatment, a person must avoid sex, overwork, and alcohol. If this condition is treatable by herbs, results should appear in 3 weeks. The lung pulse will be slippery.

Pin Yin	Latin	English	Dosage
She gan	Belamcandae Rhizoma	Belamcanda rhizome	3 g
Gan cao	Glycyrrhizae Radix	Licorice root	4.5 g
Sheng di huang	Rehmannia Radix	Fresh Chinese foxglove root, rehmannia root	9 g
Yu zhu	Polygonati Odorati Rhizoma	Solomon's seal rhizome, polygonatum	9 g
Ma bo	Fructificatio Lasiosphaera seu Calvatia	Fruiting body of puff-ball	4.5 g
Chuan bei mu	Fritillariae Cirrhosae Bulbus	Szechuan fritillaria bulb, tendrilled fritillary bulb, fritillaria	9 g
Mai men dong	Ophiopogonis Radix	Ophiopogon tuber/root	9 g
Mu hu die	Oroxyli Semen	Oroxylum seeds	4.5 g
Nan sha shen	Adenophorae seu Glehniae Radix	Adenophora root or glehnia root, ladybell root	9 g
Jie geng	Platycodi Radix	Root of balloonflower, platycodon root	6 g
Feng mi	Mel Millis	Honey	1 tsp

Hamilton Rotte   Dr. Shen indicates that a chronic sore throat is an indication of a severe condition. This formula focuses on nourishing yin, resolving phlegm, and clearing heat and toxicity.

The herbs that nourish yin include sheng di huang, yu zhu, chuan bei mu, mai men dong, and nan sha shen. Herbs that resolve phlegm include chuan bei mu and jie geng. Ma bo and she gan resolve toxicity. It is possible that these are included to prevent the development of cancer because many clear heat and toxin herbs are used in this manner.

Jie geng acts as a guide to the throat and mu hu die, a qi-regulating herb, also targets the throat.

Sore Throat, Constant

FROM DR. SHEN: The causes can be the same as in the "Sore Throat, Sudden Laryngitis" and "Sore Throat, Acute with Fever" conditions. However, the lungs may be constitutionally weak and the body condition even weaker. This condition can turn into throat and lung cancer. A person must rest for 6 months or expect a very slow recovery. The special lung pulse is very weak.

Pin Yin	Latin	English	Dosage
Sang bai pi	Mori Cortex	Mulberry root bark, morus bark	9 g
Pang da hai	Sterculiae Lychnophorae Semen	Sterculia seed	6 g
Yu zhu	Polygonati Odorati Rhizoma	Solomon's seal rhizome, polygonatum	9 g

Pin Yin	Latin	English	Dosage
Zhe bei mu	Fritillariae Thunbergii Bulbus	Zhejiang fritillaria, Thunberg fritillaria bulb, fritillaria	9 g
Jing jie	Schizonepetae Herba	Schizonepeta	4.5 g
Bai mao gen	Imperatae Cylindricae Rhizoma	Rhizome of woolly grass, imperata, white grass	9 g
Gan cao	Glycyrrhizae Radix	Licorice root	4.5 g
Mai men dong	Ophiopogonis Radix	Ophiopogon tuber/root	9 g
Fang feng	Saposhnikoviae Radix	Ledebouriella root, saposhnikoviae root, siler	4.5 g
Sheng di huang	Rehmannia Radix	Fresh Chinese foxglove root, rehmannia root	9 g
Mu dan pi	Moutan Radicis Cortex	Tree peony root bark, moutan root bark	6 g

Hamilton Rotte   This formula is for internally generated heat that lodges in the lungs. It contains herbs that clear heat and target the lungs and throat, and also those that release the exterior, which aids dispersion of heat. The herbs that clear lung heat include *sang bai pi*, *zhe bie mu*, *bai mao gen*, and *pang da hai*. *Pang da hai* in particular targets the throat. *Jing jie* and *fang feng* are included as a means to treat lung heat by releasing the exterior.

Substances that clear heat from other organs include *sheng di huang* and *mu dan pi*. These may be included to target the liver, which is often a source of internal heat.

This formula also contains tonic herbs that target the lung, especially lung *yin*. Lung *yin* tonics include *yu zhu* and *mai men dong*.

Sore Throat, Sudden Laryngitis

FROM DR. SHEN: This condition comes suddenly and is not preceded by a cough. The body is strong but tight inside from stress. The internal tightness generates heat that is trapped inside the lungs. Chinese medicine describes this as "hot inside/cold outside." This condition should not be confused with *yin* deficiency. The pulse will be a little tight.

Pin Yin	Latin	English	Dosage
Bo he	Menthae Haplocalycis Herba	Field mint, mentha, peppermint leaves	4.5 g
Pang da hai	Sterculiae Lychnophorae Semen	Sterculia seed	9 g

Hamilton Rotte   An acute sore throat is usually associated with an exterior invasion of wind-heat. In this case, the suggestion is that the heat is generated from the inside, and presumably because of the vulnerability of the lungs, the internally generated heat moves to the throat. Dr. Shen's statement that this is referred to "hot inside/cold outside," however, does suggest that an exterior pathogen may also be present.
Bo he and *pang da hai* are both cooling herbs that target the throat, and both have exterior-releasing func-

tions. *Bo he* also enters the liver channel, which may be relevant in this case. *Pang da hai* has a marked moistening effect.

Neither of these herbs should be cooked for more than 5 minutes; in fact it is likely that Dr. Shen intended this recipe to be prepared as an infusion. Generally speaking, using bulk herbs is the strongest method of treatment (compared to using prepared medicines), and one virtue of this recipe is that it utilizes bulk herbs in a manner that does not require a lengthy cooking time.

Leon Hammer

Pulse:

• The presence of an exterior pathogenic factor would be confirmed by a floating quality:
  – Exterior cold pathogen: floating, tense, and slightly slow

– Exterior heat pathogen: floating, yielding, and slightly rapid
– Exterior phlegm pathogen: add slippery to the above floating qualities depending on whether it is cold or heat

• The presence of an internal pathogenic factor: floating and tight

Tinnitus

Pin Yin	Latin	English	Dosage
Tian ma	Gastrodiae Rhizoma	Gastrodia rhizome	6 g
Shan yao	Dioscoreae Oppositae Rhizoma	Chinese yam root, dioscorea rhizome	9 g
Jue ming zi	Cassiae Semen	Fetid cassia seeds	9 g
Mu li	Ostreae Concha	Oyster shell	9 g
Gou qi zi	Lycii Fructus	Chinese wolfberry, matrimony vine fruit, lycium fruit	9 g
Tu si zi	Cuscutae Chinensis Semen	Chinese dodder seeds, cuscuta	9 g
Sheng di huang	Rehmanniae Radix	Fresh Chinese foxglove root, fresh rehmannia root	6 g

Hamilton Rotte   This formula contains kidney and liver tonic herbs in addition to descending herbs. The kidney and liver tonics include *tian ma* (especially for liver), *shan yao* (especially for kidneys), *jue ming zi*, *mu li*, *gou qi zi*, *tu si zi*, and *sheng di huang*. These herbs mainly tonify *yin*, though *shan yao*, *gou qi zi*, and *tu si zi* have *qi*- or *yang*-tonifying effects.

Tian ma, *jue ming zi* and *mu li* are descending, as tinnitus is frequently due to ascending liver energies that are not rooted because of a liver *yin* deficiency.

Leon Hammer   Liver *qi* is not rooted when liver *yin* and *yang* are separated. Liver *qi* (the lighter energy) usually escapes and rises to vulnerable organs (heart [palpitations] and lungs [asthma] and areas [breast]). The deficiency can be of liver *yin* or of liver *qi-yang*, which is more common in our time.

Endocrine Conditions

Diabetes

Leon Hammer   Diabetes, according to Dr. Shen is characterized by three "much's": drinking too much, eating too much, passing too much water, and is thus called in Chinese an "emaciation-thirst" ("wasting and thirsting") disease.

Dr. Shen ascribes the disease to the formation of an internal fire/heat from eating too much sumptuously fatty and spicy food and/or a long suppressed melancholic emotion and an inability to deal with this heat perhaps due to innate kidney *yin* deficiency. Diabetes in old age comes mainly from deficiency of kidney *yin*.

Dr. Shen states that one of the Chinese classic medical books, *Qian Jin Fang*, written in the Tang dynasty more than 1000 years ago, writes on the treatment of diabetes: "Take precautions in three ways against drinking wine, having too much sex and eating too much food made of flour which is alkaline in nature. If these three precautions are followed, the disease will be cured all by itself." (Author's note: the concept of "alkaline" 1000 years ago and even to Dr. Shen, unfamiliar with modern nutritional concepts, seems farfetched and must be attributed to one of many editors.)

Formula for "true" diabetes:

Pin Yin	Latin	English	Dosage
Sheng di huang	Rehmannia Radix	Fresh Chinese foxglove root, rehmannia root	12 g
Sheng huang qi	Astragali Radix	Fresh milk vetch root, fresh astragalus root	24 g
Sheng shan yao	Dioscoreae Oppositae Rhizoma	Fresh Chinese yam root, dioscorea rhizome	26 g
Shan zhu yu	Corni Officinalis Fructus	Asiatic Cornelian cherry fruit, cornus	16 g
Zhu yi	Pancreas Suis	Pig's pancreas	1 whole piece

FROM DR. SHEN: Boil the medicines in water. Drink one dose a day divided into three to four portions. Continue until the sugar content in the urine drops to normal level.

Hamilton Rotte   Diabetes is most commonly associated with *yin* deficiency, especially of the liver and kidneys. This is especially true of late-stage diabetes. This formula contains the tonics of the famous formula *Liu Wei Di Huang Wan* (Six Ingredient Rehmannia) with *sheng di huang* substituted for *shu di huang*, *shan yao*, and *shan zhu yu*. *Sheng di huang* is a modern favorite for the treatment of diabetes, often used as a substitute for *shu di huang* for diabetes in particular. *Huang qi* is another modern favorite for diabetes (treating "wasting and thirsting" disorder), and *qi* deficiency is also another major component of diabetes. Pig's placenta is a blood and essence tonic.

> **FROM DR. SHEN:** There is also a kind of pseudo-diabetes caused mainly by exhaustion and unchecked eating habits, which result in indigestion that causes food sugar to go directly into the urine. This sugar content varies greatly. Diet and rest must be considered. Some medicines that will help digestion and strengthen the spleen will do the patient good.

Formula for pseudo-diabetes:

Pin Yin	Latin	English	Dosage
Huo xiang	Agastaches seu Pogostemi Herba	Agastache, patchouli	9 g
Mu xiang	Saussureae Lappae Radix or Aucklandia Lappae Radix	Costus root, saussurea, aucklandia	6 g
Dang shen	Codonopsis Pilosulae Radix	Codonopsis root	9 g
Bai zhu	Atractylodis Macrocephalae Rhizoma	White atractylodes rhizome	9 g
Fu ling	Poria Cocos Sclerotium	Sclerotium of tuckahoe, poria, China root, hoelen, Indian bread	9 g
Gan cao	Glycyrrhizae Radix	Licorice root	6 g
Chen pi	Citri Reticulatae Pericarpium	Tangerine peel	6 g
Shen qu	Massa Medicata Fermentata	Medicated leaven (dough)	9 g

Boil the medicine into tea and drink a daily dose until the sugar content drops to normal.

Hamilton Rotte   Late-stage diabetes roughly corresponds to what is known in Chinese medicine as "wasting and thirsting," marked by thirst, frequent urination, and emaciation. The literature frequently describes wasting and thirsting as possible excess heat in the early stages and yin deficiency (of one of the three burners, especially lower burner) in the later stages.

We find that in the early stages of diabetes as defined by biomedicine, patients can present with damp excess and a generally overburdened digestive system. This fits with the correlation that has been made between overeating and a sedentary lifestyle with diabetes. In later stages the chronic excess heat from stagnation consumes the yin and patients fit into what is traditionally described as "wasting and thirsting."

This formula deals with excess conditions in the digestive system, including dampness, qi stagnation and food stagnation. There are also some mild tonics that address the qi deficiency that can arise from a chronically overburdened digestive system. The herbs that treat damp excess include huo xiang, mu xiang, bai zhu, fu ling, and chen pi. Herbs that regulate qi include mu xiang, chen pi, and shen qu. Herbs that relieve food stagnation include mu xiang and shen qu. Tonic herbs include dang shen, bai zhu, fu ling, and gan cao. These four herbs comprise the famous spleen qi tonic formula the Si Jun Zi Tang (Four Gentlemen Decoction).

Menopause, Nervous Tension

> **FROM DR. SHEN:** In this condition, the body is strong and the flashes will occur mainly during the day. There will usually be no other symptoms.

Pin Yin	Latin	English	Dosage
Qing hao	Artemisiae Annuae Herba	Wormwood, ching-hao	9 g
Huang qin	Scutellariae Baicalensis Radix	Baical skullcap root, scutellaria, scute	4.5 g
Tian hua fen	Trichosanthis Kirilowii Radix	Trichosanthes root	9 g

Pin Yin	Latin	English	Dosage
Di gu pi	Lycii Radicis Cortex	Cortex of wolfberry root, lycium bark	9 g
Long chi	Fossilia Dentis Mastodi	Dragon teeth, fossilized teeth	9 g
Zhi ke	Citri Aurantii Fructus	Mature fruit of the bitter orange	6 g
Chuan xiong	Chuanxiong Rhizoma	Chuanxiong root, Szechuan lovage root, cnidium	4.5 g
Yu jin	Curcumae Radix	Curcuma tuber	9 g
Chuan lian zi	Meliae Toosendan Fructus	Szechuan pagoda tree fruit, Szechuan chinaberry, melia	9 g

Hamilton Rotte In the literature, menopause is mainly attributed to kidney deficiency, either yin deficiency or yang deficiency. Menopausal syndromes are usually marked by a mixture of kidney yin- and yang-deficiency signs and symptoms. This is commonly seen in kidney deficiency in general. The literature also describes blood stasis, qi stagnation, and phlegm as other contributing factors.

Dr. Shen indicates that hot flashes that occur during the day are found in a more robust individual. It is unusual to describe menopause in these terms and therefore this formula is a valuable contribution to the literature.

This formula regulates liver qi, calms the spirit, cools the liver, and clears deficient heat. We also find that it contains many ingredients that have a markedly descending tendency. This formula demonstrates the tendency of liver qi stagnation to create heat in the liver and how heat tends to rise.

The herbs that regulate the liver qi include yu jin and chuan lian zi. The herbs that calm the spirit include long chi, a potent heavy mineral.

Herbs that cool the liver include yu jin, chuan lian zi, huang qin, and qing hao. Qing hao and di gu pi are also included to clear deficient heat, as excess heat over time progresses to yin deficiency. The herbs that have a descending tendency include huang qin, long chi, di gu pi, zhi ke, yu jin, and chuan lian zi. Clearly, directing qi downward is a major focus of this formula. A light dosage of chuan xiong, which has an ascending nature, may be included to balance the actions of the descending herbs.

Leon Hammer It is clear to me that the body's first choice is to eliminate pathogens through the bowels and urinary tract. When these avenues are not sufficient, the skin is the next and perhaps final choice that is addressed in this formula. Further comments on the menopause follow the next formula.

Menopause, Nervous Tension, and Weak Body

FROM DR. SHEN: If the body is weak menopause will cause many different symptoms. There will be night sweating and many more hot flashes than in the condition described above.

Pin Yin	Latin	English	Dosage
Ren shen	Ginseng Radix	Ginseng root	4.5 g
Fu ling	Poria Cocos Sclerotium	Sclerotium of tuckahoe, poria, China root, hoelen, Indian bread	9 g
Da zao	Zizyphi Jujubae Fructus	Chinese date, jujube	9 g
Bie jia	Carapax Amydae Sinensis	Chinese soft-shelled turtle shell	12 g
Yuan zhi	Polygalae Radix	Chinese senega root, polygala root	6 g

Pin Yin	Latin	English	Dosage
Bai shao	Paeoniae Alba Radix	White peony root	6 g
Nuo dao gen xu	Oryzae Glutinosae Radix	Glutinous rice root	30 g
Chai hu	Bupleuri Radix	Hare's ear root, thorowax root, bupleurum	3 g
Di gu pi	Lycii Radicis Cortex	Cortex of wolfberry root, lycium bark	9 g

Hamilton Rotte   Dr. Shen indicates that menopausal symptoms that occur at night indicate a deficiency syndrome. As discussed earlier, menopausal syndromes are mainly associated with either kidney *yin* or *yang* deficiency.

This formula places significant emphasis on tonifying kidney *yin* and clearing deficient heat. We also find that this formula tonifies *qi* and stops sweating. We frequently find that conditions where there is excessive sweating involve a deficiency of both *qi* and *yin*.

The ingredients that tonify *yin* include *bie jia* and *bai shao*. *Bie jia*, a potent substance, targets the liver and kidneys and *bai shao* targets the liver. *Qi* tonics include *ren shen*, *fu ling*, and *da zao*.

Di gu pi is included to clear deficient heat and *nuo dao gen xu* stops sweating. These two ingredients address the branch of the condition, rather than the root, but they are effective in symptom management.

Yuan zhi is possibly included to calm the spirit, as spirit disturbances are common in menopausal syndromes.

Leon Hammer   The origin of hot flashes and sweats are often considered *yin*-deficient conditions. The commonly used formula for this condition is *Er Xian Tang* (Two Immortal Decoction), a formula that has three *yang*-nourishing herbs and one blood-nourishing herb and two herbs to clear deficient heat.

In my opinion, hot flashes occur when *either yin* or *yang* are sufficiently deficient to cause a "separation of *yin* and *yang*." More often in our time the deficiency is in *yang*, and while the heavier *yin* tends to remain in the body, the lighter *yang* rises and leaves the body as a hot flash. When the separation becomes very severe the *yin* follows the *yang* and we have hot (*yang*) sweats (*yin*). Wandering *yang* can also interfere with function in vulnerable organs, the heart being in my opinion the most overworked and susceptible. This often leads to uncontrollable mental agitation that the usually deficient kidneys cannot counterbalance.

Though perhaps outside this discussion, Dr. Shen talked about a "separation of *qi* and blood" in the lower burner with the *qi* rising and causing headaches and menopausal symptoms in that age group. (I am told that Zhang Zhong Jing, author of the Shang Hun Lun, also wrote about the separation of *qi* and blood in the lower burner and its consequences. In their commentary, the author quotes the Su Wen: "When blood gathers in the lower [body] and *qi* gathers in the upper body [there will be] derangement and forgetfulness" (Mitchel, 1999).

Why do these hot flashes and sweats occur most during the evening and night? During the day when the sun is rising and has its maximum effect on the earth it inhibits the body's *yang* from separating from the *yin* and rising. Later in the day, in the evening, and at night the *yang* of the sun is no longer able to inhibit the *yang* of the body that "wanders." When the separation of *yin* and *yang* is profound even the sun cannot control the escaping *yang* and *yin*. (Cold day sweats are associated with heart *yang* deficiency.)

Thyroid Problems

FROM DR. SHEN:
- Local iodine problem—eyes big
- Heart enlarged, neck big, eyes not big
- Stomach and digestion
- Liver
- Emotions, for instance women "keeping emotions and anger" causing *qi* stagnation in the neck and esophagus area

Formula for enlarged heart (can cause thyroid problems):

Pin Yin	Latin	English	Dosage
Shi chang pu	Acori Tatarinowii Rhizoma	Grass-leaved sweetflag rhizome, acorus	2.4 g[a]
Chen xiang	Aquilariae Lignum	Aloeswood, aquilaria	2.1 g
Chao huang lian	Coptidis Rhizoma	Dry-fried coptis rhizome	2.1 g
Chao bai shao	Paeoniae Alba Radix	Fried white peony root	6 g
Fu shen	Poria Cocos Pararadicis Sclerotium	Poria fungus	9 g
Yuan zhi	Polygalae Radix	Chinese senega root, polygala root	4.5 g
Wu wei zi	Schisandrae Chinensis Fructus	Schisandra fruit	4.5 g
Duan mu li	Ostreae Concha	Calcined oyster shell	12 g
Mai men dong	Ophiopogonis Radix	Ophiopogon tuber/root	9 g

[a] A small amount makes the heart relax.
See "General comments about Dr. Shen's heart formulas," page 7.

Leon Hammer While Dr. Shen ascribes hyperthyroidism to "deficiency in *yin* to induce vigorous fire" or "warm ambitions so suppressed that they rise in revolt into a sort of stagnant 'fire' burning vehemently, thereby depleting the *yin* and harming both the liver and the kidneys," there is little in this formula to treat *yin* and a great deal to treat fire.

Hyperthyroidism, Graves disease and mania, the psychological pattern closely resembling it, occur when the triple burner is unable to maintain a smooth transition in the nourishing (*sheng*) cycle between water, wood, and fire. Perhaps related to repressed powerful and "hot" emotions, the wood begins to burn out of control (of the triple burner) and the fire goes to the heart beyond the ability of the water to control it. The spirit housed in the heart becomes highly agitated in the form of mania and/or Graves disease (severe acute hyperthyroidism). The heart protects itself by retaining the fire pathogen in a nonfatal yet vulnerable area of the body—in this instance, the thyroid.

This manifests as Graves disease in which the thyroid gland enlarges and its output of thyroid hormone is accentuated. In Chinese medical terms, the thyroid is the organ that produces the normal metabolic heat that is one aspect of *qi*, and when out of control produces an excess of this metabolic heat. The water is depleted attempting to control the fire and gradually the wood is consumed and the fire banks into the condition we call depression. As long as the triple burner is unable to sustain a smooth transition between the phases the pattern will begin again as soon as the wood recovers. Hyperthyroidism occurs if, in my opinion, either the lung that controls the upper part of the body or the spleen that is closely related to metabolism are deficient. Otherwise, this scenario manifests as the closely related manic phase of the bipolar disease, and rages until the wood is consumed, followed by a dampening of the fire and depression. One can also see this as a kidney–heart disharmony brought about by the failure of the triple burner to regulate that relationship.

Gastrointestinal Disturbances

FROM DR. SHEN:
- Stomach problems arise from:
  - Too many cold beverages
  - Poor eating schedule
  - Working when hungry
  - Eating too fast
  - Thinking and worrying while eating
  - Sudden emotional problems while eating
  - Eating too much
- If the stool sinks, digestion is not good (food is in the stools).
- If the stools always float, digestion is good.

Leon Hammer   Biomedicine teaches that normally feces should sink, and float only because of poor fat digestion. Fat floats in water.

FROM DR. SHEN:
- If the breath has no smell this is a good sign.
- If the breath smells sweet there is too much acid.
- If the urine is dark or there is sediment, this indicates a blood or kidney problem.
- If there are lines on the side of the tongue and the tongue is red this indicates that there is too much acid and the person should avoid sour foods.
- If a person eats and then vomits, this indicates an esophagus problem due to emotions while eating (this make the esophagus tight).
- If there is chronic diarrhea than the stomach is weak.
- If a person keeps a poor eating schedule and works while hungry and there is mild, ongoing pain, the stomach has prolapsed a little. The person should not eat too much and should eat often so the food won't pull the stomach down. After eating, the person should squat (put their back against a chair). This will pull the stomach up. Do for 10–15 minutes.

Leon Hammer   Dr. Shen had some thoughts in particular about sudden emotional problems during meal times that are briefly summarized in *Dragon Rises Red Bird Flies* (DRRBF; Hammer, 2005) as follows: An important factor in determining the outcome of sudden emotion is the activity in which the person is engaged at the time of the sudden emotional stress. For example, if a person has a great anger and happens to be physically quiet at the time, it will affect the liver. One will find a big change in the liver pulse, which will become inflated. If the person is active, the anger will affect the heart, and the heart pulse will become inflated. If the person is eating, it will affect the esophagus and stomach and, of course, the digestion; one will find an inflated pulse, frequently on the upper part of the stomach or between the lung and the stomach positions, on the right side.

Again, in DRRBF Chapter 14, there is more about the relationship between *qi*, food, and phlegm stagnation and mental illness as follows: "*qi* stagnation in the middle burner (spleen-stomach) occurs most often when the *qi* in the liver becomes stagnant. Whereas this may be the result of chemical stress, such as alcohol, or trauma, it is most often the result of suppressed feelings, especially unexpressed anger. Liver *qi* stagnation causes stagnation in the entire middle burner and is eventually accompanied by some heat, which may be likened to the heat of friction from two strongly opposing forces. The *qi* is unable to move down to the lower burner (intestines) and may either stay in the middle, causing physical discomfort, or, if the heart is vulnerable, will rise with the heat and go to the heart; because the heart controls the mind, mental symptoms will occur.

These symptoms include mental confusion that occurs periodically, clearing and clouding on and off throughout the day. There may even be days when the person is entirely well, interspersed with days when these symptoms appear. *Qi* problems generally tend to come and go, depending on whether the *qi* is stronger or weaker at any one time. And since *qi* is relatively so insubstantial, so ephemeral, its strength, and therefore stagnation, responds to influences much more readily than blood or water stagnation. This process can be likened to a fire in a house in which the windows are closed. The smoke will be unable to escape and will tend to rise with the heat to the attic.

Food stagnation:

Food stagnation is our second consideration. This occurs most often as the result of a severe emotional shock while eating, or just after, sharply curtailing digestion. The stagnation is of both food and *qi* and occurs actually in the esophageal area and is an upper burner chest distress problem. The pulse is stagnant in the form of a right diaphragm position that is more inflated and often rough, as one rolls the finger between the middle position and right distal position, than when one rolls the finger from the distal toward the middle position; and the tongue coating is thick and 'dirty.' The symptoms are the same as those mentioned under *qi* stagnation, except that the periods of confusion are more frequent, last longer, and are more severe.

Phlegm-fire:

Phlegm-fire congestion is the result of stagnant dampness from poor digestion (spleen *qi* deficiency or poor food habits), which accumulates into mucus, combined with excessive heat from liver *qi* stagnation. Since food is eighty percent water, a deficient spleen or excess food that is difficult to digest can leave the digestive tract with more dampness (water) than it can handle. Chinese medicine states that this dampness normally ascends to the lungs with spleen energy to be 'digested' or, more accurately, 'misted.' If, in addition to poor digestion, the lungs are weak and cannot digest this dampness that is normally dispersed through sweat or sent to the kidneys, the dampness accumulates into mucus. Long-standing heat from liver *qi* stagnation turns into fire and combines with the mucus to become the more viscous substance referred to as phlegm-fire, which goes to the heart where it blocks the orifices. Especially if the 'nervous system' is already compromised, we have mental confusion that is continuous and unabating. These are the severe, long-term psychoses that, according to Chinese medicine, are on a continuum with epilepsy, which is thought to represent an even greater aggregate of phlegm fire in the heart orifices. The pulse is slippery, and the tongue has some coating and mucus threads" (Hammer, 2005, Chapter 14, pp. 367–369).

Digestive System

FROM DR. SHEN: Long-term problem. Right-side pulses (distal, middle, proximal) all weak, all tight. Causes:
- Poor diet in childhood
- Adults too busy to eat
- Not eating when hungry
- Not recovering after a cold

Original formula for the digestive system:

Pin Yin	Latin	English	Dosage
Bai zhu	Atractylodis Macrocephalae Rhizoma	White atractylodes rhizome	6 g
Fu ling	Poria Cocos Sclerotium	Sclerotium of tuckahoe, poria, China root, hoelen, Indian bread	10 g
Chen pi	Citri Reticulatae Pericarpium	Tangerine peel	6 g
Shan yao	Dioscoreae Oppositae Rhizoma	Chinese yam root, dioscorea rhizome	10 g
Zhi ke	Citri Aurantii Fructus	Mature fruit of the bitter orange	2 g
Huang qin	Scutellariae Baicalensis Radix	Baical skullcap root, scutellaria, scute	2 g
Bai shao	Paeoniae Alba Radix	White peony root	6 g
Ji nei jin	Corneum Gigeriae Galli Endothelium	Chicken gizzard's inner lining	12 g
Gu ya	Oryzae Germinatus Fructus	Rice sprout	6 g
Mai ya	Hordei Germinatus Fructus	Barley sprout, malt	6 g

Hamilton Rotte   Formulas that treat the spleen and stomach fall into two broad categories: those that are sweet and tonifying and those that treat excess conditions such as damp, food stagnation, and *qi* stagnation. Frequently, elements of both approaches are required.

Dr. Shen's digestive system formula contains tonics as well as herbs that address excesses that affect the digestive system. The tonics, which are mild in nature, include *bai zhu*, *fu ling*, and *shan yao*, *mai ya* and *gu ya*. Ding Gan Ren indicated that *bai shao* tonifies the middle burner, calms the spleen, and treats fullness and distention in deficiency. None of these are the strong *qi* tonics like *ren shen* or *huang qi*, which are the chief herbs of standard tonic formulas. The digestive system formula also contains herbs for all of the excess conditions that burden the spleen and stomach. For damp excess, we find *bai zhu*, *fu ling*, *chen pi*, *zhi ke*, and *huang qin*. For heat we find *huang qin*. For *qi* stagnation we find *chen pi* and *zhi ke*. For food stagnation, we find *ji nei jin*, *mai ya*, *gu ya*, and, according to Ding Gan Ren, *bai zhu*. *Ji nei jin* and *bai zhu* are also a two-herb combination.

A method of indirectly "tonifying" the spleen and stomach apart from using the conventional sweet tonics such as *ren shen* and *huang qi* is to rid the digestive system of the excess conditions that slow down its function. This formula serves this purpose.

Additional formula for the digestive system from a lecture in October, 2000:

Pin Yin	Latin	English	Dosage
Chao bai zhu	Atractylodis Macrocephalae Rhizoma	Fried white atractylodes rhizome	6 g
Fu ling	Poria Cocos Sclerotium	Sclerotium of tuckahoe, poria, China root, hoelen, Indian bread	9 g
Shan yao	Dioscoreae Oppositae Rhizoma	Chinese yam root, dioscorea rhizome	12 g
Zhi ke	Citri Aurantii Fructus	Mature fruit of the bitter orange	4.5 g
Sha ren	Amomi Fructus	Cardamom	4.5 g
Shi hu	Dendrobii Herba	Dendrobium	9 g
Chao huang qin	Scutellariae Baicalensis Radix	Fried baical skullcap root, scutellaria, scute	4.5 g
Chao bai shao	Paeoniae Alba Radix	Fried white peony root	6 g
Ji nei jin	Corneum Gigeriae Galli Endothelium	Chicken gizzard's inner lining	12 g

Hamilton Rotte This is a more recent version of the digestive system formula that Dr. Shen conveyed in 2000. In this version of the formula we see that *chen pi* is not included, but *sha ren* is, another *qi* regulator. This version also does not include *gu ya* and *mai ya*, two herbs that tonify the spleen and resolve food stagnation.

The most substantial difference between this version of the formula and those that preceded it is the inclusion of *shi hu*, which nourishes stomach *yin*. *Shi hu*, a potent nourishing substance, offsets any drying tendencies of the *qi*-regulating and damp-resolving herbs included in the formula. According to Ding Gan Ren, *shi hu* generates flesh, correcting tissue damage from digestive problems. Ding Gan Ren also indicated that *shi hu* strengthens the intestines and stops diarrhea, making it an ideal herb for tonifying stomach *yin* when co-existing *qi* deficiency predisposes an individual to loose stools.

Leon Hammer The "digestive system" can be accessed over the entire right side of the pulse when all of the qualities on that side are approximately the same. The "digestive system" (*yang* brightness) includes the lungs, the stomach-spleen, small intestine, and the bladder-kidneys. According to Dr. Shen, the lungs digest mucus, the stomach-spleen digest food, and the kidneys digest water. Symptoms associated with digestive system disorders include fluctuating appetite and irregular bowel movements (changing from constipation to diarrhea). There is no equivalent term or condition in TCM.

There are two pulse pictures. The right side may be deep and feeble when a person eats irregularly, or it may be very tight, especially on the surface, if a person eats too rapidly.

Esophagus (from Weak Spleen)

Pin Yin	Latin	English	Dosage
Xie bai	Albi Bulbus	Bulb of Chinese chive, macrostem onion, bakeri	4.5 g
Gua lou pi	Trichosanthis Pericarpium	Peel of trichosanthes fruit	9 g
Chao huang qin	Scutellariae Baicalensis Radix	Fried baical skullcap root, scutellaria, scute	4.5 g
Zhi ban xia	Pinelliae Preparatum Rhizoma	Dried, processed pinellia rhizome	9 g
Bai zhu	Atractylodis Macrocephalae Rhizoma	White atractylodes rhizome	9 g
Cang zhu	Atractylodis Rhizoma	Black atractylodes rhizome	9 g

For stomach *yin* deficiency add:

Pin Yin	Latin	English	Dosage
Bai shao	Paeoniae Alba Radix	White peony root	6–15 g
Sheng di huang	Rehmanniae Radix	Fresh Chinese foxglove root, rehmannia root	9–15 g
Mai men dong	Ophiopogonis Radix	Ophiopogon root	6–15 g
Shi hu	Dendrobii Herba	Dendrobium	6–12 g

Hamilton Rotte This formula is indicated for esophagus problems, which may include reflux or discomfort in the area. Reflux is a rebellion of stomach *qi*, which may come from the liver "attacking" the middle burner, spleen *qi* deficiency (because the spleen is too weak to send clear *qi* upward), damp excess, stomach *yin* deficiency or stomach heat. This formula addresses reflux from spleen deficiency and damp excess. The primary method of addressing reflux is to descend stomach *qi*. In this formula, *zhi ban xia* and *huang qin* serve this purpose.

The inclusion of *gua lou shi* and *xie bai* are unusual and surprising in this formula. This two-herb combination is utilized to move *qi* in the chest. They are probably included here because of the influence that the lung *qi* has on descending *qi* in general. When lung *qi* descends, the *qi* of digestive organs descends as well.

Bai zhu and *cang zhu* address damp excess that help the spleen in its transforming and transporting functions, thereby benefiting the spleen. This formula is indicated for spleen deficiency, yet utilizing conventional sweet tonic herbs would introduce the possibility of exacerbating the stagnation that is already present.

Because the formula contains drying ingredients, herbs that are moistening are offered as possible modifications in situations where stomach *yin* deficiency is present.

Esophagus Tight

FROM DR. SHEN: If a person eats and then vomits, this indicates an esophagus problem due to emotions while eating (this makes esophagus tight).

Pin Yin	Latin	English	Dosage
Xie bai	Albi Bulbus	Bulb of Chinese chive, macrostem onion, bakeri	4.5 g
Gua lou pi	Trichosanthis Pericarpium	Peel of trichosanthes fruit	9 g
Xiang fu	Cyperi Rotundi Rhizoma	Nut grass rhizoma, cyperus	4.5 g
Chen pi	Citri Reticulatae Pericarpium	Tangerine peel	4.5 g
Yu jin	Curcumae Radix	Curcuma tuber	6 g
Zhi ke	Citri Aurantii Fructus	Mature fruit of the bitter orange	4.5 g
Bai dou kou	Amomi Kravanh Fructus	Cardamom fruit/round seed	4.5 g
Fo shou	Citri Sarcodactylis Fructus	Finger citron fruit, Buddha's hand	4.5 g

Hamilton Rotte This formula is indicated for a "rebellion" of stomach *qi* due to an "overacting" liver. This formula, like the previous esophagus formula contains the combination of *xie bai* and *gua lou pi* that descends the *qi* in the upper burner in order to treat the middle.

Here we also have many ingredients that regulate the liver *qi*: *xiang fu*, *yu jin*, and *fo shou*. These are included to move a stagnant liver, which as a result is unable to assist the stomach *qi* to move downward.

Because the liver *qi* stagnation is affecting the spleen and stomach, *qi*-regulating herbs are included to target this area: *chen pi*, *zhi ke*, *bai dou kou*, and *fo shou*. These herbs exhibit a marked descending effect on the spleen and stomach *qi*, addressing the manifestations of the condition.

Leon Hammer The term "esophagus tight" is derived from the quality "tight" on the pulse at the esophagus position in the Shen-Hammer pulse system (Hammer, 2001).

The terms "overacting" or "attacking" liver is a misconception. In keeping with a very intelligent organism the liver's survival interests lie in symbiosis and homeostasis and not in antagonism or conflict.

One of the liver's principal functions is to move and direct *qi* throughout the body. A principal area of this function is assisting the stomach to move *qi* downward (peristalsis). When liver *qi* is unable to perform this task due to stagnation or deficiency, *qi* in the digestive system moves in the wrong direction since spleen *qi* moves upward. This regurgitation of *qi* and food is again mislabeled "rebellious" stomach *qi*. The stomach does not want *qi* and food to move upward, the wrong direction (Hammer, 2009).

This is an important formula since the tight quality at the esophagus position on the pulse is a sign of possible Barrett esophagus, a dysplasia that is a precursor to esophageal cancer.

Organ System

Formula for organ system deficient:

Pin Yin	Latin	English	Dosage
Dang shen	Codonopsis Pilosulae Radix	Codonopsis root	9 g
Shan yao	Dioscoreae Oppositae Rhizoma	Chinese yam root, dioscorea rhizome	12 g
Bai zhu	Atractylodis Macrocephalae Rhizoma	White atractylodes rhizome	9 g
Shan zhu yu	Corni Officinalis Fructus	Asiatic Cornelian cherry fruit, cornus	9 g
Fu ling	Poria Cocos Sclerotium	Sclerotium of tuckahoe, poria, China root, hoelen, Indian bread	9 g
Yuan zhi	Polygalae Radix	Chinese senega root, polygala root	6 g
Da zao	Zizyphi Jujubae Fructus	Chinese date, jujube	9 g
Ji nei jin	Corneum Gigeriae Galli Endothelium	Chicken gizzard's inner lining	12 g
Sang ji sheng	Taxilll Herba	Mulberry mistletoe stems, loranthus, taxillus, mistletoe	9 g
Yu jin	Curcumae Radix	Curcuma tuber	6 g
Bai shao	Paeoniae Alba Radix	White peony root	6 g
Rou gui	Cinnamomi Cassiae Cortex	Inner bark of Saigon cinnamon	3 g

Hamilton Rotte While Dr. Shen indicated that the organ system involves the heart, liver, and kidneys, this formula primarily focuses on spleen, liver, and kidneys. It is primarily geared toward tonifying *qi* and *yang*.

Herbs that tonify spleen *qi* include *dang shen*, *shan yao*, *bai zhu*, *fu ling*, and *da zao*. *Ji nei jin*, a substance that resolves food stagnation indirectly strengthens the spleen by resolving the excesses that burden the spleen. Herbs that tonify liver include both *yin*-blood tonics as well as *qi-yang* tonics. *Yin*-blood tonics for the liver include *bai shao* and *sang ji sheng*. *Shan zhu yu* is considered to be both a *qi* and *yin* tonic for the liver.

Herbs that tonify the kidneys include *rou gui* and *shan zhu yu*. According to Ding Gan Ren, *yuan zhi* tonifies the kidneys and benefits the essence. *Yu jin* is included to regulate the *qi* and blood, in order to prevent stagnation from tonic herbs.

Formula for organ system from February 2000:

Pin Yin	Latin	English	Dosage
Chao huang qi	Astragali Radix	Fried milk vetch root, fried astragalus root	9 g
Bai zhu	Atractylodis Macrocephalae Rhizoma	White atractylodes rhizome	6 g
Shan zhu yu	Corni Officinalis Fructus	Asiatic Cornelian cherry fruit, cornus	12 g
Bai shao	Paeoniae Radix Alba	White peony root	6 g
Fu ling	Poria Cocos Sclerotium	Sclerotium of tuckahoe, poria, China root, hoelen, Indian bread	9 g
Yuan zhi	Polygalae Radix	Chinese senega root, polygala root	4.5 g
Da zao	Zizyphi Jujubae Fructus	Chinese red date, jujube	7 pieces
Tu si zi	Cuscutae Chinensis Semen	Chinese dodder seeds, cuscuta	12 g
Chuan bei mu	Fritillaria Cirrhosae Bulbus	Szechuan fritillaria bulb, tendrilled fritillary bulb, fritillaria	9 g
Zhe bei mu	Fritillariae Thunbergii Bulbus	Zhejiang fritillaria, Thunberg fritillaria bulb, fritillaria	9 g

FROM DR. SHEN:
- Pulse on the left side is weak.
- If the *qi* is very low add *dang shen*.
- *Huang qi* helps *qi* build blood.
- If blood is very deficient add *dang gui*.
- *Shan zhu yu* and *bai shao* are for the middle.
- *Tu si zi* and *da zao* are for the kidneys and heart.

Hamilton Rotte   Here is another version of the organ system formula. This formula is very similar to the original formula, though it contains herbs that focus on the lungs, notable *chuan bei mu* and *zhe bie mu*. Both of these herbs clear heat and resolve phlegm in the lungs, and *chuan bei mu* is also nourishing to lung *yin*.

Leon Hammer   The "organ system" (greater, lesser, and absolute *yin*) includes the *yin* solid organs, especially the heart, liver, and kidneys that are accessed on the left side of the pulse when all of the pulse qualities on the left side are approximately the same and with varying degrees of deficiency. The pathological condition associated with deficiency of this system is primarily *yang* deficiency. These include spontaneous cold, beady perspiration, being easily fatigued, frequent pale urination, aversion to cold and preference for warmth, diarrhea with undigested food or infrequent bowel movements, and an extreme vulnerability to chronic illness and infections from which it is difficult to recover. There is no equivalent term or condition in TCM (Hammer, 1990, Chapter 14, p. 303).

Pain in the Stomach from Cold

FROM DR. SHEN: This pain can be brought on by eating or drinking too much cold or raw food. The tongue will be white and the stomach pulse will be weak or strong depending on the individual's constitution.

Formula I for pain in the stomach from cold:

Pin Yin	Latin	English	Dosage
Huang lian	Coptidis Rhizoma	Coptis rhizome	1.5 g
Wu zhu yu	Evodiae Fructus	Evodia fruit	1.8 g
Gan jiang	Zingiberis Rhizoma	Dried ginger	4.5 g
Fu ling	Poria Cocos Sclerotium	Sclerotium of tuckahoe, poria, China root, hoelen, Indian bread	9 g
Zhi shi	Aurantii Immaturus Fructus	Immature bitter orange, unripe bitter orange, chih-shih	4.5 g
Sha ren	Amomi Fructus	Cardamom	4.5 g
Shen qu	Massa Medicata Fermentata	Medicated leaven (dough)	9 g
Chuan lian zi	Meliae Toosendan Fructus	Szechuan pagoda tree fruit, Szechuan chinaberry, melia	9 g
Bai shao	Paeoniae Radix Alba	White peony root	6 g

Hamilton Rotte This formula regulates and descends stomach *qi*, relieves pain, warms the middle burner, treats damp excess, and resolves food stagnation.

Huang lian and *wu zhu yu* are a two-herb combination (called *Zou Jin Wan* or Left Metal Pill) and one of the most effective combinations in Chinese medicine at descending stomach *qi*. According to Ding Gan Ren, *wu zhu yu* is the only herb which is very good at treating distention caused by cold.

Gan jiang is the most widely used substance for removing cold from the middle burner.

Fu ling drains dampness through the urine, commonly combined with substances that target the middle burner more directly.

Qi regulators in this formula include *zhi shi*, *sha ren*, *shen qu*, and *chuan lian zi*. *Chuan lian zi* is particularly effective at relieving pain.

Shen qu is included to relieve food stagnation. Dr. Shen commonly used herbs for food stagnation as a means of aiding in the relief of other excesses that burden the middle burner.

Bai shao is included because of its pain-relieving effects.

Leon Hammer Sucking on ice, ice cream, and cold drinks in excess was very common until recently when caffeinated beverages seem to have replaced them and become ubiquitous. The consequences of imbibing cold substances, especially in women, went beyond *qi* and food stagnation and created blood stagnation in the lower burner and severe menstrual pain.

Pulse:
- Entire pulse: tense-tight (3–4) (the tight aspect is due to pain):
  - Right middle position (RMP): tense-tight (3–5)
  - Stomach-pylorus extension (SPEP): tense (3–5); slippery; (3–5); rough vibration; muffled
  - Pelvic lower body (PLB): muffled; tense-tight; choppy

Tongue:
Wide; moderate white coat; gray sides; center swollen

Formula II for pain in the stomach from cold

FROM DR. SHEN: This pain is caused by alternating too quickly between hot and cold food. Often this problem develops from drinking ice water with hot food. In this condition, there will also be pain in the intestines because the whole digestive system is weakened. Often there is diarrhea. The lower right pulse can be either weak or tight. The coating on the tongue can be a little yellow or gray.

Pin Yin	Latin	English	Dosage
Huang lian	Coptidis Rhizoma	Coptis rhizome	1.8 g
Wu zhu yu	Evodiae Fructus	Evodia fruit	2.4 g
Mu xiang	Saussureae Lappae Radix or Aucklandia Lappae Radix	Costus root, saussurea, aucklandia	6 g
Gan jiang	Zingiberis Rhizoma	Dried ginger	4.5 g
Can sha	Bombycis Faeces	Silkworm feces	9 g
Da fu pi	Arecae Catechu Pericarpium	Betel husk, areca peel	9 g
Qing pi	Citri Reticulatae Pericarpium Viride	Unripe tangerine peel, green tangerine peel, blue citrus	6 g
Huang qin	Scutellariae Baicalensis Radix	Baical skullcap root, scutellaria, scute	4.5 g
Shan zha tan	Crataegi Fructus	Charred hawthorn fruit	12 g

Pain in the Stomach from Eating Too Much

FROM DR. SHEN: This pain occurs only when a person eats too much. There will be a feeling of pressure in the chest, and the coating of the tongue will be thick. Take this formula, eat very lightly, and rest well until the pain goes away.

Pin Yin	Latin	English	Dosage
Chuan xiong	Chuanxiong Rhizoma	Chuanxiong root, Szechuan lovage root, cnidium	4.5 g
Xiang fu	Cyperi Rotundi Rhizoma	Nut grass rhizoma, cyperus	4.5 g
Hou po	Magnoliae Officinalis Cortex	Magnolia bark	4.5 g
Zhi shi	Aurantii Immaturus Fructus	Immature bitter orange, unripe bitter orange, chih-shih	4.5 g
Huang qin	Scutellariae Baicalensis Radix	Baical skullcap root, scutellaria, scute	4.5 g
Bai tou weng	Pulsatillae Radix	Pulsatilla, Chinese anemone root, anemone	4.5 g
Da fu pi	Arecae Catechu Pericarpium	Betel husk, areca peel	9 g
Gua lou pi	Trichosanthis Pericarpium	Peel of trichosanthes fruit	9 g
Shen qu	Massa Medicata Fermentata	Medicated leaven (dough)	9 g

Hamilton Rotte Dr. Shen attributes pain in the chest to food stagnation, in addition to the more conventional symptoms. It is interesting to note that biomedicine correlates overeating with heart attacks ("holiday heart").

This formula regulates *qi* of the spleen and stomach, liver, intestines, and chest. It also clears heat and resolves food stagnation. It is similar to *Yue Ju Wan* (Escape Restraint Pill), in that *Yue Ju Wan* has similar treatment principles and contains *chuan xiong* and *xiang fu*.

The ingredients that regulate *qi* in the spleen and stomach include *hou po*, *zhi shi*, *da fu pi*, and *shen qu*. *Xiang fu* is included to regulate the liver. It also enters the triple burner, giving it the ability to regulate *qi* in the whole body. Dr. Shen probably included it here to influence the chest (*xiang fu* is contained in Dr. Shen's formula for "Move *Qi* in the Chest"; see above). *Gua lou pi* is included to regulate *qi* in the chest. *Zhi shi* and *da fu pi* regulate *qi* in the intestines. *Hou po*, *zhi shi*, *da fu pi*, *gua lou pi* and *xiang fu* all descend *qi*, aiding in the movement of food through the body.

Heat develops as a result of the stagnant food and *qi*. *Huang qin* is included to clear heat in the middle burner and *bai tou weng* is included to clear heat in the intestines.

The herbs that resolve food stagnation include *shen qu* and *da fu pi*.

Compared to the most commonly utilized formula for food stagnation, *Bao He Wan* (Preserve Harmony Pill), this formula utilizes milder ingredients to resolve food stagnation and emphasizes regulating *qi* to a much greater degree. This formula provides a nice alternative to *Bao He Wan* because *Bao He Wan* contains very strong substances for dissolving food stagnation that can be damaging to the *qi*.

Leon Hammer One explanation for the effect of excess food on the heart is the passage of the stomach divergent channel through the heart.

Pulse:
- First impressions of entire pulse: tense.
  - RMP: muffled (2); tense-light (3); rough vibration; robust pounding (3)
  - SPEP: tense; slippery (4); choppy (3); robust pounding (3)

Tongue:
Wide; thicker yellowish coat; gray sides; center swollen with deep cracks, bright red on inside of crack

Spleen Like Stomach

FROM DR. SHEN: Blood platelets low, anemia. Spleen enlarged. Poor eating and overwork, platelets drop, always a body condition problem. Cook one batch of the following formula three separate times and sip all day. Folk remedy: give peanut skins on their own, cooked for a long time. Infection is likely if pulse is thin, tight, and slightly fast and eyelid is red (this indicates organ or blood problem). If the pulse is weak there is no infection.

Pin Yin	Latin	English	Dosage
Gao li shen	Ginseng Coreensis Radix	Korean ginseng	12 g
Xi yang shen	Panacis Quinquefolii Radix	American ginseng root	18 g
Huang qi	Astragali Radix	Milk vetch root, astragalus root	24 g
Dang gui	Angelicae Sinensis Radix	Chinese angelica root, *tang-kuei*	24 g
Bai zhu	Atractylodis Macrocephalae Rhizoma	White atractylodes rhizome	24 g
Shu di huang	Rehmanniae Preparata Radix	Prepared Chinese foxglove root (cooked in red wine), cooked rehmannia rhizome	24 g
Sheng di huang	Rehmannia Radix	Fresh Chinese foxglove root, rehmannia root	24 g

Pin Yin	Latin	English	Dosage
Shan yao	Dioscoreae Oppositae Rhizoma	Chinese yam root, dioscorea rhizome	24 g
Shan zhu yu	Corni Officinalis Fructus	Asiatic Cornelian cherry fruit, cornus	24 g
Fu ling	Poria Cocos Sclerotium	Sclerotium of tuckahoe, poria, China root, hoelen, Indian bread	24 g
Chi shao	Paeoniae Rubra Radix	Red peony root	15 g
Mu dan pi	Moutan Radicis Cortex	Tree peony root bark, moutan root bark	15 g
Huang qin	Scutellariae Baicalensis Radix	Baical skullcap root, scutellaria, scute	15 g
Duan mu li	Ostreae Concha	Calcined oyster shell	24 g
Duan long gu	Fossilia Ossis Mastodi	Calcined fossilized dragon's bone, fossilized vertebrae and bones of the extremities (usually of mammals)	24 g
Mai men dong	Ophiopogonis Radix	Ophiopogon tuber/root	24 g
Yan hu suo	Corydalis Yanhusuo Rhizoma	Corydalis rhizome	15 g
Lu lu tong	Liquidambaris Fructus	Sweetgum fruit, liquidambar fruit	18 g
Ji nei jin	Corneum Gigeriae Galli Endothelium	Chicken gizzard's inner lining	18 g

Hamilton Rotte   When Dr. Shen referred to the spleen being like the stomach, he probably meant that the spleen was behaving like the stomach, consuming the body's resources. The spleen becomes enlarged and consumes red blood cells excessively. It is a qi-, blood-, and yin-deficient condition that occurs from the body consuming itself. From a biomedical point of view, this is likely an autoimmune disorder.

Herbs in this formula that tonify qi include gao li shen, si yang shen, huang qi, bai zhu, shan yao, and fu ling. Blood tonics include dang gui, and shu di huang. This formula contains the ingredients in Liu Wei Di Huang Wan (Six Ingredient Rehmannia) except for ze xie, a famous formula for tonifying kidney yin.

There are also herbs to reduce masses (and therefore reduce the size of an enlarged organ). Mu li, long gu, and mai men dong are a three-herb combination to serve this purpose. Ji nei jin is also a modern favorite to dissolve masses, in addition to aiding in digestion by resolving stagnation of food. Yan hu suo and lu lu tong, both qi- and blood-invigorating ingredients, are probably included to reduce the size of the enlarged spleen that indicates the use of this formula.

The large dosages in this formula suggest that this formula was intended for about 5 days of treatment.

Stomach Pain

FROM DR. SHEN: From working while hungry, pain and burning. Person should rest and eat lightly. Drink coconut juice, rest 1 week, then no problems.

Pin Yin	Latin	English	Dosage
Shi hu	Dendrobii Herba	Dendrobium	9 g
Chao huang lian	Coptidis Rhizoma	Dry-fried coptis rhizome	2 g
Wu zhu yu	Evodiae Fructus	Evodia fruit	2 g
Shan yao	Dioscoreae Oppositae Rhizoma	Chinese yam root, dioscorea rhizome	9 g

Pin Yin	Latin	English	Dosage
Fu ling	Poria Cocos Sclerotium	Sclerotium of tuckahoe, poria, China root, hoelen, Indian bread	9 g
Zhi ke	Citri Aurantii Fructus	Mature fruit of the bitter orange	4.5 g
Bai bian dou	Lablab Semen Album	White hyacinth bean	4.5 g
Chao huang qin	Scutellariae Baicalensis Radix	Fried baical skullcap root, scutellaria, scute	4.5 g
Chao mai ya	Hordei Germinatus Fructus	Fried barley sprout	12 g
Chao gu ya	Oryzae Germinatus Fructus	Fried rice sprout	12 g
Fo shou	Citri Sarcodactylis Fructus	Finger citron fruit, Buddha's hand	6 g

Hamilton Rotte This formula, similar to his formulas for ulcers below and his "Digestive System" formula above, is indicated for acute stomach pain. Ding Gan Ren indicates that *shi hu* nourishes stomach *yin* and generates flesh, restoring the stomach tissue from damage caused by irregular eating. In this formula we also find the highly effective two-herb combination of *huang lian* and *wu zhu yu* (a classic formula called *Zou Jin Wan* or Left Metal Pill), which is very good at descending rebellious stomach *qi* and treating acid reflux.

Shan yao is a mild *qi* tonic, but otherwise we find herbs that counteract the excesses that become stagnant in the spleen and stomach.

For *qi* stagnation there is *zhi ke, wu zhu yu*, and *fo shou*. For damp stagnation there is *fu ling, bai bian dou, zhi ke*, and *huang qin*. For food stagnation there is *mai ya* and *gu ya* . For heat there is *huang qin*.

Ulcers

FROM DR. SHEN: Ulcers are caused by irregular eating, eating too quickly, or having emotions while eating. In ulcers:
- Eat soft, light foods
- Eat on time
- No alcohol or spicy food
- Do not work too hard

Formula for a bleeding ulcer:

Pin Yin	Latin	English	Dosage
Shi hu	Dendrobii Herba	Dendrobium	9 g
Wu zhu yu	Evodiae Fructus	Evodia fruit	1.8 g
Fu ling	Poria Cocos Sclerotium	Sclerotium of tuckahoe, poria, China root, hoelen, Indian bread	9 g
Zhi ke	Citri Aurantii Fructus	Mature fruit of the bitter orange	4.5 g
Chao huang lian	Coptidis Rhizoma	Dry-fried coptis rhizome	1.8 g
Chao huang qin	Scutellariae Baicalensis Radix	Fried baical skullcap root, scutellaria, scute	4.5 g
Mai ya	Hordei Germinatus Fructus	Barley sprout, malt	12 g
Gu ya	Oryzae Germinatus Fructus	Rice sprout	12 g
Ou jie	Nelumbinis Nodus Rhizomatis	Node of lotus rhizome, lotus root node	12 g
Xian he cao	Agrimoniae Herba	Hairy vein agrimony	9 g
Dan shen	Salviae Miltiorrhizae Radix	Salvia root	6 g

Hamilton Rotte   Peptic ulcers are marked by pain that begins 30 minutes to 2 hours after eating. There may also be nausea, regurgitation, and distension.

In the literature, peptic ulcers are associated with blood stagnation, cold in the stomach, stomach heat, liver *qi* stagnation, spleen *qi* deficiency, and stomach *yin* deficiency. All of these pathologies would involve a rebellion of *qi*. Typically, ulcers will occur with a combination of these factors.

This formula descends stomach *qi*, treats damp excess, nourishes stomach *yin*, clears stomach heat, reduces food stagnation, stops bleeding, and moves blood. Based on these treatment principles, we can assume that these are the conditions that Dr. Shen considered to be the main causes of ulcers.

The herbs that descend stomach *qi* include the two-herb combination of *wu zhu yu* and *huang lian* (called *Zou Jin Wan* or Left Metal Pill), *huang qin*, and *zhi ke*. *Whu zhu yu* and *huang lian* are particularly effective at descending stomach *qi*, especially indicated for reflux. The herbs that treat damp excess include *zhi ke* and *fu ling*.

The herb that nourishes stomach *yin* is *shi hu*, the strongest substance in the pharmacy for achieving this aim. *Shi hu* also generates flesh, regenerating damaged stomach tissue.

Huang lian and *huang qin* clear stomach heat. Herbs in their charred form are especially good for stopping bleeding.

Herbs that stop bleeding include *ou jie* and *xian he cao*. *Mai ya* and *gu ya* reduce food stagnation and mildly tonify the spleen. Dr. Shen frequently included these in his formulas for the digestive system.

Dan shen is included to move the blood.

Leon Hammer
Not immediately dangerous:
Pulse:
- RMP, SPEP; SI:
  – Slippery, tight, hollow and rapid; the rapid rate indicates inflammation, the slippery quality at the organ depth has been associated with *H. pylori*, the hollow quality may suggest some bleeding
  – A slower rate is a sign that the ulcer is more chronic due to *qi* stagnation from deficiency with pain due to an accumulation of hydrochloric acid

Tongue:
Marked by many deep cracks in the middle of the tongue that are very red inside the cracks

Dangerous—requires emergency measures:
Pulse:
- Leather—hard at *qi* depth (surface)
- Completely hollow blood depth (middle)
- Normal organ (deep) depth
- Rapid rate—imminent hemorrhage
- Slow rate—past hemorrhage—can recur

Tongue:
Very pale and dry

Formula for ulcer, nonbleeding:

Pin Yin	Latin	English	Dosage
Shi hu	Dendrobii Herba	Dendrobium	3 g
Huang lian	Coptidis Rhizoma	Coptis rhizome	1.8 g
Wu zhu yu	Evodiae Fructus	Evodia fruit	1.8 g
E zhu	Curcumae Rhizoma	Zedoary rhizoma, zedoaria	2.4 g
Fu ling	Poria Cocos Sclerotium	Sclerotium of tuckahoe, poria, China root, hoelen, Indian bread	9 g
Zhi ke	Citri Aurantii Fructus	Mature fruit of the bitter orange	4.5 g
Bai dou kou	Amomi Kravanh Fructus	Cardamom fruit/round seed	4.5 g
Huang qin	Scutellariae Baicalensis Radix	Baical skullcap root, scutellaria, scute	4.5 g
Mai ya	Hordei Germinatus Fructus	Barley sprout, malt	12 g
Gu ya	Oryzae Germinatus Fructus	Rice sprout	12 g
Yu jin	Curcumae Radix	Curcuma tuber	6 g
Yan hu suo	Corydalis Yanhusuo Rhizoma	Corydalis rhizome	9 g

Hamilton Rotte This formula addresses similar pathologies to the previous formulas: stomach *yin* deficiency, rebellious stomach *qi*, stomach heat, damp excess, food stagnation, and blood stagnation. It does not stop bleeding, but instead warms the stomach and strongly relieves pain.

There is significantly less emphasis on nourishing stomach *yin* in this formula because the dosage of *shi hu* is 3 g instead of 9 g as in the previous formula. According to Ding Gan Ren, *shi hu* and *yu jin* generate flesh, regenerating damaged stomach tissue.

The ingredients to descend stomach *qi* are similar: the combination of *wu zhu yu* and *huang lian*, *huang qin*, and *zhi ke*. *Qi*-regulating ingredients include *zhi ke*, *wu zhu yu*, and *bai dou kou*. Herbs for damp excess include *fu ling* and *zhi ke*. Herbs for food stagnation include *mai ya* and *gu ya*, also slightly tonifying to the spleen. *Bai dou kou* is included to warm the stomach and stop pain.

A lot of emphasis is placed on moving blood and relieving pain with *e zhu*, *yu jin*, and *yan hu suo* (the most effective herb in Chinese medicine for relieving stomach pain). These would be contraindicated if a person were bleeding because moving blood is generally contraindicated when bleeding is present.

Genitourinary Conditions

Male Infertility

FROM DR. SHEN: In Chinese medicine, male infertility is seen from two respects. From the physiological point of view, it may be from hereditary weakness of the kidneys and as such is an innate deficiency. Indulgence in masturbation in adolescence causes deficiency of the kidneys, resulting in weak, inactive sperm. Also at the time of adolescence, a man may have sustained an unobserved external trauma. If such a case is overlooked for a long time, a disruption in circulation of the *qi* and blood will result in infertility. In addition, if a man overworks or overindulges in sex to the point of exhaustion he will impair himself.
The result is a deficiency of *jing* and *qi*, the essence and vitality, which can lead to infertility and a weak constitution. Overindulgence in sex can be easily discerned by a recurrent feeling of exhaustion after intercourse. According to Chinese medical theory, 40 drops of blood make one drop of sperm. Since men are "*qi*" and women "blood," men are lacking in the blood necessary to make sperm. That is why sexual overindulgence is inadvisable for men. Generally speaking, masturbation should be entirely avoided in adolescence.
Male infertility may also have psychological factors. Sexual nerves, brain nerves, and heart nerves are closely interwoven. Indulgence in masturbation could result in a palpitating weak heart and dizziness. The same is true for a man with heart disease, who may also become impotent and infertile. Industrious young men often overwork themselves and become impotent and infertile.
Different cases of male infertility should be tackled with different formulas. It depends upon the degree of weakness of the sperm and the kidneys. The following formulas are good for these patients. They are contraindicated if a patient has a severe cold or diarrhea.

Leon Hammer Dr. Shen's crossing over to allopathic terminology is vaguely informative as with "sexual nerves, brain nerves, and heart nerves are closely interwoven." These are only common language metaphoric allusions to a more exact science.

Formula for male infertility:

Pin Yin	Latin	English	Dosage
Wu wei zi	Schisandrae Chinensis Fructus	Schisandra fruit	20 g
Tu si zi	Cuscutae Chinensis Semen	Chinese dodder seeds, cuscuta	20 g
Che qian zi	Plantaginis Semen	Plantago seeds	20 g
She chuang zi	Cnidii Fructus	Cnidium seed	20 g
Fu pen zi	Rubi Fructus	Palm leaf raspberry fruit	20 g
Rou cong rong	Cistanches Herba	Cistanche, fleshy stem of the broomrape	20 g
Zhi yuan zhi	Polygalae Radix	Prepared Chinese senega root, polygala root	20 g
Zhong ru shi	Stalactitum	Stalactite	40 g
Lu rong	Cornu Cervi Parvum	Velvet of young deer antler, cervi	20 g

This formula should be taken in powder form, 3 g twice daily, to improve male sexual function.

Hamilton Rotte Male infertility is normally associated with kidney *yang* essence deficiency (as *yang* essence is viewed as the motive force that drives reproduction). This formula mainly tonifies kidney *yang*, but includes, as all kidney *yang* tonics do, some herbs that tonify the *yin*. It is important to tonify kidney *yin* when tonifying kidney *yang* because of the intimate relationship between *yin* and *yang* in the kidneys.

This formula also contains many ingredients that stabilize the essence, very commonly utilized in kidney tonic formulas that especially address sexual function. Stabilizing the essence improves sexual function and aids the body in building essence because it prevents loss of essence.

Kidney *yang* tonics include *tu si zi*, *she chuang zi*, *rou cong rong*, *zhong ru shi*, and *lu rong*. *She chuang zi* is especially indicated for male infertility and *zhong ru shi* and *lu rong* are especially indicated for poor sexual function.

Kidney *yin* tonics include *wu wei zi* and *tu si zi*, providing balance to the *yang* tonics.

Herbs that stabilize the essence include *wu wei zi*, *tu si zi*, and *fu pen zi*.

Wu wei zi and *zhi yuan zhi* are a two-herb combination, used to harmonize heart and kidneys, common in both kidney and heart tonic formulas. The sour, stabilizing effect of *wu wei zi* is balanced by the acrid, moving effect of *zhi yuan zhi*.

Che qian zi is used to promote urination. It is used in combination with kidney essence-stabilizing herbs, partially because when one promotes urination this causes essence to be retained. Also, it rids the body of excesses that can damage the kidneys.

According to Ding Gan Ren, *che qian zi* benefits the essence.

Gynecologic Conditions

Amenorrhea from Tense Nervous System

Pin Yin	Latin	English	Dosage
Shi chang pu	Acori Tatarinowii Rhizoma	Grass-leaved sweetflag rhizome, acorus	3 g
Chuan xiong	Chuanxiong Rhizoma	Chuanxiong root, Szechuan lovage root, cnidium	4.5 g
Dang gui	Angelicae Sinensis Radix	Chinese angelica root, tang-kuei	6 g
Sheng di huang	Rehmannia Radix	Fresh Chinese foxglove root, rehmannia root	9 g
Dan shen	Salviae Miltiorrhizae Radix	Salvia root	6 g
Huai niu xi or niu xi	Achyranthis Bidentatae Radix	Ox-knee root from Huai	9 g
Yan hu suo	Corydalis Yanhusuo Rhizoma	Corydalis rhizome	9 g
Yi mu cao	Leonuri Herba	Chinese motherwort, leonurus	9 g
Lu lu tong	Liquidambaris Fructus	Sweetgum fruit, liquidambar fruit	12 g

Hamilton Rotte Nervous tension compromises the liver function of regulating the menses. It causes stagnation of qi and blood. This formula, which bears some similarity to Dr. Shen's "Nervous System Tense" formulas, is aimed at regulating qi and blood. Ingredients that are commonly included in Dr. Shen's "Nervous System Tense" formulas include shi chang pu, chuan xiong, and lu lu tong.

Other than these ingredients, his formula contains mostly blood-invigorating ingredients. These include dang gui, dan shen, niu xi, yan hu suo, and yi mu cao. Dang gui, niu xi, and yi mu cao are widely used in gynecology. Dr. Shen also especially liked to use dan shen and yan hu suo for moving blood in gynecologic conditions. Niu xi is strongly descending and therefore especially indicated for amenorrhea.

Sheng di huang and dang gui are included to offset drying tendencies of other herbs in the formula.

Breast Qi and Blood Stagnation with Enlarged Lymph Nodes

Pin Yin	Latin	English	Dosage
Chao dang gui	Angelicae Sinensis Radix	Fried Chinese angelica root, tang-kuei	6 g
Zhi xiang fu	Cyperi Rotundi Rhizoma	Honey-fried nutgrass rhizome, cyperus	6 g
Hong hua	Carthami Tinctorii Flos	Safflower flower, carthamus	6 g
Si gua lou	Fasciculus Vascularis Luffae	Dried skeleton of vegetable sponge	6 g
Hou po	Magnoliae Officinalis Cortex	Magnolia bark	6 g
Sang ji sheng	Taxilli Herba	Mulberry mistletoe stems, loranthus, taxillus, mistletoe	9 g
Huai niu xi or niu xi	Achyranthis Bidentatae Radix	Ox-knee root from Huai	9 g

Pin Yin	Latin	English	Dosage
Mu xiang	Saussureae Lappae Radix or Aucklandia Lappae Radix	Costus root, saussurea, aucklandia	4.5 g
Yu jin	Curcumae Radix	Curcuma tuber	9 g
Chao bai shao	Paeoniae Alba Radix	Fried root of white peony	9 g
Chao chi shao	Paeoniae Rubra Radix	Fried red peony root	9 g

Hamilton Rotte This formula, which bears significant resemblance to "Move *Qi* in the Chest," is strongly moving to both *qi* and blood and targets the upper burner and breasts. Circulation of *qi* and blood in the breasts mainly depends on circulation in the upper burner (heart and lungs) as well as the liver. *Qi*-moving herbs in this formula include *xiang fu, hou po, mu xiang,* and *yu jin.* The focus is on the liver (*xiang fu, mu xiang, yu jin*), lungs (*hou po*), heart (*yu jin*), and triple burner (*xiang fu* and *mu xiang*). Swelling of the lymph nodes is associated with a disturbance of the triple burner's ability to circulate fluids throughout the body.

Blood-invigorating ingredients include *dang gui, hong hua, si gua lou, niu xi, yu jin,* and *chi shao.* These herbs all treat the liver. *Hong hua* is light, ascending, and affects the upper burner. *Niu xi* and *yu jin* are descending, very important in the treatment of stagnation in the upper burner. *Si gua lou* opens channels and collaterals and is especially indicated for stagnation in the breasts.

Dang gui and *bai shao* tonify blood. It is essential to include blood tonics along with blood-moving herbs in order not to damage the blood.

Delayed Menses

Formula for belated menses arising from coldness in the womb:

Pin Yin	Latin	English	Dosage
Dang gui	Angelicae Sinensis Radix	Chinese angelica root, *tang-kuei*	6 g
Xiang fu	Cyperi Rotundi Rhizoma	Nutgrass rhizome, cyperus	4.5 g
Dan shen	Salviae Miltiorrhiziae Radix	Salvia root	9 g
Gan jiang	Zingiberis Rhizoma	Dried ginger	3 g
Mu xiang	Saussureae Lappae Radix or Aucklandia Lappae Radix	Costus root, saussurea, aucklandia	6 g
Jiao ai ye	Artemisiae Argyi Folium	Calcined mugwort leaf	3 g
Huai niu xi or niu xi	Achyranthis Bidentatae Radix	Ox-knee root from Huai	12 g
Rou gui	Cinnamomi Cassiae Cortex	Inner bark of Saigon cinnamon	3 g

Hamilton Rotte Excess cold easily lodges in the uterus from exposure to cold or ingesting cold foods, especially during menses when the uterus is open. This causes pain and delayed menses because of the effect that cold has in slowing down circulation. The excess cold causes stagnation of *qi* and blood. This formula removes cold from the uterus and moves *qi* and blood in the uterus.

The herbs that expel cold from the uterus include *gan jiang* (Dr. Shen especially liked ginger products for menstrual problems), *ai ye,* and *rou gui.* Herbs

that move blood include *dang gui, dan shen, huai niu xi,* and *rou gui. Huai niu xi* exerts a particularly descending effect, especially for unblocking menstruation. *Dang gui* may also be included to offset the drying effects of the warming ingredients. *Qi* regulators include *xiang fu* and *mu xiang,* both targeting the liver channel and descending *qi.*

Delayed menses is also commonly caused by deficiency of kidney *yang* essence and liver blood. In such a case a tonic formula would be indicated.

Female Infertility

FROM DR. SHEN: Infertility of a woman should not be assumed to be so based entirely on Western medical methods. Consider the following three cases:
- Infertility due to a cold womb
- Infertility due to a womb that is too warm
- Infertility due to deficiency in the womb

When sperm enters the womb, it arrives in much the same way that a stranger enters a new room. If the room temperature is too cold or warm, the stranger will feel uncomfortable. If the room is without ventilation, the stranger will also feel uneasy. In both cases the visitor will find the room inhospitable. Only with the use of these Chinese medical diagnostic considerations can one effectively treat a patient's particular fertility issue.

Treatment of a Cold Womb

FROM DR. SHEN: Coldness in the womb comes from two factors. First, an acquired factor, is one in which a woman has been fond of cold drinks before and after her adolescence. This can produce a "cold womb." Second, a woman may have a congenital deficiency, such as childhood anemia, which can also result in a "cold womb." Both these situations may make a woman infertile.

A "cold womb" may be indicated by the following symptoms: stomach pain before and during menstruation, pale red menstrual blood, sometimes coagulating into little pale-colored clots. First, she should be advised to stop drinking all cold beverages. Generally speaking, most Chinese women dislike cold drinks. They tend to be clad in warm clothes and drink warm drinks. They understand that during their periods cold drinks and great fatigue tend to impair their physique and cause a "cold womb."

Hot compression upon the abdomen will relieve pain, and in some cases, rid the belly of itching and a cold womb. When children have a stomach ache arising from consuming too many cold drinks or ice cream, the following formula is very effective to treat an ordinary stomach ache (gastroenteritis).

Stir-fry 1 or 2 lb of rough sea-salt until it turns gray. Then put it on a thick cloth (or into a thick sock) to make a small pack. Be sure to check the temperature of the pack before placing it on the abdomen to avoid burning the skin (**Fig. 5**). Then massage the skin at the location of pain until it is relieved.

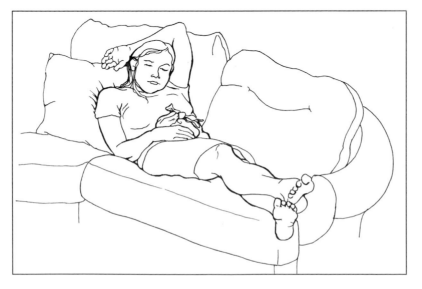

Fig. 5 Salt pack.

Formula for a cold womb:

Pin Yin	Latin	English	Dosage
Jiu dang gui	Angelicae Sinensis Radix	Chinese angelica root, *tang-kuei* prepared with 1 tsp wine	6 g
Ai ye	Artemisiae Argyi Folium	Mugwort leaf, artemesia	3 g
Gan jiang	Zingiberis Rhizoma	Dried ginger	3 g
Dan shen	Salviae Miltiorrhiziae Radix	Salvia root	9 g
Yi mu cao	Leonuri Herba	Chinese motherwort, leonurus	6 g
Lu lu tong	Liquidambaris Fructus	Sweetgum fruit, liquidambar fruit	12 g
Rou gui	Cinnamomi Cassiae Cortex	Inner bark of Saigon cinnamon	0.3 g

FROM DR. SHEN: The Chinese angelica root should be stir-fried with some wine for several seconds. The formula is taken three times a week until the pain subsides. Discontinue the formula when the period starts. If it is a case of severe cold in the womb, a dose should be taken daily for 3 to 4 months until pain is relieved and the menstrual cycle becomes regular.

Hamilton Rotte   This formula is devised for mostly excess cold that has lodged in the uterus. As Dr. Shen suggested, this can occur because of intake of cold beverages or vulnerability of the uterus because of innate deficiency. The excess cold causes stagnation of *qi* and blood and this prevents the uterus from functioning properly.

The herbs that remove cold from the uterus include *dang gui*, *ai ye*, *gan jiang*, and *rou gui*. Dr. Shen highly valued ginger products for menstrual disorders. Herbs that address stagnation of blood include *dang gui*, *dan shen*, *yi mu cao*, and *lu lu tong*, one of Dr. Shen's favorite herbs. Both *dan shen* and *yi mu cao* are cooling in nature, possibly to offset the warming tendencies of other herbs in the formula. *Yi mu cao* particularly targets the blood stagnation in the uterus, which accounts for its inclusion in this formula. *Lu lu tong* is also included because of its pronounced *qi*-regulating effect.

Dang gui is also an important blood tonic, addressing the underlying deficiency (anemia as Dr. Shen called it) that made the uterus vulnerable before the excess cold was able to enter the body.

This formula contains mostly warming or blood-invigorating herbs that target the uterus. *Rou gui*, *yi mu cao*, *ai ye*, and *dang gui* have a direct effect on the uterus and the other herbs in the formula support these ingredients in warming or moving blood.

If we compare this to formulas in the standard repertoire that warm the uterus such as *Jiao Ai Tang* (Asshide Gelatin and Mugwort Decoction) we find that this formula is less tonifying than either of these. We find that individuals who are *yang* deficient are frequently predisposed to cold in the uterus so this could be integrated with tonics if necessary.

Leon Hammer   With regard to the etiology from imbibing cold substances, the pulse and tongue information listed under "Pain in the Stomach from Cold" would apply here except that the choppy quality in the pelvic lower body would be greater and would appear also in the proximal positions.

Treatment of a Warm Womb

FROM DR. SHEN: In contrast to a "cold womb," when the womb is a bit too warm it is not caused by taking in too much warm food or drinks. It is mainly caused by overwork that leads to nervous tension, especially during periods. This leads to irregular circulation of blood and thus to irregular periods. In Chinese medicine we call this "heat." The menstrual flow is dark and scanty, often mixed with dark clots accompanied by slight pain. Some women experience abdominal spasms 1 or 2 days before the period, which cease with the onset of menses.

It is advised to relax the nerves with herbal medicine. Rest is of utmost importance. I suggest that patients stop working 1 or 2 days before the period and rest throughout the cycle in the same way we would stop a hot machine to allow it cool down.

Formula for an overly warm womb:

Pin Yin	Latin	English	Dosage
Sheng di huang	Rehmannia Radix	Fresh Chinese foxglove root, rehmannia root	9 g
Dang gui	Angelicae Sinensis Radix	Chinese angelica root, tang-kuei	6 g
Chuan xiong	Chuanxiong Rhizoma	Chuanxiong root, Szechuan lovage root, cnidium	4.5 g
Bai shao	Paeoniae Alba Radix	White peony root	6 g
Fu ling	Poria Cocos Sclerotium	Sclerotium of tuckahoe, poria, China root, hoelen, Indian bread	9 g
Dan shen	Salviae Miltiorrhiziae Radix	Salvia root	6 g
Mu dan pi	Moutan Radicis Cortex	Tree peony root bark, moutan root bark	6 g
Chi shao	Paeoniae Rubra Radix	Red peony root	9 g
Hei shan zhi zi	Gardeniae Jasminoidis Fructus	Charred cape jasmine fruit, gardenia fruit	9 g

FROM DR. SHEN: Put the herbal medicine into water and boil slowly for 20 to 25 minutes. Then filter the solution. Drink the filtrate twice a day, one cup each time.

The dosage and duration of treatment are determined by the seriousness of the illness. If the menstrual flow is dark with dark clots and pain, then the medicine should be taken daily until the symptoms subside. If the imbalance is only slightly advanced and the blood does not appear dark, take the medicine three times a week. If only slight pain is felt during the period, take the medicine 3 days consecutively before the period. If a woman is deficient and has a womb that is a bit too warm and rather long periods with pale blood, the following formula is used.

Hamilton Rotte   In the literature infertility is usually associated with kidney deficiency or cold, but Dr. Shen demonstrates that excess heat can also be a cause. This excess heat causes stagnation of blood and the condition includes pain and clots.

This formula is designed to cool the blood and treat stagnation of blood that results from the heat. It is similar to *Gui Zhi Fu ling Wan* (Cinnamon and Poria Pill), except that it does not include the warming *gui zhi* and or the descending *tao ren*.

The ingredients that cool the blood include *sheng di huang*, *dan shen*, *mu dan pi*, and *zhi zi*.

The ingredients that move the blood include *dang gui*, *chuan xiong*, *dan shen*, *mu dan pi*, and *chi shao*.

This formula also contains *dang gui* and *bai shao*, two herbs to tonify liver blood. Blood tonic ingredients are customarily included in formulas to move the blood in order to protect the blood from damage caused by moving ingredients. *Bai shao* is also included to address the "nervous tension" that leads to the heat in the blood.

Formula for a deficient, slightly warm womb:

Pin Yin	Latin	English	Dosage
Dang gui	Angelicae Sinensis Radix	Chinese angelica root, tang-kuei	6 g
Dan shen	Salviae Miltiorrhiziae Radix	Salvia root	6 g
Hong hua	Carthami Tinctorii Flos	Safflower flower, carthamus	6 g
Chao sheng di huang	Rehmannia Radix	Dry-fried fresh root of rehmannia, fried Chinese foxglove root	9 g
Chao huang qi	Astragali Radix	Fried milk vetch root, fried astragalus root	4.5 g
Yu jin	Curcumae Radix	Curcuma tuber	9 g
Chuan xiong	Chuanxiong Rhizoma	Chuanxiong root, Szechuan lovage root, cnidium	4.5 g
Yan hu suo	Corydalis Yanhusuo Rhizoma	Corydalis rhizome	9 g
Xi yang shen	Panacis Quinquefolii Radix	American ginseng root	4.5 g
Di gu pi	Lycii Radicis Cortex	Cortex of wolfberry root, lycium bark	6 g

FROM DR. SHEN: Soak herbs before boiling, then simmer for 30 to 40 minutes. Filter the solution and drink twice a day, once in the morning and once in the evening.
The dosage depends on the severity of the condition. It is advisable to take the formula even during the periods. If the case is rather serious, go on taking it for quite some time, or take it only three times a week.

Hamilton Rotte This formula is indicated for a condition where there is excess heat occurring against the ground of qi and blood deficiency. The "long periods with pale blood" occur because of the deficiencies.
As in the previous formula indicated for excess heat, the heat is causing stagnation. In addition to cooling herbs, blood-invigoration ingredients are also included. In this formula the herbs that cool the blood include dan shen, sheng di huang, yu jin, and di gu pi. Blood-invigorating ingredients include dang gui, dan shen, hong hua, yu jin, chuan xiong, and yan hu suo. Dang gui is included partially to tonify the blood. Huang qi and xi yang shen are qi tonics contained within the formula.

Leon Hammer
Pulse:
When more than one condition exists at the same time in one organ or area of the body the pulse exhibits only the most acute (usually an excess condition), which when resolved reveals the other, usually a deficient condition. The conditions associated with excess have qualities such as robust pounding that, with regard to sensation, override those qualities associated with deficiency (feeble).
Or at times, especially if the condition is more chronic, both qualities may exist at the same time, changing from one to the other. In this instance qualities appearing simultaneously but changing back and forth in the proximal positions would be signs of excess heat (robust pounding) and of kidney yang-essence deficiency (reduced substance, diffuse, feeble-absent). As one palpates the proximal positions one can feel the change from one set to the other set of qualities.
The pulse findings accompanying this formula that treats heat in the blood are at the blood depth. As one releases the pressure from the organ depth to the qi depth the vessel fills out rather than diminishes the normal condition.

Deficiency in the Womb

FROM DR. SHEN: There are three causes of a deficient womb. The first is hereditary, if the patient's parents have weak constitutions. Second, if a woman was inadequately nourished as a child, possibly due to poverty, this could lead to a deficient womb condition. Another cause is an irregular life in adolescence that results in physical weakness. All of these can make a woman deficient in *qi* and blood so she will tend to miscarry. Even though she can become pregnant rather easily, she may have habitual miscarriages. In my experience I have seen many such cases. However, with correct diagnosis and appropriate treatment, fertility can be achieved.

A woman with a deficient womb shows signs of blood deficiency in that the cycle is usually shorter than 3 days with the blood being either pale or dark and the interval between periods is 30 days or longer. Sometimes the onset of menses is 3 days earlier or later by 3 days. When the period does start she may experience spasms, trembling as if from cold, dizziness, and poor vision. Other signs of a deficient womb are when a woman feels relieved when something warm is pressed on her belly or if the woman feels as if the womb is trying to contract during the period. If she feels slightly exhausted after her periods, this is a sign of physical deficiency. Frequent hard labor will lead to deficiency of both the womb and constitution in women.

The question of deficiency in Chinese medicinal theory includes consideration of both the whole body and a single organ system at the same time. A single organ exerts influence on the entire body's well-being, just as the patient's constitutional health will be expressed. Consideration only of an isolated part and not of the whole will often bring the recurrence of the malady. Only a sound body acting as a whole system can uproot the latent threat.

Formula for deficiency of the womb:

Pin Yin	Latin	English	Dosage
Huang qi	Astragali Radix	Milk vetch root, astragalus root	15 g
Dang shen	Codonopsis Pilosulae Radix	Codonopsis root	15 g
Dang gui	Angelicae Sinensis Radix	Chinese angelica root, *tang-kuei*	15 g
Shu di huang	Rehmanniae Preparata Radix	Prepared Chinese foxglove root (cooked in red wine), cooked rehmannia rhizome	15 g
Da zao	Ziziphi Jujubae Fructus	Chinese date, jujube	7 pieces
Tu si zi	Cuscutae Chinensis Semen	Chinese dodder seeds, cuscuta	12 g
Shu nu zhen zi	Ligustri Lucidi Fructus	Prepared fruit of glossy privet	12 g

FROM DR. SHEN: Soak the medicine in water, then boil on low heat for 25 minutes. Each dose can be boiled and taken twice. Repeat the process two to three times a week.

It is also advisable to put the first five kinds of herbal medicines into a Chinese Yunnan steam pot, together with two skinned chicken legs as well as some ginger and onion and boil it for 3 to 4 hours on slow heat and drink the soup; repeat the process two to three times a week. Start taking it when the period comes to end.

Hamilton Rotte This formula addresses *qi* and blood deficiency, and also includes herbs to tonify the kidneys. All of these essential substances contribute to the functioning of the uterus.

Qi tonics include *huang qi, dang shen,* and *da zao. Huang qi* exerts a lifting effect, which is beneficial in protecting a fetus. Blood tonics include *dang gui, shu di huang,* and *da zao. Dang gui* and s*hu di huang* particularly target the liver.

Kidney tonics in this formula include *tu si zi* and *nu zhen zi.* These tonics are mild and between the two of them strike a balance between tonifying kidney *yin* and *yang. Tu si zi* also stabilizes the kidneys and is a valuable substance for preventing miscarriage.

The typical features during periods of the above-mentioned cases of infertility are listed in the table below.

Condition	Pain in Periods	Color	Quantity	Pulse	Other Symptoms
Cold womb	Pain in the belly	Pale, dark	Little	Deep	With clots in blood, dislikes tight clothing, prefers warm dress and drinks
Warm womb strong body	Slight pain 1–2 days before	Dark	Much	Fine	Dark clots in blood
Warm womb	No pain	Pale	A bit more	Fine	A longer period
Weak womb	Feeling pain	Pale red	Little	Very weak	Feeling cold, dizzy at the end of period, dim-sighted, short periods (3 days)

Miscarriage

Leon Hammer Dr. Shen successfully predicted a miscarriage several times based on two vertical black lines on the tongue parallel to the center crack about halfway between the crack and the outer edge (**Fig. 6**).

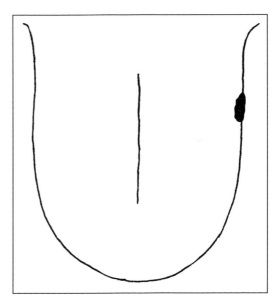

Fig. 6 Miscarriage tongue.

FROM DR. SHEN: The likelihood of miscarriage is increased for the pregnant mother if she has too much sex, lifts heavy loads, jumps, consumes alcohol, or is constitutionally weak. If she feels a soreness in her waist, has untimely bleeding, and she feels the fetus falling as if she's unable to hold it, these are all signs of an impending miscarriage. In these instances, she must immediately lie flat and GV-26 *shui gou/ren zhong* should be stimulated. With a couple of days' rest she should feel better. For a woman with a weak constitution and a history of miscarriage, use the following formula. If these warning signals are neglected and the amount of bleeding increases, miscarriage will ensue.

Leon Hammer   While stimulating GV-26 will help in avoiding an impending miscarriage, I found that Dr. Shen's recommendation of repeated moxa on a needle at GV-20 was even more useful for the purposes of avoiding a miscarriage or for women who had repeated miscarriages.

Formula for the prevention of miscarriage:

Pin Yin	Latin	English	Dosage
Chao bai zhu	Atractylodis Macrocephalae Rhizoma	Dry-fried white atractylodes rhizome	6 g
Shan yao	Dioscoreae Oppositae Rhizoma	Chinese yam root, dioscorea rhizome	12 g
Chao bai shao	Paeoniae Alba Radix	Fried root of white peony	6 g
Fu ling	Poria Cocos Sclerotium	Sclerotium of tuckahoe, poria, China root, hoelen, Indian bread	9 g
Yuan zhi	Polygalae Radix	Chinese senega root, polygala root	4.5 g
Tu si zi	Cuscutae Chinensis Semen	Chinese dodder seeds, cuscuta	9 g
Nu zhen zi	Ligustri Lucidi Fructus	Privet fruit, ligustrum	9 g
Zhu huang qi	Astragali Radix	Dried milk vetch root, astragalus root	4.5 g

FROM DR. SHEN: The patient should rest in bed for 1 week and take the medicine twice a day in the morning and afternoon until bleeding ceases.

Hamilton Rotte   The substances that nourish a fetus include *qi*, blood, and kidney *yang* essence. In order to protect a fetus it is also beneficial to utilize stabilizing and lifting herbs.
This formula primarily includes *qi* tonics as well as kidney *yin* and *qi-yang* tonics. The *qi* tonics in this formula include *bai zhu*, *shan yao*, *fu ling*, and *huang qi*. *Bai shao* tonifies the blood.
Herbs that tonify the kidneys include *shan yao*, *tu si zi*, and *nu zhen zi*, and, according to Ding Gan Ren, *yuan zhi*. These herbs are mild and balanced in tonifying kidney *yin* and *yang*. *Yin* tonics include *shan yao*, *tu si zi*, and *nu zhen zi*. *Yang* tonics include *shan yao* and *tu si zi*.
Herbs that are stabilizing include *shan yao*, *tu si zi*, and *bai shao*. *Huang qi* is lifting.
The warm, acrid *yuan zhi* is used to balance the stabilizing ingredients.

Leon Hammer   In terms of "lifestyle" Dr. Shen pointed out that it is the lifestyle of our parents that determines so much of our destiny as follows.

Suitable choice of partner:
The assault on our constitution begins with our parents' choice of a partner. In nature the female of most species chooses to mate with the male who demonstrates the strongest constitution whether it be through physical competition, the ability to build a nest, or the colors of their plumage.
As a child psychiatrist and a parent and even as a child I observed this to hold true in human children until puberty when the endocrine system replaces this atavis-

tic sorting system. However "chemistry" was interceded by pragmatism sometime in the past when children became pawns in a chess game operated by parents in a game called "power."

Procreation and union based upon physical attraction became liberated in the 20th century when power shifted from the family to individual initiative and has been the primary basis for union for the past 100 years. It has proven no better and perhaps worse than the arranged marriages of the past for the progeny we are concerned with here, with broken families everywhere and the loss of the support of the extended family.

With the advent of the nuclear family, education at home except by example, and in school regarding marriage or the opposite sex, is mostly absent, even where there is no outright objection by puritan religious factions. The age and health of one's partner as well as the ability to provide is little understood in face of the hormonal cascade.

Pre-conception and conception:

Either parent or both can affect the viability of sperm and ova due to a compromised constitution. Poor nutrition, even in childhood and adolescence, drugs, alcohol and tobacco, exercise, work and sex beyond capacity, can seriously curtail the possibility of conception. Dr. Shen placed great emphasis on excessive masturbation in adolescent males as a determent to sperm vitality, to which he added lower burner trauma as caused by vigorous sports.

Age is an important factor. The sperm of a man of 25 is considerably more active than that of a man of 35. We can imagine the sperm activity of considerably older men who are starting families and the consequences for their children.

The same personal abuse will compromise the sperm and the ova at the time of conception, including exhaustion, especially due to intercourse. Furthermore the mental state of both parents, especially the mother, affects the vitality of both. Abuse, physical and emotional, in particular rape, will compromise the vitality of the fetus. Excessive or repressed emotion and shock of any kind will affect the heart and circulation and the development and function of the placenta. War and natural disasters are catastrophic to incipient life.

Temperature at conception is an unexpected factor according to Dr. Shen for which he gave examples. In one, the combination of the woman's body condition (terrain), the sexual act, and cold substances (he cites pomegranate in one instance), caused her death. Furthermore, according to Dr. Shen, for the fetus to be healthy the conceptual act must be enjoyable.

Comment:

Why is the lifestyle of one's parents an important topic in this context? The principal purpose is to alert you as potential parents of how your lifestyle will affect the life of your most precious possession, your child. Attention to the above discussion can make your life and that of your children much more of a joy and much less of a burden.

Formula for repeated miscarriage:

Pin Yin	Latin	English	Dosage
Ren shen	Ginseng Radix	Ginseng root	45 g
Xi yang shen	Panacis Quinquefolii Radix	American ginseng root	30 g
Chao huang qi	Astragali Radix	Fried milk vetch root, fried astragalus root	30 g
Zi he che or tai pan	Placenta Hominis	Human placenta, placenta	30 g

Leon Hammer This formula contains *qi* and *yang* essence tonics to assist a woman in carrying a baby successfully. *Qi* tonics include *ren shen*, *xi yang shen*, and *huang qi*. Dr. Shen was fond of combining Chinese and American ginseng. *Yang* tonics include *zi he che* and *tu si zi*. *Zi he che* is also a very potent liver blood tonic and *tu si zi* mildly tonifies *yin*.

This formula is also lifting (with the inclusion of *huang qi*) and stabilizing (with the inclusion of *tu si zi*).

This formula was gleaned from Dr. Shen's records in treating patients and it was not specified how many days this formula was intended to last. Given the standard dosages of the ingredients, it is reasonable to assume that the specified dosages were intended to provide several days of treatment.

Formula to benefit conception:

Pin Yin	Latin	English	Dosage
Shu di huang	Rehmanniae Preparata Radix	Prepared Chinese foxglove root (cooked in red wine), cooked rehmannia rhizome	9 g
Jing jie	Schizonepetae Herba	Schizonepeta	4.5 g
Chuan xiong	Chuanxiong Rhizoma	Chuanxiong root, Szechuan lovage root, cnidium	4.5 g
Gan cao	Glycyrrhizae Radix	Licorice root	4.5 g
Mu dan pi	Moutan Radicis Cortex	Tree peony root bark, moutan root bark	6 g
Jin yin hua	Lonicerae Flos	Honeysuckle flower	6 g
Yi yi ren	Coicis Semen	Seeds of Job's tears, coix seeds	9 g
Lu lu tong	Liquidambaris Fructus	Sweetgum fruit, liquidambar fruit	12 g
Mu xiang	Saussureae Lappae Radix or Aucklandia Lappae Radix	Costus root, saussurea, aucklandia	4.5 g
Gu ya	Oryzae Germinatus Fructus	Rice sprout	9 g
Mai ya	Hordei Germinatus Fructus	Barley sprout, malt	9 g

FROM DR. SHEN: First put the medicine in water and boil for 20 to 35 minutes. Filter and drink. If the woman's body is free of chemical contaminants, the *jin yin hua* can be omitted from the formula. One bag of herbs should be divided into two parts and taken twice daily. The patient should take two to three doses per week until conception is confirmed. The medicine will help clear the body of heat while it readjusts and harmonizes the internal organs by balancing *qi* and blood, which will improve overall health.

Some women become so weak they lose too much blood during their menstrual flow, which exacerbates the weakness. If they overwork at the same time, dizziness and palpitations may be experienced. A simple treatment is to drink ginger tea made in the following way: cut three thin pieces of fresh ginger (approximately the thickness of a nickel) and boil them for 10 minutes to make a cup of ginger tea. Sweeten with a little red rock sugar. The rock sugar should not be average brown sugar, it should be the kind of sugar bought at a Chinese grocery store.

Sometimes, even if too much blood is not lost with menstruation, stomach pain is sometimes felt, which may be caused by stagnant blood in the abdomen. In this case improvement may be made by drinking several cups of hot ginger tea. Put several slices of peeled fresh ginger in water and boil it on a slow heat, sweeten it with a small cube of white rock sugar (the thickness of a nickel), and drink before each period, one cup a day for several days.

Already alluded to above, when a couple is ready to have a baby, they must be aware of several important considerations. They should never have sex when drunk or exhausted. Any sort of irritation or tension, such as great anger, would constitute an unfavorable condition for conception.

Alcohol and other chemicals are harmful to the blood. These substances have an adverse effect on both the semen and the egg, and in turn on the fetus, which can lead to natal diseases. Exhaustion, especially due to intercourse, lowers one's immunity and harms the health of both partners. Any sort of drastic changes in emotion should be avoided as they will act unfavorably on fetal development.

Hamilton Rotte This formula contains a balance between tonifying and moving herbs, but favors more moving, heat-clearing, and detoxifying herbs. Liver blood and kidney essence deficiency and both prominent and well-known causes of infertility and more excess conditions are often overlooked.

An interesting theme in this formula is the presence of "exterior-releasing" herbs that tend to move energy upward. A thorough evaluation of the materia medica reveals that exterior-releasing substances seem to bring energy upward in the body's effort to bring energy to the exterior (consider, *ge gen*, *chai hu*, and

qiang huo, common additions in formulas to preserve a fetus). Here we see chuan xiong and jing jie that serve this purpose.
According to Ding Gan Ren, mu xiang calms a restless fetus, making it an ideal qi-regulating ingredient before and during pregnancy.
We have to consider whether Dr. Shen viewed mai ya and gu ya as tonics as they frequently appear in formulas for the digestion that are generally tonifying in nature. Utilizing herbs that dissolve food stagnation, especially those of a mild nature, are a means of strengthening the digestive system in order to unburden the spleen and stomach.
Formulas that are more strongly tonifying should also certainly be considered for the treatment of infertility.

Leon Hammer According to Dr. Shen, the gender of the child is decided upon at the instant of the climax. When the woman's climax comes first, the child will be a boy, when the man's climax comes before that of the woman it will be a girl.

Painful Periods

Hamilton Rotte Dr. Shen stated the following with regard to the menstrual cycle.

Intervals:
- Short cycles: liver-kidney *yin* deficiency
- Long cycle: kidney *yang* essence deficiency
- Skip periods: liver *qi* stagnation
- Period starts and stops: blood stagnation

Length of period:
- Prolonged period:
  - Light flow and pale blood: kidney *yang* essence deficiency
  - Heavy flow and bright red blood: heat in the blood
  - Heavy flow with purple clots: blood stagnation

Pain:
- Before period: liver *qi* stagnation
- During period: blood stagnation
- After period: kidney *yang* essence deficiency

Pain after Period

FROM DR. SHEN: This condition comes from a weakened uterus. Weakness comes from a combination of body condition and lifestyle. After the period, an aching sensation will occur as the uterus closes.

Pin Yin	Latin	English	Dosage
Dang gui	Angelicae Sinensis Radix	Chinese angelica root, *tang-kuei*	6 g
Gan jiang	Zingiberis Rhizoma	Dried ginger	4.5 g
Niu xi or huai niu xi	Achyranthis Bidentatae Radix	Ox-knee root from Huai	9 g
Long gu	Fossilia Ossis Mastodi	Dragon bone, fossilized vertebrae and bones of the extremities (usually of mammals)	12 g
Bai shao	Paeoniae Alba Radix	White peony root	6 g
Yan hu suo	Corydalis Yanhusuo Rhizoma	Corydalis rhizome	9 g
Tu si zi	Cuscutae Chinensis Semen	Chinese dodder seeds, cuscuta	9 g
Huang qin	Scutellariae Baicalensis Radix	Baical skullcap root, scutellaria, scute	3 g
Nu zhen zi	Ligustri Lucidi Fructus	Privet fruit, ligustrum	9 g

Hamilton Rotte Pain after periods occurs because of deficiency of the liver blood or kidneys. This formula contains *dang gui* and *bai shao* in order to tonify liver blood. The following herbs are kidney tonics, addressing both *yin* and *yang* deficiency: *niu xi*, *tu si zi*, and *niu zhen zi*. *Yan hu suo*, *niu xi*, and possibly *gan jiang* are included because of their pain-relieving effects.

In addition, we find many consolidating and stabilizing herbs in this formula. *Tu si zi*, *bai shao*, and *long gu* are stabilizing, and *huang qin* may be included to exert a similar effect, and it is known to calm a restless fetus. It is notable that there are no widely known formulas for pain from deficiency in standard texts.

Pain before Period

FROM DR. SHEN: In this condition, pain comes 3 or 4 days before the period. If the body is weak, the increased menstrual circulation hurts the body.

Pin Yin	Latin	English	Dosage
Dang shen	Codonopsis Pilosulae Radix	Codonopsis root	6 g
Fu ling	Poria Cocos Sclerotium	Sclerotium of tuckahoe, poria, China root, hoelen, Indian bread	9 g
Hong hua	Carthami Tinctorii Flos	Safflower flower, carthamus	6 g
Niu xi or *huai niu xi*	Achyranthis Bidentatae Radix	Ox-knee root from Huai	9 g
Dang gui	Angelicae Sinensis Radix	Chinese angelica root, *tang-kuei*	6 g
Yuan zhi	Polygalae Radix	Chinese senega root, polygala root	6 g
Yan hu suo	Corydalis Yanhusuo Rhizoma	Corydalis rhizome	9 g
Ze lan	Lycopi Herba	Lycopos, bugleweed leaf	6 g
Bai shao	Paeoniae Alba Radix	White peony root	6 g
Yi mu cao	Leonuri Herba	Chinese motherwort, leonurus	6 g
Lu lu tong	Liquidambaris Fructus	Sweetgum fruit, liquidambar fruit	12 g

Hamilton Rotte Pain that occurs before periods is mostly due to excess conditions, primarily stagnation of *qi* and blood. The blood-moving ingredients in this formula include *hong hua*, *niu xi*, *dang gui*, *yan hu suo*, and *ze lan*. As usual it is important to include blood tonics when utilizing blood-moving herbs. The blood tonics include *dang gui* and *bai shao*. *Qi*-moving ingredients in this formula include *yuan zhi* and *lu lu tong*. The presence of *yuan zhi* is admittedly somewhat mysterious because it does not target the liver or the uterus.

Also there is the suggestion that this condition can also involve *qi* deficiency. This is evidenced by the inclusion of *dang shen* and *fu ling*. This is a slightly unconventional approach, though it suggests that *qi* tonics should be included when using *qi* or blood-moving herbs.

Leon Hammer The liver stores the blood and is responsible for supplying blood to muscles, ligaments, tendons, and peripheral nerves as well as supplying it to other organs, especially the heart. The liver is also known to initiate the menstrual cycle when it begins to move stored blood out of the uterus.
The liver is also the master of *qi* both for moving *qi*, as well as containing it, and, as explained in DRRBF, it

also controls the direction of *qi*. The liver recovers the *qi* and is known as the "second wind," when at the end of the day one is tired (around 4 p.m.) and experiences a resurgence of energy. It is my contention that the exigencies of this premenstrual period are primarily a function of the integrity of liver *qi*.
The premenstrual period is associated with mental-emotional turmoil. Premenstrual symptoms include

tension, anxiety, irritability, crying, mood swings, parietal headaches, abdominal bloating and cramps, breast tenderness, insomnia, joint and/or muscle pain, fatigue, acne, and eye problems. Pain in Chinese medicine is due to stagnation of substances. Pain before the period as well as during is due to the inability of liver *qi* to move the blood from the uterus. While most of the preceding symptoms have been attributed to stagnation of liver *qi*, the issue raised here is what is causing this stagnation. The principal liver problem in Chinese medicine in our time is liver *qi-yang* deficiency and not liver stagnation due to excess (Hammer, 2009). It is my contention that the stagnation, in our time, is more often due the deficiency of liver *qi* to move the *qi* than the inhibition of that movement due to repression of liver *qi*. Liver *qi*, as with the *qi* in any organ will determine the viability of all of its other functions. Even the capacity to stagnate *qi* or store the blood and liver blood deficiency depends upon the strength of liver *qi*.

The process of beginning to move blood out the uterus in the premenstrual phase of the cycle supersedes all other liver function at that time. From nature's point of view, the perpetuation of the species is paramount, and depends on the integrity of liver *qi*. If that *qi* is deficient, blood does not move sufficiently out of the uterus as well as to all of the other areas that depend on liver blood. Let us examine premenstrual symptoms from that perspective.

With regard to the emotional issues listed above, most of which I believe occur or are exacerbated at this time due to deficient liver *qi* being so drained by its work of beginning to move blood out of the uterus, that it is unable to serve one of its main functions of containment of emotion and their appropriate expression through the medium of heart *qi* and blood. When liver *qi* is unable to move *qi* and blood in the heart the ensuing stagnation requires heat to move the resulting stagnation and fluid to balance the heat. The result is an increase in "phlegm misting the orifices" and consequential emotional instability associated with this condition accounting for the presence of *yuan qi* in the above formula. The presence of a phlegm-moving herb (*fu ling*) in this formula is in concordance with my clinical experience that much emotional turmoil is due to "phlegm misting the orifices" of the heart that I always treat with orifice-opening herbs including acorus (*shi chang pu*) and senega root (*yuan zhi*).

Blood stagnation in the uterus and associated pain is again the result of the reduced ability of deficient liver to move the blood out of the uterus, leading to blood clots and dysmenorrhea.

Pain during Period

FROM DR. SHEN: This pain comes from cold in the uterus. This cold develops from drinking too much cold water, which stagnates the blood and *qi*. This pain can also come from tumors or fibroids.

Pin Yin	Latin	English	Dosage
Dang gui	Angelicae Sinensis Radix	Chinese angelica root, *tang-kuei*	6 g
Gan cao	Glycyrrhizae Radix	Licorice root	4.5 g
Chi shao	Paeoniae Rubra Radix	Red peony root	6 g
Sha ren	Amomi Fructus	Cardamom	4.5 g
Shu di huang	Rehmanniae Preparata Radix	Prepared Chinese foxglove root (cooked in red wine), cooked rehmannia rhizome	9 g
Dan shen	Salviae Miltiorrhiziae Radix	Salvia root	6 g
Mu xiang	Saussureae Lappae Radix or Aucklandia Lappae Radix	Costus root, saussurea, aucklandia	6 g
Sheng di huang	Rehmannia Radix	Fresh Chinese foxglove root, rehmannia root	9 g
Ze lan	Lycopi Herba	Lycopos, bugleweed leaf	6 g
Wang bu liu xing	Vaccariae Segetalis Semen	Vaccaria seeds	6 g

Hamilton Rotte   Pain during the period occurs because of *qi* and blood stagnation. This formula contains *qi* and blood-invigorating herbs, as well as herbs that tonify the blood. Warming herbs in this formula include *dang gui, mu xaing, sha ren,* and *ze lan.*
The herbs that tonify the blood include *dang gui, chi shao, dan shen, ze lan,* and *wang bu liu xing.*
This formula contains many blood tonic herbs as well, including *dang gui* and *shu di huang. Sheng di huang* is sometimes used as a blood tonic. Blood tonics are advisable when utilizing blood-moving herbs to prevent damage to the blood.
Sha ren and *mu xiang* are included to aid in the digestion of the blood tonics, which can be hard to digest. *Sha ren* is commonly combined with *shu di huang* for this purpose.

Leon Hammer   I have also observed this condition in women who swim in very cold water (see "Dr. Shen's Life-cycle Formulas", p. 172).

Pain (Menstrual) for Just One Day

FROM DR. SHEN: This is a mild condition that develops when the body is just a little weak. Steep a slice of fresh peeled ginger and drink as a tea.

Hamilton Rotte   Dr. Shen has a slightly unusual view of fresh ginger, which is usually utilized to relieve exterior conditions or detoxify other herbs. The literature does not mention that it is indicated for menstrual pain. It is interesting to consider that *pao jiang,* a quick-fried prepared form of ginger is used to relieve pain and invigorate blood in the uterus (as it is utilized in the formula *Sheng Hua Tang* [Generating and Transforming Decoction]).

Painful Periods, Periods Not On Time, Endometriosis

FROM DR. SHEN: Endometriosis is always from a weak body condition. It can develop from birth control pills, not resting after surgery, working too much, or standing too long.

Pin Yin	Latin	English	Dosage
Dang gui	Angelicae Sinensis Radix	Chinese angelica root, *tang-kuei*	9 g
Shu di huang	Rehmanniae Preparata Radix	Prepared Chinese foxglove root (cooked in red wine), cooked rehmannia rhizome	9 g
Dan shen	Salviae Miltiorrhiziae Radix	Salvia root	9 g
Yi mu cao	Leonuri Herba	Chinese motherwort, leonurus	6 g
Tu si zi	Cuscutae Chinensis Semen	Chinese dodder seeds, cuscuta	12 g
Yan hu suo	Corydalis Yanhusuo Rhizoma	Corydalis rhizome	9 g
Bai shao	Paeoniae Alba Radix	White peony root	6 g
Mu xiang	Saussureae Lappae Radix or Aucklandia Lappae Radix	Costus root, saussurea, aucklandia	6 g

Hamilton Rotte This formula is indicated for blood stagnation in a liver blood- and kidney essence-deficient individual. Frequently, blood stagnation occurs in kidney deficiency because the kidneys govern all of the organs in the lower burner.

Herbs that move blood include *dan shen, yi mu cao,* and *yan hu suo. Yan hu suo* is particularly effective at relieving pain. *Mu xiang* is included as a *qi* regulator to assist in moving blood. It also has strong pain-relieving effects.

Herbs that tonify liver blood include *dang gui, bai shao,* and *shu di huang.*

Tu si zi nourishes both the *yin* and *yang* of the kidneys, and is a favorite of Dr. Shen's in treating deficiencies that lead to gynecological problems.

Leon Hammer As mentioned above, in my clinical experience "stagnation from deficiency" far exceeds "stagnation from excess" in our time when we now observe deficiency in younger and younger people.

Pregnancy ("Good for Pregnant Lady")

FROM DR. SHEN: During pregnancy:
- Keep a clean body
- No drugs or alcohol
- No emotional problems

After 3 months, a little sex; no sex after 5 months.

Taken after fifth month until delivery. Start by taking two to three times weekly and increase until delivery. Take daily toward end of pregnancy to make an easy delivery and healthy baby. This formula can also turn a baby when in the wrong position.

Pin Yin	Latin	English	Dosage
Dang gui	Angelicae Sinensis Radix	Chinese angelica root, *tang-kuei*	3 g
Bai zhu	Atractylodis Macrocephalae Rhizoma	White atractylodes rhizome	3 g
Chuan xiong	Chuanxiong Rhizoma	Chuanxiong root, Szechuan lovage root, cnidium	3 g
Hong hua	Carthami Tinctorii Flos	Safflower flower, carthamus	1.5 g
Tu si zi	Cuscutae Chinensis Semen	Chinese dodder seeds, cuscuta	4.5 g
Qiang huo	Notopterygii Rhizoma et Radix	Notopterygium root and rhizome, *chiang-huo*	3 g
Gan jiang	Zingiberis Rhizoma	Dried ginger	2.4 g
Huang qin	Scutellariae Baicalensis Radix	Baical skullcap root, scutellaria, scute	3 g
Ai ye	Artemisiae Argyi Folium	Mugwort leaf, artemesia	2.4 g
Bai shao	Paeoniae Alba Radix	White peony root	3 g
Jing jie	Schizonepetae Herba	Schizonepeta	3 g
Shan yao	Dioscoreae Oppositae Rhizoma	Chinese yam root, dioscorea rhizome	4.5 g

Hamilton Rotte The practice of taking herbs during pregnancy in order to promote a healthy baby is a common one in TCM. Commonly, *qi*, blood, and kidney tonic herbs are used, especially those that have a stabilizing function or those that "calm a restless fetus" to prevent miscarriage.

Here the tonics include *dang gui, bai zhu, tu si zi, bai shao,* and *shan yao. Tu si zi, bai shao,* and *shan yao* all have stabilizing effects.

Herbs within the formula that treat a restless fetus include *huang qin* and *ai ye.*

Also common among formulas that are administered during pregnancy are herbs that move upward. We find that many of the herbs that move upward are among the herbs that release the exterior. In this formula *qiang huo* and *jing jie* act in this way.

It is possible that *gan jiang* is included because it has an effect of stopping bleeding, especially uterine bleeding. However, the quick-fried version of the herb (*pao jiang*) is normally used for this purpose. Blood-invigorating substances are normally used with extreme caution during pregnancy. In this for-

mula, the blood-moving herbs (*chuan xiong* and *hong hua*) are used in very light dosages. Also, *chuang xiong* and *hong hua* have distinct upward-moving effects, making them suitable for use during pregnancy. These blood-invigorating herbs facilitate a smoother delivery (just as acupuncture points that have a moving effect also facilitate a smooth delivery).

Formula for induction of labor:

Pin Yin	Latin	English	Dosage
Dang gui	Angelicae Sinensis Radix	Chinese angelica root, *tang-kuei*	4.5 g
Chuan xiong	Chuanxiong Rhizoma	Chuanxiong root, Szechuan lovage root, cnidium	3 g
Hong hua	Carthami Tinctorii Flos	Safflower flower, carthamus	3 g
Tu si zi	Cuscutae Chinensis Semen	Chinese dodder seeds, cuscuta	3 g
Hou po	Magnoliae officinalis Cortex	Magnolia bark	1.8 g
Qiang huo	Notopterygii Rhizoma et Radix	Notopterygium root and rhizome, *chiang-huo*	4.5 g
Gan jiang	Zingiberis Rhizoma	Dried ginger	3 g
Huang qin	Scutellariae Baicalensis Radix	Baical skullcap root, scutellaria, scute	3 g
Bai shao	Paeoniae Alba Radix	White peony root	4.5 g
Bai zhu	Atractylodis Macrocephalae Rhizoma	White atractylodes rhizome	4.5 g
Yi mu cao	Leonuri Herba	Chinese motherwort, leonurus	4.5 g
Sheng di huang	Rehmanniae Radix	Fresh Chinese foxglove root, fresh rehmannia root	4.5 g
Ai ye	Artemisiae Argyi Folium	Mugwort leaf, artemesia	3 g

Hamilton Rotte This formula, described in Giovanni Maciocia's book *Obstetrics and Gynecology in Chinese Medicine* (1997), is related to the "Pregnancy" formula above. It is used to induce labor if it is delayed. Compared to the "Pregnancy" formula, it contains slightly higher dosages of some of the blood-invigorating ingredients. It also includes additional

moving herbs *hou po* (a *qi* regulator that has a marked descending effect) and *yi mu cao* (a blood-invigoration ingredient that focuses on the uterus).

Sheng di huang, an important addition to this formula, is described by Ding Gan Ren as "resolving stagnation" and "facilitating delivery."

Reactions in Pregnancy

FROM DR. SHEN: During the first 3 months of pregnancy the woman tends to vomit and can find taking food intolerable. Slippery and comparatively rapid pulses are felt in different degrees for different physiques. It is also possible that some women don't show these signs.

If a woman has very severe symptoms, drop several drops of ginger juice on her tongue and these signs will soon subside. If the ginger juice is not effective, then use the following formula.

Serious pregnancy reactions can be treated with the following formula:

Pin Yin	Latin	English	Dosage
Bai zhu	Atractylodis Macrocephalae Rhizoma	White atractylodes rhizome	4.5 g
Bai shao	Paeoniae Alba Radix	White peony root	4.5 g
Bai dou kou	Amomi Kravanh Fructus	Cardamom fruit/round seed	3 g
Chen pi	Citri Reticulatae Pericarpium	Tangerine peel	3 g
Zhu ru	Bambussae in Taeniis Caulis	Bamboo shavings	4.5 g
Gu ya	Oryzae Germinatus Fructus	Rice sprout	9 g
Ban xia	Rhizoma Pinelliae	Pinellia rhizome	4.5 g
Sheng jiang	Zingiberis Officinalis Recens Rhizoma	Fresh ginger rhizome	3 slices

Hamilton Rotte This formula is a modification of *Wen Dan Tang* (Warm the Gallbladder Decoction), a famous formula for treating nausea and vomiting in an individual who has a damp condition. Dr. Shen suggested that it is especially indicated for women who have a slippery pulse.

Herbs that dry dampness include *bai zhu*, *bai dou kou*, *chen pi*, *zhu ru*, and *zhi ban xia*. The herbs that descend stomach *qi* include *zhi ban xia*, *zhu ru*, *sheng jiang*, *chen pi*, and *bai dou kou*.

Gu ya mildly tonifies the spleen and resolves food stagnation.

Bai shao is included possibly because it strongly relieves stomach pain and offsets the drying tendencies of the other herbs in the formula. Dr. Shen included *bai shao* in many of his formulas for digestive difficulties.

This modification of *Wen Dan Tang* is closer to neutral in temperature compared to the original with the addition of *bai dou kou*, which warms the middle burner.

Uterine Bleeding from Fibroids

FROM DR. SHEN: Why uterus problem?
- Period comes and goes because uterus moves
- Life no good causes *qi* stagnation
- Working too much
- Emotions cause *qi* stagnation
- Water metabolism no good

In uterus problems: for 1 week before period, during, and 1 week after period don't work too hard, no cold drinks, no sex. Sex makes uterus open and often causes excessive uterine bleeding.

Fibroids weaken the uterus and keep it from functioning properly.

Pin Yin	Latin	English	Dosage
Dang gui	Angelicae Sinensis Radix	Chinese angelica root, *tang-kuei*	6 g
Dan shen	Salviae Miltiorrhiziae Radix	Salvia root	6 g
Yan hu suo	Corydalis Yanhusuo Rhizoma	Corydalis rhizome	9 g
Shu di huang	Rehmanniae Preparata Radix	Prepared Chinese foxglove root (cooked in red wine), cooked rehmannia rhizome	6 g
Ai ye	Artemisiae Argyi Folium	Mugwort leaf, artemesia	3 g

Pin Yin	Latin	English	Dosage
E zhu	Curcumae Rhizoma	Zedoary rhizoma, zedoaria	2.4 g
Bai shao	Paeoniae Alba Radix	White peony root	6 g
Tu si zi	Cuscutae Chinensis Semen	Chinese dodder seeds, cuscuta	9 g
Nu zhen zi	Ligustri Lucidi Fructus	Privet fruit, ligustrum	9 g

Hamilton Rotte   Dr. Shen frequently referred to a "weak uterus" as a cause of uterine bleeding. In the formulas that address this condition, he utilized kidney tonics and liver blood tonics, especially those that are stabilizing (astringent). This formula contains liver blood tonics (*dang gui, shu di huang*, and *bai shao*) and kidney tonics (*shu di huang, tu si zi*, and *nu zhen zi*). *Tu si zi* is a stabilizing herb, which has an indirect effect on stopping bleeding. *Ai ye*, a warming herb, has a direct effect on stopping bleeding.

A fibroid is a mass and therefore is a form of stagnation. This formula contains ingredients that move the blood (*dang gui, dan shen, yan hu suo*, and *e zhu*). *E zhu* also dissolves masses.

In this formula there is a balance between tonic and blood-moving herbs because the condition involves simultaneous deficiency and stagnation. Both deficiency and stagnation need to be addressed without going too far in either direction.

Uterine Bleeding from Sex During Period

FROM DR. SHEN: Sex stimulates the uterus. Because the uterus is already working hard during the period, sex puts too much pressure on it and keeps it from closing properly.

Pin Yin	Latin	English	Dosage
Mai men dong	Ophiopogonis Radix	Ophiopogon tuber/root	9 g
Dang gui	Angelicae Sinensis Radix	Chinese angelica root, *tang-kuei*	6 g
Fu ling	Poria Cocos Sclerotium	Sclerotium of tuckahoe, poria, China root, hoelen, Indian bread	9 g
Dan shen	Salviae Miltiorrhiziae Radix	Salvia root	6 g
Bai shao	Paeoniae Alba Radix	White peony root	6 g
Yuan zhi	Polygalae Radix	Chinese senega root, polygala root	6 g
Yi mu cao	Leonuri Herba	Chinese motherwort, leonurus	6 g
Zi he che or tai pan	Placenta Hominis	Human placenta, placenta	9 g
Tu si zi	Cuscutae Chinensis Semen	Chinese dodder seeds, cuscuta	12 g
Mu li	Ostreae Concha	Oyster shell	9 g

Hamilton Rotte   This formula tonifies kidney *yang* essence and liver blood, moves blood and contains herbs that are astringent. Dr. Shen frequently associated excessive bleeding with deficient conditions of the uterus, related to kidney *yang* essence and liver blood deficiency. Kidney *yang* tonics include *zi he che* and *tu si zi*. Some sources indicate that *yuan zhi* is a kidney tonic. Liver blood tonics include *dang gui* and *bai shao*.

Dr. Shen may have viewed sex during the period as trauma, which causes blood stagnation. The herbs that move blood include *dang gui, dan shen*, and *yi mu cao*.

Herbs that are stabilizing (and intended to stop bleeding) include *tu si zi* and *mu li*. According to Ding Gan Ren, *mu li* treats excessive bleeding.

The reason for his inclusion of *mai men dong* is unclear.

Uterine Bleeding from Weak Body Condition

FROM DR. SHEN: In this case, the woman is constitutionally weak. When the period comes, sometimes, depending on the lifestyle, the uterus cannot close completely.

Pin Yin	Latin	English	Dosage
Gao li shen	Ginseng Coreensis Radix	Korean ginseng	24 g
Ren shen	Ginseng Radix	Ginseng root	3 g
Ge jie	Gekko Gecko Linnaeus	Gecko	3 g
Zi he che or tai pan	Placenta Hominis	Human placenta, placenta	9 g

Hamilton Rotte Bleeding can occur from excessive heat in the blood, blood stasis or *qi* deficiency. When bleeding occurs from *qi-yang* deficiency, herbs that directly stop bleeding become less relevant. This formula stops bleeding with tonic herbs. The uterus derives its energy from the kidneys. Kidney *yang* tonics include *ge jie* and *zi he che*. This formula also contains two types of ginseng, which are effective for stopping bleeding due to deficiency. *Ge jie* and *zi he che* are blood tonics and address blood deficiency that results from excessive bleeding.

Leon Hammer A Dr. Shen formula with the same herbs, except for *ge jie*, has been used to boost *qi* and *yang* and recover energy especially when one is tired and has to perform. I have used it for 30 or more years to stay alert when I teach. It was my impression that except for *ge jie*, these herbs also tonify the heart.

Uterine Bleeding from Working Too Hard

FROM DR. SHEN:
- Too much work drains energy from the body that is already tired from the period.
- Use "Uterine Bleeding From Sex During Period" formula.

Uterine Fibroids from Tense Nervous System

Pin Yin	Latin	English	Dosage
Dang gui	Angelicae Sinensis Radix	Chinese angelica root, *tang-kuei*	6 g
Chuan xiong	Chuanxiong Rhizoma	Chuanxiong root, Szechuan lovage root, cnidium	4.5 g
Bai shao	Paeoniae Alba Radix	White peony root	6 g
Yi mu cao	Leonuri Herba	Chinese motherwort, leonurus	6 g
Dan shen	Salviae Miltiorrhizae Radix	Salvia root	6 g
Yan hu suo	Corydalis Yanhusuo Rhizoma	Corydalis rhizome	9 g
Niu xi or huai niu xi	Achyranthis Bidentatae Radix	Ox-knee root from Huai	9 g
E zhu	Curcumae Rhizoma	Zedoary rhizome, zedoaria	2.4 g
Mu xiang	Saussureae Lappae Radix or Aucklandia Lappae Radix	Costus root, saussurea, aucklandia	6 g
Lu lu tong	Liquidambaris Fructus	Sweetgum fruit, liquidambar fruit	9 g

Hamilton Rotte   This following formula is very similar in treatment principles and ingredients to the formula for uterine bleeding from fibroids on p. 84. This formula contains lu lu tong, a common ingredient in formulas for nervous tension. E zhu is included because it moves blood and is especially indicated for abdominal masses.

Formula for uterus weak, heavy bleeding (possibly but not necessarily tumor or endometriosis):

Pin Yin	Latin	English	Dosage
Dang gui	Angelicae Sinensis Radix	Chinese angelica root, tang-kuei	9 g
Shu di huang	Rehmanniae Preparata Radix	Prepared Chinese foxglove root (cooked in red wine), cooked rehmannia rhizome	9 g
Dan shen	Salviae Miltiorrhiziae Radix	Salvia root	9 g
Yi mu cao	Leonuri Herba	Chinese motherwort, leonurus	6 g
Tu si zi	Cuscutae Chinensis Semen	Chinese dodder seeds, cuscuta	12 g
Yan hu suo	Corydalis Yanhusuo Rhizoma	Corydalis rhizome	9 g
Nu zhen zi	Ligustri Lucidi Fructus	Privet fruit, ligustrum	9 g
San qi	Notoginseng Radix	Noto ginseng root, root of pseudo-ginseng	1.8 g
Xian he cao	Agrimoniae Herba	Hairy vein agrimony	12 g
Rou cong rong	Cistanches Herba	Cistanche, fleshy stem of the broomrape	9 g
Mu xiang	Saussureae Lappae Radix or Aucklandia Lappae Radix	Costus root, saussurea, aucklandia	6 g

Hamilton Rotte   Dr. Shen clearly related "weakness of the uterus" with deficiency of kidney yang and liver blood. This formula contains the following tonics for kidney yang: tu si zi and rou cong rong. Kidney yin tonics include shu di huang and nu zhen zi. When tonifying the kidneys, it is customary to include tonics for both yin and yang.

Liver blood tonics include dang gui and shu di huang. Rou cong rong is also a mild blood tonic.

Bleeding can also occur from stagnation of blood. This formula is indicated for tumors and endometriosis, both of which involve stagnation of blood. Blood-moving ingredients include yi mu cao, yan hu suo, dang gui, dan shen, and san qi.

We also find ingredients to stop bleeding, namely san qi and xian he cao. Yi mu cao is considered to "regulate the menses," and is an ideal blood-moving ingredient when heavy bleeding is also present.

Tu si zi, a stabilizing herb, is a favorite of Dr. Shen to treat excessive menstrual bleeding. Mu xiang, which is astringent, is indicated for diarrhea and may be included here because Dr. Shen utilized its astringent effects on the uterus as well.

Health Maintenance

Balance the Body

This makes "all nervous system relax":

Pin Yin	Latin	English	Dosage
Fang feng	Saposhnikoviae Radix	Ledebouriella root, saposhnikoviae root, siler	3 g
Qiang huo	Notopterygii Rhizoma et Radix	Notopterygium root and rhizome, chiang-huo	4.5 g
Xiang fu	Cyperi Rotundi Rhizoma	Nut grass rhizoma, cyperus	4.5 g
Chuan xiong	Chuanxiong Rhizoma	Chuanxiong root, Szechuan lovage root, cnidium	4.5 g
Yu jin	Curcumae Radix	Curcuma tuber	9 g
Chao huang qin	Scutellariae Baicalensis Radix	Fried baical skullcap root, scutellaria, scute	4.5 g
Bai dou kou	Amomi Kravanh Fructus	Cardamom fruit/round seed	4.5 g
Chao bai shao	Paeoniae Alba Radix	Dry-fried white peony root	6 g
Chao gu ya	Oryzae Germinatus Fructus	Fried rice sprout	12 g
Chao mai ya	Hordei Germinatus Fructus	Fried barley sprout	12 g
Chuan lian zi	Meliae Toosendan Fructus	Szechuan pagoda tree fruit, Szechuan chinaberry, melia	9 g

Hamilton Rotte One of the ways that herbs can be utilized is to preserve health in the absence of disease or symptoms. This formula was presented by Dr. Shen as a means to accomplish this.

The suggestion is that this formula is suitable for an individual who tends toward nervous tension. Many of the herbs in this formula are included in his formulas for a "nervous system tense" individual, including, xiang fu, chuang xiong, yu jin, huang qin, and bai shao. This formula contains herbs that target the various tissues: fang feng for the skin, qiang huo for the muscles, xiang fu for the qi, chuan xiong for the blood, bai shao for the muscles, huang qin and yu jin for the liver, gu ya and mai ya for the digestive system.

Leon Hammer It is my experience and contention that liver blood nourishes muscles (and peripheral nerves) as well as ligaments and tendons, hence, the use in this formula of bai shao. In the textbooks control of the muscles is attributed to the spleen. I find instead that the spleen controls connective tissue where excess fluid is stored when the spleen is unable to "digest" water.

Clear Stagnant *Qi*, Damp and Food

FROM DR. SHEN: Even if there is no problem, you can take these herbs for 3 to 4 days out of every month, or even more frequently. These herbs are safe.

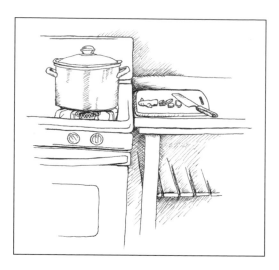

Fig. 7   Preparing a ginger bath. Cooking the ginger.

Sun Heat

Pin Yin	Latin	English	Dosage
Pei lan	Eupatorii Herba	Eupatorium	9 g
He ye	Nelumbinis Folium	Lotus leaf	1 corner
Sheng yi yi ren	Coicis Semen	Fresh seeds of Job's tears, fresh coix seeds	12 g
Sheng gan cao	Glycyrrhizae Radix	Fresh licorice root	3 g
Gu ya	Oryzae Germinatus Fructus	Rice sprout	12 g
Mai ya	Hordei Germinatus Fructus	Barley sprout, malt	12 g

Hamilton Rotte   This formula is indicated for excessive exposure to heat from the sun, especially in the presence of humidity. *Pei lan* and *he ye* treat summer heat (with dampness). Heat and dampness often affect the middle burner, as the spleen loathes dampness. *Ma ya* and *gu ya* are included to treat excess in the middle burner. Exterior heat and dampness also frequently affect the bladder and this is addressed with *yi yi ren*.

Hematologic Conditions

Blood Deficiency

FROM DR. SHEN: There are two causes of anemia from a Chinese medical perspective. First, poor early life nourishment or upbringing resulting in the ineffective functioning of the internal organs leads to insufficiency of blood that arises either from the circulation or supplying mechanism. The second cause is an adult life that is consumed by overwork. This wears down the blood circulation system, resulting in anemia. In Chinese medicine, anemia can be improved by supplying the patient with enough "*qi*" to pump up the circulation system. Preventive measures must also be taken, such as sufficient rest and agreeable nourishment to fortify one's body condition.

Formula for anemia:

Pin Yin	Latin	English	Dosage
Huang qi	Astragali Radix	Milk vetch root, astragalus root	30 g
Dang gui	Angelicae Sinensis Radix	Chinese angelica root, *tang-kuei*	15 g
Da zao	Zizyphi Jujubae Fructus	Chinese date, jujube	5 g
Ji xiong pu	Gallus	Skinless chicken breast	2 pieces

FROM DR. SHEN: Put the medicines in a Yunnan steam pot and steam for 4 to 5 hours; eat one or two bowls of the soup a day two to three times a week to effectively promote the circulation of blood. If the case is serious consume each day. For gestational blood deficiency, add three kinds of livers to the soup.

Hamilton Rotte This formula is designed to treat blood deficiency (see **Fig. 8a, b** for how blood deficiency manifests in the eyes). *Huang qi* and *dang gui* are a widely utilized two-herb combination. *Huang qi* tonifies *qi* to produce blood. Its ability to do so is greatly accentuated when it is combined with *dang gui*, a blood tonic. *Da zao*, a blood tonic, is a food-level herb, also highly regarded for its ability to make formulas and food remedies more palatable.

San qi is included to move the blood, making blood tonic herbs more effective. Since blood does not have its own volition to move, utilizing moving herbs aids in tonifying blood.

Chicken, especially the dark meat, is an effective dietary remedy for blood deficiency. Cooking tonics with food over a long period of time enhances their effectiveness.

Leon Hammer Yunnan steam pot cooking with herbs and chicken and drinking the distillate in the upper part of the pot along with the chicken was one of Dr. Shen's favorite ways to deliver the herbs for chronic conditions.

With regard to blood each organ plays a part:
• A global blood deficiency will create blood deficiency in all organs and tissues.

• Specific blood deficiencies:
  – Kidney: kidney blood deficiency is associated with the ability of the kidney to support the marrow where half of the blood is produced.
  – Liver: liver blood deficiency is associated with its ability to store the blood and deliver it to the tendons, ligaments, muscles, and peripheral nerves. It also detoxifies the blood.

– Heart: heart blood deficiency is associated with the ability of heart *qi* to circulate blood through the heart (coronary arteries) and the brain.
– Spleen: the spleen contributes to the formation of blood to the entire organism and spleen *qi* deficiency reduces its ability to provide blood.

– Lungs: the lungs contribute *qi* (oxygen) to the formation of blood when *zong qi* combines with *gu qi* (from spleen) and body fluids to form blood and eliminates CO_2.
• Psychological: blood is emotion and gives us meaning and purpose in life.

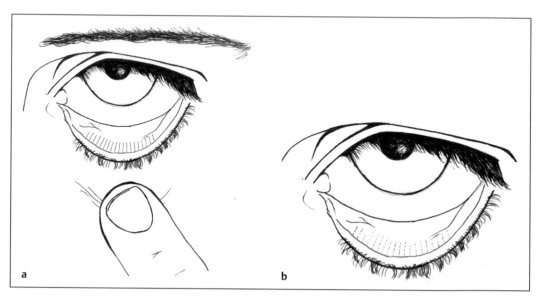

Fig. 8a, b
a Normal: arteries appear as uniform, thin, red, straight lines.
b Blood deficiency: artery lines appear pale and faded.

Blood Unclear

Pin Yin	Latin	English	Dosage
Dang gui	Angelicae Sinensis Radix	Chinese angelica root, *tang-kuei*	6 g
Sheng di huang	Rehmanniae Radix	Fresh Chinese foxglove root, rehmannia root	9 g
Chi shao	Paeoniae Rubra Radix	Red peony root	9 g
Gan cao	Glycyrrhizae Radix	Licorice root	4.5 g
Xia ku cao	Prunellae Spica Vulgaris	Self-heal spike, prunella	9 g
Yi yi ren	Coicis Semen	Seeds of Job's tears, coix seeds	12 g
Mu dan pi	Moutan Radicis Cortex	Tree peony root bark, moutan root bark	6 g
Luo han guo	Momordicae Fructus	Grosvenor momordica fruit	9 g
Ze xie	Alismatis Rhizoma	Water plantain rhizome, alisma rhizome	9 g

Hamilton Rotte "Blood unclear" is a pulse quality that indicates the presence of inhaled toxins. The pulse is also deep and a very slow rate is a pulse quality associated with the accumulation of chemical toxins in the blood.

To address this situation we must cool and move the blood in order to release the toxins from the blood. We then use herbs that promote urination to discharge the toxins from the body.

Herbs that cool the blood include *sheng di*, *chi shao*, *xia ku cao*, and *mu dan pi*. Some sources also indicate that *luo han guo* cools the blood. Herbs that move the blood include *dang gui*, *chi shao*, and *mu dan pi*. *Yi yi ren* and *ze xie* promote urination to discharge the toxins. *Luo han guo* targets the lungs and may address the common situation where toxicity enters the body through inhalation.

Leon Hammer This is Dr. Shen's term for a condition in which the blood depth just barely increases (rather than normally decreases) in size as one raises the finger from the organ depth toward the *qi* depth. Occasionally the pulse is also slightly slippery. There is no equivalent term in TCM. The most common cause of this quality is exposure to environmental toxins. I first encountered it with artists using highly toxic solvents, often in poorly ventilated rooms, and with the use of acetylene torches, both in art and industry (welders).

Skin symptoms (eczema, psoriasis) are one obvious way that the body attempts to discharge that toxicity. Another common symptom is fatigue. Dr. Shen likens this condition to a glass of water in which dirt is suspended: the quality of the blood is not good. A related origin is a stagnant or deficient liver that does not properly detoxify. In addition to storing the blood itself, the liver also stores the blood toxins that are not metabolized by the liver. These toxins contaminate the blood and ultimately the entire organism that it nourishes. (See also **Fig. 9a, b** for manifestation of toxicity in the eyes.)

Another cause of this pattern is a *qi*-deficient spleen that does not build the blood well due to poor absorption and digestion of food, especially protein. The protein is only partially digested into short-chain polypeptides the size of viruses, instead of being completely digested down to amino acids. The short-chain polypeptides are absorbed and the body reacts to them as if they were viruses by inappropriately mobilizing the immune system. Eventually, autoimmune diseases develop.

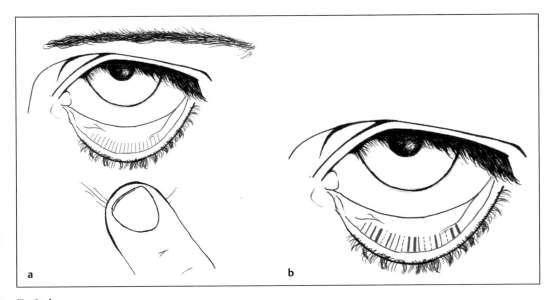

Fig. 9a, b
a Normal: arteries appear as uniform, thin, red, straight lines.
b Toxicity: artery lines are irregular varying in thickness and color.

Blood Heat

Pin Yin	Latin	English	Dosage
Dang gui	Angelicae Sinensis Radix	Chinese angelica root, tang-kuei	6 g
Sheng di huang	Rehmanniae Radix	Fresh Chinese foxglove root, rehmannia root	9 g
Chi shao	Paeoniae Rubra Radix	Red peony root	9 g
Gan cao	Glycyrrhizae Radix	Licorice root	4.5 g
Xia ku cao	Prunellae Spica Vulgaris	Self-heal spike, prunella	9 g
Mu dan pi	Moutan Radicis Cortex	Tree peony root bark, moutan root bark	6 g
Luo han guo	Momordicae Fructus	Grosvenor momordica fruit	9 g
Ze xie	Alismatis Rhizoma	Water plantain rhizome, alisma rhizome	9 g
Shan dou gen	Menispermi Rhizoma/Sophorae Tonkinensis Radix	Bushy sophora	9 g

Hamilton Rotte Blood heat develops because of heat from one of the organs in the body, often the liver or stomach or the transmission of an external pathogen into the blood. This excess heat also causes stagnation of the blood. In this formula the following ingredients cool the blood: *sheng di*, *chi shao*, *xia ku cao*, *mu dan pi*, and, according to some sources, *luo han guo*. *Dang gui*, *chi shao*, and *mu dan pi* move the blood. Blood heat is frequently discharged through the urine. A standard formula, *Long Dan Xie Gan Tang* (Gentiana Decoction to Drain the Liver) also utilizes this approach.

Shan dou gen may be included in the blood heat formula because of its ability to address skin conditions, common symptoms of a blood heat condition.

This formula contains many cold substances and should be used with great caution in *qi*-deficient conditions. (See **Fig. 10a, b** for manifestation of excess heat in the eyes.)

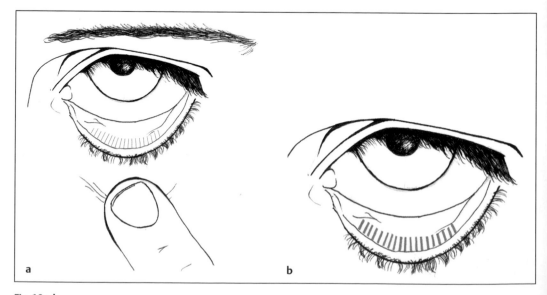

Fig. 10a, b
a　Normal: arteries appear as uniform, thin, red, straight lines.
b　Excess heat: artery lines appear dark red and thickened.

Leon Hammer As one lifts one's finger from the organ depth the pulse expands even more in the blood depth than is the case with "blood unclear." This is a sign of excess heat in the blood. Often the blood depth is also slippery. (According to Dr. Shen, "blood heat" without slipperiness is due to overworking the nervous system, while "blood heat" with slipperiness is associated with inadequate digestion and metabolism of lipids. I equate the slipperiness with turbulence in the blood.) Dr. Shen likens this pattern to a glass containing hot water, in contrast to one containing dirty water, his metaphor for the "blood unclear" condition.

Two patterns can give rise to this pulse, often simultaneously. The first pattern, increasingly common in our time, is one of excess heat that is associated with an extremely tense nervous system ("nervous system tense"), one working beyond its capacity. Over a very long period of time the accumulated heat can lead to a hypertensive condition if the body cannot eliminate the heat. Ultimately, kidney *yin* depletion ensues in the organism's attempt to balance the heat with fluid.

The second is excess heat associated with such foods as spices, wine, shellfish, coffee, chocolate, and other heat-inducing items. The organs that are directly affected are the liver and stomach and secondarily the heart and lungs.

Blood Thick

Pin Yin	Latin	English	Dosage
Dang gui	Angelicae Sinensis Radix	Chinese angelica root, *tang-kuei*	6 g
Sheng di huang	Rehmanniae Radix	Fresh Chinese foxglove root, rehmannia root	9 g
Chi shao	Paeoniae Rubra Radix	Red peony root	9 g
Gan cao	Glycyrrhizae Radix	Licorice root	4.5 g
Xia ku cao	Prunellae Spica Vulgaris	Self-heal spike, prunella	9 g
Mu dan pi	Moutan Radicis Cortex	Tree peony root bark, moutan root bark	6 g
Luo han guo	Momordicae Fructus	Grosvenor momordica fruit	9 g
Dan shen	Salviae Miltiorrhiziae Radix	Salvia root	6 g
Hong hua	Carthami Tinctorii Flos	Safflower flower, carthamus	4.5 g

Hamilton Rotte The "blood thick" condition is marked by heat and turbidity of the blood. In this case the primary concern is to cool and move the blood. Herbs that cool and move the blood are the same as in "blood heat" and "blood unclear," but additional substances are included to move the blood: *dan shen* and *hong hua*.

Leon Hammer As one lifts one's finger from the organ depth the pulse expands at the blood depth and continues to expand to and at the *qi* depth. With this pattern the pulse has become extremely wide, often slippery and sometimes with rough vibration, indicating damage to the intima (wall) of the vessels. Biomedically we are in the realm of "inflammation." Later, it often develops into a tense hollow full-overflowing wave, a sign of the later stages of the "blood thick" process in that the heat in the blood has entered a dangerous phase associated with hypertension, cardiovascular disease, and stroke. Con-

comitantly, a ropy quality may appear, a sign of more severe damage to the walls of the vessels that we call arteriosclerosis and atherosclerosis. (According to Dr. Shen, an early sign of the "blood thick" condition can be persistent acne after adolescence.)

"Blood thick" has several etiologies and courses, often simultaneous. Again, in our time, the most important explained by "blood heat" is an overworking nervous system ("nervous system tense"). Another is a damp-heat condition involving heat from the liver (repressed emotions) interfering with efficient metabolism of fat and sugar, dampness from the gallbladder accumulating and balancing liver heat and the spleen's inability to digest both fat and sugar as well as fluids.

Excessive intake of fat and sugar is a stress on both systems, leading to elevated levels of serum glucose, cholesterol, and triglycerides. The pulse shows more slipperiness (phlegm and turbulence), especially where the dampness predominates. Excess heat associated with foods such as spices, wine, shellfish, coffee, chocolate, and other heat-inducing items are also factors.

Chemicals in the Blood

FROM DR. SHEN: Vertical lines under eyes, alternating light and dark brown. A darker brown color indicates a greater presence of toxins or chemicals in the blood. Depending on body condition, chemicals or toxins will stay longer.
Snake meat is good for chemicals in the blood. Snake skin is good for skin disease. Snake venom is good for cancer. Snake gallbladder is good for the eyes, and is not bitter.

Pin Yin	Latin	English	Dosage
Mu dan pi	Moutan Radicis Cortex	Tree peony root bark, moutan root bark	6 g
Ban zhi lian	Scutellariae Barbatae Herba	Barbat skullcap, scutellaria	9 g
Di gu pi	Lycii Radicis Cortex	Cortex of wolfberry root, lycium bark	9 g
Bai hua she she cao	Heydyotis Diffusae Herba	Heydyotis, oldenlandia	9 g
Yi yi ren	Coicis Semen	Seeds of Job's tears, coix seeds	12 g
Ze xie	Alismatis Rhizoma	Water plantain rhizome, alisma rhizome	9 g
Tong cao	Tetrapanacis Medulla	Rice paper plant pith, tetrapanax	4.5 g
Mu tong	Akebiae Caulis	Akebia caulis	3 g

Hamilton Rotte   The alternating light and dark colors under the eyes mentioned by Dr. Shen are specific to toxicity when it is causing joint pain. This formula utilizes cold herbs that especially target the liver in order to remove toxins: *mu dan pi* and *ban zhi lian, di gu pi* and *bai hua she she cao*. It may also be significant that *mu dan pi* and *ban zhi lian* also invigorate the blood in order to help the drawing of toxins out of the body. Dr. Shen's blood unclear formula, which is also detoxifying, also contains many blood-moving substances. *Di gu pi* is an herb that enters the lung, liver, and kidney channels and it may be significant that it has a distinct downward-moving action, which may aid in eliminating toxins.

The second set of herbs are also heat-clearing herbs that promote urination. These herbs aid the body in excreting the toxins from the body, an essential aspect of any detoxification protocol. In this formula, *bai hua she she cao, yi yi ren, tong cao,* and *mu tong* all promote urination. Interestingly, we can see a precedent for utilizing herbs that promote urination in order to aid the body in discharging liver heat in formulas such as *Long Dan Xie Gan Tang* (Gentiana Decoction to Drain the Liver).

This formula, like others that address chemical toxicity, is draining and cooling and would not be well tolerated by the highly *qi*-deficient individual. For the treatment of toxicity, Dr. Shen also used a combination of the bitter and cold Western herb goldenseal with licorice (*gan cao*). The dosage is 4 g of goldenseal and 1 g of licorice. He considered this treatment to be extremely effective.

Leon Hammer
Etiology, Signs, and Symptoms:
Today we are inundated with all forms of toxicity, chemicals, airborne toxins, toxins in food, water, fabrics and medications, and radiation from electromagnetic field devices. There are said to be objects in our blood, primarily short-chain hydrocarbons, that did not exist in blood prior to 1950 and are products produced from oil.

As mentioned above, my initial experience with toxicity was in the 1970s with artists who were using solvents in poorly ventilated spaces. The principal complaint was extreme fatigue.

Pulse:
- Fl:
  - Deep; very slow
  - Blood depth: unclear

Tongue:
Very thick brown or black and dry

Gulf War Syndrome, denied for so long by the military, exploded in our clinic in the form of patients with extreme fatigue, headaches, dizziness, loss of memory and concentration, joint pains, and muscle weakness among other symptoms. Ascribed now to pyridostigmine bromide, organophosphate pesticides, and depleted uranium (used in shells) we found the following then and increasingly so now in most patients to one extent or another.

Choppy, a pulse sign of blood stagnation, once rare is now common. Puzzled by this finding, investigation showed that many poisonous snake bites that are not neurotoxic kill by coagulating blood.

Pulse:
- Fl:
  - LMP; blood depth; organ depth (organ *qi*, blood, substance): very choppy

Tongue:
Purple

Eyes:
- Blood vessels inside lower eyelids alternating dark and light
- Alternating brighter and darker lines in the lower eyelid was associated with what Dr. Shen claimed was a new type of arthritis due to toxins—he was very excited by this finding (**Fig. 11a, b**)

Reframed in other Chinese medical terms, Dr. Shen found an additional sign indicating what has been described as a "retained pathogen" diverted from vital organs by the divergent channels to parts of the body such as joints where they are not an immediate threat to life.

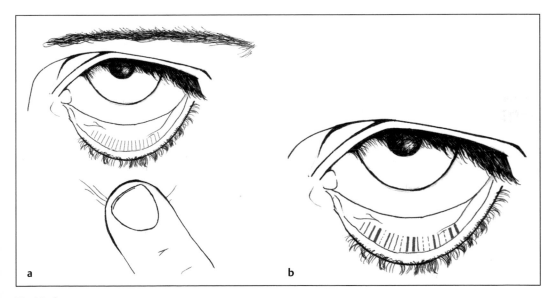

Fig. 11a, b
a Normal: arteries appear as uniform, thin, red, straight lines.
b Toxicity: artery lines are irregular varying in thickness and color.

Poison

Pin Yin	Latin	English	Dosage
Jin yin hua	Lonicerae Flos	Honeysuckle flower, lonicera	15 g
Sheng gan cao	Glycyrrhizae Radix	Fresh licorice root	4.5 g

Hamilton Rotte   It was not specified in Dr. Shen's records which type of poison this formula was intended to treat, but this may be considered in cases of toxic exposure. Both ingredients are known to clear heat and toxicity.

Hepatic and Biliary Tract Conditions

Cirrhosis

Pin Yin	Latin	English	Dosage
Chai hu	Bupleuri Radix	Hare's ear root, thorowax root, bupleurum	3 g
Chuan xiong	Chuanxiong Rhizoma	Chuanxiong root, Szechuan lovage root, cnidium	4.5 g
Chao bai shao	Paeoniae Alba Radix	Dry-fried white peony root	6 g
Chao huang qin	Scutellariae Baicalensis Radix	Fried baical skullcap root, scutellaria, scute	4.5 g
Fu ling	Poria Cocos Sclerotium	Sclerotium of tuckahoe, poria, China root, hoelen, Indian bread	9 g
Mu xiang	Saussureae Lappae Radix or Aucklandia Lappae Radix	Costus root, saussurea, aucklandia	4.5 g
Yu jin	Curcumae Radix	Curcuma tuber	9 g
Yuan zhi	Polygalae Radix	Chinese senega root, polygala root	6 g
Chuan lian zi	Meliae Toosendan Fructus	Szechuan pagoda tree fruit, Szechuan chinaberry, melia	9 g
Yan hu suo	Corydalis Yanhusuo Rhizoma	Corydalis rhizome	9 g
Ji nei jin	Corneum Gigeriae Galli Endothelium	Chicken gizzard's inner lining	12 g
Wa leng zi	Arcae Concha	Cockle shell	15 g
Chao hei jing jie	Schizonepetae Herba	Fried, charred schizonepeta	4.5 g
Tan fang feng	Saposhnikoviae Radix	Charred ledebouriella root, saposhnikoviae root, siler	4.5 g

Hamilton Rotte   This formula contains herbs that move *qi* and blood and reduce masses. *Qi* movers include *chai hu, chuan xiong, mu xiang, yu jin, yuan zhi, chuan lia zi,* and *yan hu suo.* Blood movers include *chuan xiong, yu jin, yan hu suo, wa leng zi* and (according to Ding Gan Ren) *jing jie* and *huang qin.*
Fu ling is used to treat stagnation in the abdomen because it promotes urination and eliminates damp excess.

Bai shao is well known for its ability to "soften" the liver by tonifying liver blood and *yin. ji nei jin* reduces masses (as many herbs for food stagnation do). *Wa leng zi* is especially useful in treating masses because, in addition to moving blood, its salty property softens hardness.

Hepatitis C

Pin Yin	Latin	English	Dosage
Chai hu	Bupleuri Radix	Hare's ear root, thorowax root, bupleurum	3 g
Chuan xiong	Chuanxiong Rhizoma	Chuanxiong root, Szechuan lovage root, cnidium	4.5 g
Chao bai shao	Paeoniae Alba Radix	Dry-fried white peony root	6 g
Chao huang lian	Coptidis Rhizoma	Dry-fried coptis rhizome	1.8 g[a]
Mu xiang	Saussureae Lappae Radix or Aucklandia Lappae Radix	Costus root, saussurea, aucklandia	4.5 g
Yan hu suo	Corydalis Yanhusuo Rhizoma	Corydalis rhizome	9 g
Yu jin	Curcumae Radix	Curcuma tuber	12 g
Gou qi zi	Lycii Fructus	Chinese wolfberry, matrimony vine fruit, lycium fruit	12 g
Zhi ke	Citri Aurantii Fructus	Mature fruit of the bitter orange	4.5 g
Fo shou	Citri Sarcodactylis Fructus	Finger citron fruit, Buddha's hand	6 g

[a] 2.4 g if the left middle pulse is very "tense."

Hamilton Rotte   The TCM literature generally describes the following patterns in chronic hepatitis C infection. In the early stages there is liver *qi* stagnation, spleen–stomach disharmony, excess heat and phlegm. In later stages there is liver blood stasis and liver-kidney *yin* deficiency.

This formula is appropriate in the early stages of hepatitis. The following herbs regulate liver *qi* and constitute the primary focus of the formula: *chai hu*, *mu xiang*, *yu jin*, and *fo shou*. *Bai shao* interacts synergistically with *chai hu*, a combination originating from *Si Ni San* (Frigid Extremities Powder) and *Xiao Yao San* (Rambling Powder).

We also find herbs that move blood and affect the liver, suggesting that the process of *qi* stagnation has evolved into blood stasis. These include *chuan xiong* and *yan hu suo*.

Huang lian may be included to remove heat from the liver, though other herbs are frequently used for this purpose as well.

There is significant focus on the spleen and stomach, with *qi*-regulating and pain-relieving substances to address these organs. The herbs that target the spleen and stomach include *mu xiang*, *yan hu suo*, *zhi ke*, and *fo shou*.

Although this formula is primarily focused on moving and cooling the liver, the tendency of hepatitis to progress to *yin* deficiency is addressed with *gou qi zi*, one of the primary liver *yin* tonics in Chinese medicine.

Hepatitis C, Building the Liver

FROM DR. SHEN: After hepatitis C is "better," build liver energy. Take for 2 weeks then take a break (for 3 days to 1 week). Repeat this for 1 to 3 months, maybe longer.

Pin Yin	Latin	English	Dosage
Chao bai zhu	Atractylodis Macrocephalae Rhizoma	Fried white atractylodes rhizome	6 g
Chao bai shao	Paeoniae Alba Radix	Dry-fried white peony root	9 g
Shan yao	Dioscoreae Oppositae Rhizoma	Chinese yam root, dioscorea rhizome	12 g
Chao huang qin	Scutellariae Baicalensis Radix	Fried baical skullcap root, scutellaria, scute	4.5 g
Fu ling	Poria Cocos Sclerotium	Sclerotium of tuckahoe, poria, China root, hoelen, Indian bread	9 g
Yuan zhi	Polygalae Radix	Chinese senega root, polygala root	4.5 g
Shan zhu yu	Corni Officinalis Fructus	Asiatic Cornelian cherry fruit, cornus	9 g
Yu jin	Curcumae Radix	Curcuma tuber	9 g
Yan hu suo	Corydalis Yanhusuo Rhizoma	Corydalis rhizome	9 g

Hamilton Rotte   The suggestion is that hepatitis C can be cleared with herbs and lifestyle changes. This formula is the second of two that Dr. Shen provided for the condition. His previous formula is for the early stages when the excess conditions prevail. This formula contains tonic herbs for the liver and spleen and blood-invigorating substances.

The tonics for the liver in this formula include *bai shao* and *shan zhu yu*. There is also a significant focus on tonifying the spleen and stomach with *bai zhu*, *shan yao*, and *fu ling*. These tonics are included to assist the separation of pure and impure that results in the production of blood. Many of the most valuable liver blood tonic formulas within Chinese medicine contain herbs that tonify spleen *qi* (such as *Ba Zhen Tang* [Eight Treasure Decoction] and related formulas). We find herbs in this formula that move liver blood, including *yu jin* and *yan hu suo*. *Yuan zhi* may also be included because of its moving tendencies. In the later stages of hepatitis, liver blood stasis is one of the primary patterns described in the literature.

The presence of light dosage of *huang qin* suggests that there is still some lingering excess heat, though certainly not to the degree that one would find in earlier stages of the disease.

Liver Blood Deficiency

Pin Yin	Latin	English	Dosage
Chai hu	Bupleuri Radix	Hare's ear root, thorowax root, bupleurum	2.4 g
Chuan xiong	Chuanxiong Rhizoma	Chuanxiong root, Szechuan lovage root, cnidium	4.5 g
Dang gui	Angelicae Sinensis Radix	Chinese angelica root, *tang-kuei*	6 g
He shou wu	Radix Polygoni Multiflori	Fleece-flower root, polygonum hosuwu	9 g
Bai shao	Paeoniae Alba Radix	White peony root	6 g

Pin Yin	Latin	English	Dosage
Bai zhu	Atractylodis Macrocephalae Rhizoma	White atractylodes rhizome	6 g
Yan hu suo	Corydalis Yanhusuo Rhizoma	Corydalis rhizome	9 g
Yu jin	Curcumae Radix	Curcuma tuber	6 g
Huang qin	Scutellariae Baicalensis Radix	Baical skullcap root, scutellaria, scute	4.5 g

Hamilton Rotte Formulas that tonify the blood always contain blood-moving ingredients to balance the tonic herbs because unlike *qi*, blood does not have its own volition to move. For instance, in the famous liver blood tonic formula *Si Wu Tang* (Four Substance Decoction), the ingredients *chuan xiong* and *dang gui* function as blood movers.

Like standard liver blood tonic formulas, this formula also contains blood movers, including *dang gui*, *chuan xiong*, *yan hu suo*, and *yu jin*. Unlike the standard formulas, however, it contains *qi*-moving ingredients, including *chai hu*, *yan hu suo*, and *yu jin*. Experience has shown that when the liver blood is deficient, it is unable to carry out its important *qi*-regulating function. In the standard formulas, this situation is addressed with the two-herb combination of *bai shao* and *chai hu*, which is present in this formula.

Dr. Shen avoids the most cloying blood tonic, *shu di huang*, which is present in most of the liver blood tonic formulas. *Shu di huang* is famously difficult to digest, and can be especially problematic in modern society where people are mostly over-fed and harbor excesses in the digestive system. Instead we find blood tonics that are easier to digest, including *dang gui*, *he shou wu*, and *bai shao*.

In this formula we find *bai zhu* to tonify the spleen and dry dampness. Some of the most valuable blood tonic formulas contain spleen tonics (such as *Ba Zhen Tang* [Eight Treasure Decoction] and related formulas and *Gui Pi Tang* [Restore the Spleen Decoction]), as these aid the spleen in producing blood. The drying nature of *bai zhu* offsets the moistening tendency of the tonic herbs.

Huang qin is an unexpected ingredient here, which may be included for its descending tendency in order to bring blood back to the liver. *Huang qin* may also be included to offset the warming tendencies of the tonic herbs.

Infectious Diseases

Lyme Disease

Pin Yin	Latin	English	Dosage
Wei ge gen	Puerariae Radix	Roasted kudzu root, pueraria	4.5 g
Chao jing jie	Schizonepetae Herba	Dry-fried schizonepeta	4.5 g
Chao fang feng	Saposhnikoviae Radix	Fried ledebouriella root, saposhnikoviae root, siler	4.5 g
Gui zhi	Ramulus Cinnamomi Cassiae	Cinnamon twig, cassia twig	4.5 g
Gan cao	Glycyrrhizae Radix	Licorice root	4.5 g
Jin yin hua	Lonicerae Flos	Honeysuckle flower	9 g
Mu dan pi	Moutan Radicis Cortex	Tree peony root bark, moutan root bark	9 g
Mu gua	Chaenomelis Fructus	Chinese quince fruit, chaenomeles	9 g
Tong cao	Tetrapanacis Medulla	Rice paper plant pith, tetrapanax	4.5 g
Yi yi ren	Coicis Semen	Seeds of Job's tears, coix seeds	12 g

Hamilton Rotte   In the early stages of Lyme disease, the condition is one of heat or heat toxicity entering the body from the exterior. The treatment principles are to release the exterior and to clear heat and toxicity. Lyme disease also frequently involves joint pain, and removing wind-dampness from the channels is also very relevant.

As the disease progresses, the retained pathogen consumes the body's resources, notably the *qi* and *yin*.

This formula is indicated for the early stages of Lyme disease.

Surface-relieving herbs include *ge gen*, *jing jie*, *fang feng*, *gui zhi*, and *jin yin hua*. These are mostly cooling, with the exception of *gui zhi*. As heat pathogens frequently transmit to the blood, *mu dan pi* is included to cool the blood.

Tong cao and *yi yi ren* are included as a means to remove heat from the body through the urine.

Musculoskeletal Conditions

Arthritis, Bath

FROM DR. SHEN: There are many different forms of arthritis. Some forms are caused by an old injury, some by body condition, and some by chemicals in the blood. These formulas treat rheumatic arthritis, which causes aching throughout the whole body. Arthritis is caused by impaired circulation and can be treated by the formulas that treat external injuries. These two formulas can be taken together; one is taken internally and one is used as a bath.
Add this formula to hot bath water. A person should soak in this solution until they feel ready to sweat. At that point they should get out, towel dry, and go to sleep.

Pin Yin	Latin	English	Dosage
Ma huang	Ephedrae Herba	Ephedra stem	30 g
Fang feng	Saposhnikoviae Radix	Ledebouriella root, saposhnikoviae root, siler	30 g
Hong hua	Carthami Tinctorii Flos	Safflower flower, carthamus	30 g
Mo yao	Myrrha	Myrrh	30 g
Ma qian zi	Strychni Semen	Nux-vomica seeds	30 g[a]
Qiang huo	Notopterygii Rhizoma et Radix	Notopterygium root and rhizome, chiang-huo	30 g
Wang bu liu xing	Vaccariae Segetalis Semen	Vaccaria seed	30 g
Ge gen	Puerariae Radix	Kudzu root, pueraria	30 g
Mu gua	Chaenomelis Fructus	Chinese quince fruit, chaenomeles	30 g
Ru xiang	Gummi Olibanumi	Frankincense, mastic	30 g

[a] Toxic and obsolete.

Hamilton Rotte This formula contains ingredients that release the exterior, expel wind-dampness, move blood, and relieve pain. It is indicated for a cold, "painful obstruction" syndrome.
Herbs that release the exterior include *ma huang*, *fang feng*, *qiang huo*, and *ge gen*. Herbs that expel wind-dampness include *fang feng*, *ma qian zi*, *qiang huo*, *mu gua*, and *ru xiang*.
Herbs that move blood and relieve pain include *hong hua*, *mo yao*, and *ru xiang*.

Leon Hammer
Ginger bath:
Another rather simple procedure that was recommended by Dr. Shen that was very effective for arthritis was the "ginger bath." See "Using Ginger, Ginger Bath" above, page 92, for instructions.

Arthritis, Internal

Pin Yin	Latin	English	Dosage
Dang gui	Angelicae Sinensis Radix	Chinese angelica root, *tang-kuei*	9 g
Ge gen	Puerariae Radix	Kudzu root, pueraria	9 g
Fang feng	Saposhnikoviae Radix	Ledebouriella root, saposhnikoviae root, siler	6 g
Si gua luo	Fasciculus Vascularis Luffae	Dried skeleton of vegetable sponge	6 g
Han fang ji	Stephaniae Tetrandrae Radix	Stephania, four stamen stephania root	9 g
Mu gua	Chaenomelis Fructus	Chinese quince fruit, chaenomeles	9 g
Qiang huo	Notopterygii Rhizoma et Radix	Notopterygium root and rhizome, *chiang-huo*	6 g
Dan shen	Salviae Miltiorrhiziae Radix	Salvia root	6 g
Sang ji sheng	Taxilli Herba	Mulberry mistletoe stems, loranthus, taxillus, mistletoe	12 g

Hamilton Rotte Inflammation of the joints corresponds to what is known in Chinese medicine as "painful obstruction" or *bi* syndrome. A painful obstruction involves wind, damp, and either heat or cold lodged in the channels. Pain occurs at the joints because they are naturally more difficult for energy to pass through. In the vast majority of cases there is a history of trauma to the affected joint (overuse of a joint is a form of trauma).

Formulas that address "painful obstruction" syndrome address the particular pathogens that are present, target the affected area, and may also release the exterior, move blood, or address underlying deficiencies.

This formula contains the following surface-releasing herbs: *ge gen*, *fang feng*, and *qiang huo*.

This formula contains the following herbs for wind-damp: *fang feng*, *si gua luo*, *han fang ji*, *mu gua*, *qiang huo*, and *sang ji sheng*. *Fang feng* is especially good for wind, *han fang ji* is especially good for heat, and *si gua luo*, *mu gua*, and *qiang huo* are especially good for dampness. Overall, the formula is close to neutral with slightly more emphasis on expelling wind-damp-cold. The formula also contains blood-moving ingredients, *dang gui* and *dan shen*, often very useful for intractable painful obstruction. Blood tonics include *dang gui* and *sang ji sheng* that aid in the repair of the sinews.

Arthritis, Rheumatoid

Pin Yin	Latin	English	Dosage
Ge gen	Puerariae Radix	Kudzu root, pueraria	9 g
Gui zhi	Ramulus Cinnamomi Cassiae	Cinnamon twig, cassia twig	3 g
Mu gua	Chaenomelis Fructus	Chinese quince fruit, chaenomeles	9 g
Qiang huo	Notopterygii Rhizoma et Radix	Notopterygium root and rhizome, *chiang-huo*	6 g
Fang feng	Saposhnikoviae Radix	Ledebouriella root, saposhnikoviae root, siler	9 g
Dan shen	Salviae Miltiorrhiziae Radix	Salvia root	6 g
Mu dan pi	Moutan Radicis Cortex	Tree peony root bark, moutan root bark	6 g
Wei ling xian	Clematidis Radix	Chinese clematis root	9 g
Chi shao	Paeoniae Rubra Radix	Red peony root	9 g
Sang zhi	Ramulus Mori Albae	Mulberry twig, morus twig	12 g

Hamilton Rotte   Rheumatoid arthritis is also classified as a "painful obstruction" syndrome in Chinese medicine. Compared to osteoarthritis, it is a more severe condition that can progressively lead to joint deformity, also in younger people. In the later stages it tends to involve pronounced deficiency, of either the kidney *yin* or *yang*. According to the literature it often begins as a cold condition, develops into a heat condition, and then later involves deficiency.

This formula addresses a situation where exterior wind-damp-cold is transforming into heat in the blood. The herbs that address the wind-damp-cold condition include *gui zhi*, *mu gua*, *qiang huo*, *fang feng*, *wei ling xian*, and *sang zhi*. *Ge gen* aids in releasing the exterior to expel the pathogens.

This formula contains the following ingredients to cool the blood: *dan shen*, *mu dan pi*, and *chi shao*. These address the pathogen that has moved into the interior, causing blood heat.

In the later stages of rheumatoid arthritis, herbs that tonify the kidneys and repair the sinews and bones are indicated, in addition to herbs to clear heat.

Leon Hammer   Childhood rheumatic fever, a streptococcus infection almost always in childhood before the age of 16, can result in serious cardiac sequelae at the time and last a lifetime.

That aspect of the infection and the toxic waste from the bacteria that is not completely resolved at the time is removed from immediate threat to vital organs by the divergent channels, using *yuan qi*, to the joints where the divergent channels begin.

Divergence also occurs to skin, causing chronic skin problems; to conjunctiva, teeth, bone, and "curious organs." Original (*yuan*) *qi* is gradually drained moving the pathogen through the divergent channels and essence *qi* is drained, maintaining the latency. As these are depleted the pathogen begins to move back toward the solid (*zang*) organs and other mechanisms come into play by the protective (*wei*) *qi* diverting the pathogen to the hollow (*fu*) organs, the digestive system and the connecting (*luo*) channels, draining blood to more superficial joints like the hands, fingers, feet, and toes.

Injury to Wrist or Ankle

Pin Yin	Latin	English	Dosage
Fen zhi zi	Gardeniae Jasminoidis Fructus	Powdered cape jasmine fruit, gardenia fruit	28 g
Mai fen	Tritici Fructus	Wheat flour	7 g
Ji dai qing	n. a.	Egg white	1
Gao liang jiu	n. a.	Vodka or Chinese rice wine	1 tsp

Hamilton Rotte   In Chinese medicine injuries are divided into three stages. All three stages include *qi* and blood stagnation and pain. In the first stage there is heat toxicity present, in the second stage there is still residual heat and wind-damp pathogens are beginning to invade, and in the third stage there is pronounced wind-damp-cold.

This formula is indicated for the first stage of trauma, when heat signs are pronounced. *Fen zhi zi* clears heat toxicity and moves blood (especially when used topically). It is the primary ingredient to address the trauma.

Flour is probably included in this formula to provide a desirable consistency. Egg white is used to bring the herbs to the soft tissues. It can be used by itself in injuries to soft tissue, but this recipe yields better results. Vodka, which is usually 40 % alcohol, has two functions: the alcohol carries the herbs through the skin and has a blood-moving, pain-relieving effect.

This recipe could be applied anywhere on the body, but because the mixture needs to be covered with a cellophane wrap and bandage it would be less convenient to apply it to other areas.

FROM DR. SHEN: Mix together to form a paste and apply to swollen area. Cover with bandage and cellophane to keep it moist. Leave in place for 24 hours and rest. When the plaster is removed the skin will be very green or blue, but the pain will be much reduced. This treatment can be used one or two times.

Pain in the Back

Pin Yin	Latin	English	Dosage
Xi xin	Asari Herba cum Radice	Chinese wild ginger, asarum	1.8 g
Sheng di huang	Rehmanniae Radix	Fresh Chinese foxglove root, fresh rehmannia root	12 g
Du zhong	Eucommiae Cortex	Eucommia bark	12 g
Xu duan	Dipsaci Asperi Radix	Japanese teasel root, dipsacus	12 g
Gou qi zi	Lycii Fructus	Chinese wolfberry, matrimony vine fruit, lycium fruit	12 g
San qi	Notoginseng Radix	Noto ginseng root, root of pseudo-ginseng	6 g
Gou ji	Cibotii Rhizoma	Cibotium rhizome, chain fern	9 g

Hamilton Rotte   This formula contains very similar ingredients to the formula for pain in the lower back from kidney weakness below, with the addition of *san qi*, which excels at moving blood and relieving pain.

Pain in the Low Back from Damaged Circulation Due to Injury

FROM DR. SHEN: Many times a person hurts their back from falling down, lifting too much, or from many other day-to-day activities. After the initial pain fades the local circulation is still weak. On days when a person works too hard or gets sick, the pain can flare up. It can also appear as the person gets older, and is often diagnosed as arthritis.
Use the formula for "Pain in the Low Back from a Spinal Curve" plus *Yunnan Baiyao* (Yunnan White Powder) (three capsules for 5 days).

Pain in the Low Back from Kidney Weakness

FROM DR. SHEN: This pain will be either on the left or right side of the back. The conditions described above (related to trauma) tend to cause pain in the middle. The kidneys become weak from overwork, too much sex, or genetics.

Pin Yin	Latin	English	Dosage
Du zhong	Eucommiae Cortex	Eucommia bark	12 g
Xu duan	Dipsaci Asperi Radix	Japanese teasel root, dipsacus	12 g
Sheng di huang	Rehmannia Radix	Fresh Chinese foxglove root, rehmannia root	12 g
Xi xin	Asari Herba cum Radice	Chinese wild ginger, asarum	3 g
Bu gu zhi	Psoraleae Corylifoliae Fructus	Psoralea fruit	9 g[a]
Ba ji tian	Morindae Officinalis Radix	Morinda root	9 g

Pin Yin	Latin	English	Dosage
Gou ji	Cibotii Rhizoma	Cibotium rhizome, chain fern	12 g
Shu di huang	Rehmanniae Preparata Radix	Prepared Chinese foxglove root (cooked in red wine), cooked rehmannia rhizome	9 g
Tu si zi	Cuscutae Chinensis Semen	Chinese dodder seeds, cuscuta	12 g

Hamilton Rotte   Back pain from kidney deficiency can occur in yin or yang deficiency. This formula is suitable for back pain that occurs from yang deficiency.

As in standard kidney yang tonic formulas such as Jin Gui Shen Qi Wan (Golden Cabinet Kidney Qi Pill) or Zou Gui Wan (Restore the Right Pill), this formula contains ingredients to tonify the kidney yin and the kidney yang. Yin tonics include sheng di huang and shu di huang, and to a lesser degree tu si zi. Yang tonics in this formula include du zhong, xu duan, bu gu zhi, bai ji tian, gou ji, and tu si zi. Also, as in the aforementioned standard formulas to tonify kidney yang, Dr.

Shen's formula includes ingredients to warm the interior, in particular xi xin and bu gu zhi.

This formula differs from standard kidney tonic formulas in that it contains ingredients that "strengthen the sinews and bones" and those that have a blood-moving and pain-relieving effect.

Herbs that strengthen sinews and bones include du zhong and xu duan (a two-herb combination), bai ji tian and gou ji. These herbs are especially useful for painful conditions from deficiency.

Du zhong and xu duan are also blood-moving ingredients that aid in their pain-relieving effects.

Pain in the Low Back from a Spinal Curve

FROM DR. SHEN: This formula is used when there is pain caused by a curvature in the spine. This condition can be genetic or brought on by excessive exercise when a person is young. Since you cannot change the spine, you must strengthen it and relax the surrounding muscles. A person with this condition must also be careful not to exercise excessively.

Pin Yin	Latin	English	Dosage
Du zhong	Eucommiae Cortex	Eucommia bark	12 g
Gou ji	Cibotii Rhizoma	Cibotium rhizome, chain fern	12 g
Bu gu zhi	Psoraleae Corylifoliae Fructus	Psoralea fruit	9 g
San qi	Notoginseng Radix	Noto ginseng root, root of pseudo-ginseng	12 g
Xu duan	Dipsaci Asperi Radix	Japanese teasel root, dipsacus	2.4 g
Xi xin	Asari Herba cum Radice	Chinese wild ginger, asarum	1–3 g
Qiang huo	Notopterygii Rhizoma et Radix	Notopterygium root and rhizome, chiang-huo	6 g
Dan shen	Salviae Miltiorrhiziae Radix	Salvia root	6 g

Hamilton Rotte   A curve in the spine usually develops in a person who is inherently kidney yang essence deficient who exercises excessively early in life (overuse of the body is a form of trauma). Frequently, herbs that "strengthen the sinews and bones" are

beneficial to treat musculoskeletal problems in kidney yang essence-deficient individuals. These ingredients prevent further damage to the spine. Blood-moving and pain-relieving herbs are also applicable.

In this formula the ingredients that strengthen sinews and bones and tonify kidney *yang* include *du zhong*, *gou ji*, *bu gu zhi*, and *xu duan*. *Xi xin*, an ingredient that warms the interior and reaches the level of the bones, is included to assist the *yang* and help carry the herbs to the bones.
Blood-invigorating ingredients include *dan shen* and

san qi. *San qi* is particularly effective for relieving pain and treating trauma (including trauma from overuse), which usually contributes to this condition.
Qiang huo focuses its actions on the spine, addressing the location of the problem. It also expels wind-dampness, which tends to lodge in areas where there has been a history of trauma.

Pain in the Neck and Shoulder from Early Injury

FROM DR. SHEN: Formulas for the neck can also be used for pain in other joints such as the wrist and knee.
This condition can be severe and is caused by an injury, such as whiplash that never healed properly. In this case, herbs that help the body's strength must be used in conjunction with local treatment. It may take a while for the body condition and circulation to improve. Use 7-star needle.

Pain in the Neck and Shoulder Due to Injury

FROM DR. SHEN: This problem is caused by an injury in the shoulder that, over time, causes a reaction in the neck. This reaction occurs because a person compensates for their lack of mobility by putting more stress on the neck. The tendons and muscles become tight, which damages local circulation. This formula is used in conjunction with massage and a special Chinese heat lamp.

Pin Yin	Latin	English	Dosage
Dang gui	Angelicae Sinensis Radix	Chinese angelica root, *tang-kuei*	6 g
Xu duan	Dipsaci Asperi Radix	Japanese teasel root, dipsacus	9 g
Xiang fu	Cyperi Rotundi Rhizoma	Nut grass rhizoma, cyperus	6 g
Qiang huo	Notopterygii Rhizoma et Radix	Notopterygium root and rhizome, *chiang-huo*	9 g
Hong hua	Carthami Tinctorii Flos	Safflower flower, carthamus	6 g
San qi	Notoginseng Radix	Noto ginseng root, root of pseudo-ginseng	6 g
Sang ji sheng	Taxilli Herba	Mulberry mistletoe stems, loranthus, taxillus, mistletoe	9 g

Hamilton Rotte Dr. Shen suggests that this situation develops gradually and is therefore not an acute injury. Because it is not an acute injury the treatment principles do not include clearing heat, instead they are to move blood, relieve pain, expel wind-damp, and strengthen sinews and bones.
The herbs that move blood include *dang gui*, *xu duan*, *hong hua*, and *san qi*. All of these exert significant pain-relieving effects.
Herbs that expel wind-damp include *qiang huo* and *sang ji sheng*.

Herbs that strengthen sinews and bones include *xu duan* and *sang ji sheng*.
This formula also has herbs that target the affected areas. *Hong hua* affects the upper body in general while *qiang huo* targets the neck. *Xiang fu* may be included because of its affinity for the triple burner channel, which runs through the shoulder and neck. *Xiang fu* also moves *qi* and relieves pain, beneficial for this condition.

Pain in the Neck and Shoulder, Rheumatoid Arthritis in the Neck

FROM DR. SHEN: This is caused by infection in the joints or chemicals in the blood that damage the disks. This formula clears the blood and overcomes infection so the circulation can improve.

Pin Yin	Latin	English	Dosage
Ge gen	Puerariae Radix	Kudzu root, pueraria	9 g
Qiang huo	Notopterygii Rhizoma et Radix	Notopterygium root and rhizome, chiang-huo	9 g
Sang zhi	Ramulus Mori Albae	Mulberry twig, morus twig	9 g
Fang feng	Saposhnikoviae Radix	Ledebouriella root, saposhnikoviae root, siler	6 g
Dan shen	Salviae Miltiorrhiziae Radix	Salvia root	6 g
Sang ji sheng	Taxilli Herba	Mulberry mistletoe stems, loranthus, taxillus, mistletoe	6 g
Mu gua	Chaenomelis Fructus	Chinese quince fruit, chaenomeles	9 g
Chuan shan jia	Mantis Pentadactylae Squama	Pangolin scales	No dose mentioned

Hamilton Rotte   Rheumatoid arthritis fits into the category of a *bi* syndrome or "painful obstruction" syndrome in Chinese medicine. It tends be a hot *bi* syndrome (wind-damp-heat). It also tends to be a relatively severe condition, and severe *bi* syndromes usually involve blood stasis in addition to the wind-damp pathogens.

The treatment principles of this formula are to expel wind-damp and move blood. The herbs that expel wind-damp include *qiang huo, sang zhi, fang feng, sang ji sheng,* and *mu gua* and *chuan shan jia. Chuan shan jia* is obsolete because it comes from an endangered species.

Blood-invigorating ingredients include *dan shen* and *chuan shan jia.*

This formula also contains herbs that target the neck, notably *ge gen* and *qiang huo.* Dr. Shen also seemed to utilize *fang feng* to target the upper body in *bi* syndromes.

Leon Hammer   Around 1979 Dr. Shen told me that he had found a new cause of arthritis: toxicity.

He made the diagnosis by observing the vertical blood vessels on the inside of the lower eyelid. A sign of toxic arthritis was when the vessels varied from one to the other between being bright and being dark (perhaps thinner and less straight).

I believe that this formula emerged from that observation. The arthritis was not confined to the neck. It could be anywhere.

In my opinion, this form of arthritis is a function of the body diverting pathogens from vital organs (retained pathogen) through the divergent and connecting channels.

Pain in the Neck and Shoulder Due to Sleeping Wrong

FROM DR. SHEN: This is a mild problem caused by sleeping in an incorrect position. The body may be constitutionally weak or the muscles may get cold. The muscles tighten, making movement painful. Use local spray.

Leon Hammer
Etiology:
Exposure of that part to wind-cold from open window/air-conditioning fan, driving in a car with an open window.

Treatment:
Gua sa and cupping; 7-star needle.

Pain in the Neck and Shoulder from Work, Positional

FROM DR. SHEN: This is similar in cause to sleeping wrongly. Instead of sleeping, however, it is repetitive motion that aggravates the neck. This condition is more chronic than one caused by sleeping wrongly. This formula is used on the outside of the muscle with massage. A 7-star needle can also be used to improve circulation.

Pin Yin	Latin	English	Dosage
Rou gui	Cinnamomi Cassiae Cortex	Inner bark of Saigon cinnamon	3 g
Dang gui	Angelicae Sinensis Radix	Chinese angelica root, *tang-kuei*	9 g
Fang feng	Saposhnikoviae Radix	Ledebouriella root, saposhnikoviae root, siler	6 g
Hong hua	Carthami Tinctorii Flos	Safflower flower, carthamus	6 g
Shen jin cao	Lycopodii Herba	Ground pine, common club moss, "stretch sinew herb"	9 g
Qiang huo	Notopterygii Rhizoma et Radix	Notopterygium root and rhizome, *chiang-huo*	6 g
Ru xiang	Gummi Olibanumi	Frankincense, mastic	6 g
Mo yao	Myrrha	Myrrh	6 g
Dan shen	Salviae Miltiorrhiziae Radix	Salvia root	6 g

Hamilton Rotte This is a topical formula for pain from overuse of the neck and shoulder. Overuse of a joint constitutes a trauma, one of the most common forms of trauma.

This formula is for a condition that is not acute. In the later stages of trauma wind-damp-cold pathogens lodge in the affected area. Because the cause is trauma there will invariably be blood stasis and pain.

The herbs that move blood and relieve pain include *dang gui*, *hong hua*, *ru xiang*, *mo yao*, and *dan shen*.

Ru xiang and *mo yao* are hard on the digestive system, but extremely important for topical applications.

Herbs that expel wind-damp-cold pathogens include *rou gui*, *fang feng*, *shen jin cao*, and *qiang huo*, *ru xiang*, and *mo yao*. According to Ding Gan Ren, *fang feng* is especially indicated for pain in the spine and stiffness of the neck. Among these, *rou gui* is especially indicated for cold, *shen jin cao* (literally "stretch sinew herb") is indicated for stiffness and *qiang huo* especially targets the neck.

Leon Hammer
Pulse:
- Pain in parts of the body is accessed by rolling one's fingers toward the radius, where a very tight quality will be felt in the following areas:

  – Neck–head–shoulder pain: rolling radially from the distal positions
  – Hip–lower back pain: rolling radially from the middle positions
  – Knee–ankle: rolling radially from the proximal positions

Scoliosis

Pin Yin	Latin	English	Dosage
Xi xin	Asari Herba cum Radice	Chinese wild ginger, asarum	0.3 g
Dang gui	Angelicae Sinensis Radix	Chinese angelica root, tang-kuei	6 g
San qi	Notoginseng Radix	Noto ginseng root, root of pseudo-ginseng	3 g
Xu duan	Dipsaci Asperi Radix	Japanese teasel root, dipsacus	12 g
Tao ren	Persicae Semen	Peach kernel, persica	6 g
Qiang huo	Notopterygii Rhizoma et Radix	Notopterygium root and rhizome, chiang-huo	6 g
Sang ji sheng	Taxilli Herba	Mulberry mistletoe stems, loranthus, taxillus, mistletoe	12 g
Mu gua	Chaenomelis Fructus	Chinese quince fruit, chaenomeles	9 g
Dan shen	Salviae Miltiorrhiziae Radix	Salvia root	6 g

Hamilton Rotte   This formula contains tonic herbs that strengthen the sinews and bones, including *xu duan* and *sang ji sheng*. These herbs are used when a joint or the spine becomes misshapen, as in Jiao Shu De's formulas for joint deformity *bi* syndrome (Jiao Shu-De, 2005).

This formula contains many herbs that move the blood, including *dang gui*, *san qi*, *xu duan*, *tao ren*, and *dan shen*. The blood-moving aspect of this formula is the single most prominent treatment principle, suggesting that trauma to the spine is the predominant factor that contributes to the development of scoliosis.

We also find a number of herbs that expel wind-damp-cold. In the vast majority of cases when these pathogens are present there is a history of trauma to an area. The herbs that expel wind-damp-cold include *xi xin*, *qiang huo*, *sang ji sheng*, and *mu gua*. *Mu gua* is also very good for cramping and is used here in order to relax the muscles so that the spine is allowed to straighten. Muscles are largely responsible for structural problems because if they are too tense they pull structures out of place.

Leon Hammer   Throughout my career I encountered many children driven at first by their parents and later by themselves to ignore the obvious developing disabilities associated with extreme acrobatics and ballet, including severe debilitating scoliosis. I recall one young girl age 14, who after having a rod placed next to her spine to counteract her severe scoliosis after 8 years of ceaseless and extensive competitive acrobatics would not desist, with the assent and approval of her parents.

Dr. Shen repeatedly and strongly advised against children engaging in violent body bending/stretching exercise, especially acrobatics and ballet. Structural damage by these practices, especially to bone, in an organism that requires all of its kidney essence for growth and development is inevitable, even in children with the strongest "terrain."

Structure along with stability is the single most important determinant of normal development of all organs and areas of the body including the mind. One can assess the spirit of the *qi* and of a person's frame of mind by body posture. I emphasize this centrality of structure in my article: "The concept of 'blocks': structure" (Hammer, 2006) where I discuss the assessment of the long leg syndrome and treatment with acupuncture and especially adjustment of the spine (subluxations and fixations).

Neurological Conditions

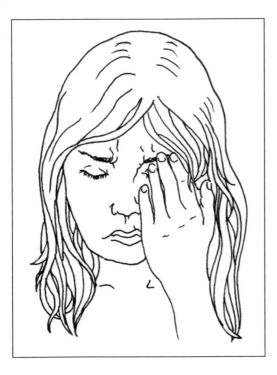

Fig. 12 Headache.

Headache from Blood Deficiency

Pin Yin	Latin	English	Dosage
Tian ma	Gastrodiae Rhizoma	Gastrodia rhizome	9 g
Dang gui	Angelicae Sinensis Radix	Chinese angelica root, *tang-kuei*	9 g
Chuan xiong	Chuanxiong Rhizoma	Chuanxiong root, Szechuan lovage root, cnidium	4.5 g
Shu di huang	Rehmanniae Preparata Radix	Prepared Chinese foxglove root (cooked in red wine), cooked rehmannia rhizome	12 g
Bai zhi	Angelicae Dahuricae Radix	Angelica root	4.5 g
Shan yao	Dioscoreae Oppositae Rhizoma	Chinese yam root, dioscorea rhizome	12 g
Gou qi zi	Lycii Fructus	Chinese wolfberry, matrimony vine fruit, lycium fruit	9 g
Bai ji li	Tribuli Terrestris Fructus	Caltrop fruit, puncture-vine fruit, tribulus	9 g

FROM DR. SHEN:
- If bowels are loose use *sheng di huang*.
- If you have to use *shu di huang* add 2.4 g of *sha ren*.
- Cook *sha ren* and *shu di huang* first for 10 minutes before adding other herbs. *Tian ma* is for weak headaches: for example, anemia, slightly high blood pressure.

Hamilton Rotte   Headaches (**Fig. 12**) from liver blood deficiency are generalized and dull. The headaches tend to be worse around menstruation. They occur in the context of other liver blood deficiency signs and symptoms (described in the TCM literature).
This formula contains the following tonic herbs for liver blood: *dang gui*, *shu di huang*, and *gou qi zi*.
Shan yao, a spleen and kidney tonic, aids in the production of blood indirectly. The spleen contributes to liver blood by transforming and transporting food and fluid, and the kidneys support the *yin* aspects of the liver.
The following herbs have pain-relieving functions and target the head: *chuan xiong*, *tian ma*, *bai zhi*, and *bai ji li*. Although *chuan xiong* and *bai zhi* can be somewhat drying in nature, the dosages of these substances are kept at a minimum and are offset by the tonic herbs that are included in the formula.

Leon Hammer   As already mentioned, the principal liver problem in Chinese medicine in our time is liver *qi-yang* deficiency and not liver *qi* stagnation (Hammer, 2009) or even liver blood deficiency. Liver *qi*, as with the *qi* in any organ will determine the viability of all of its other functions. Even the capacity to stagnate *qi* or store the blood depends upon the strength of liver *qi*.
In fact the commonly used formula for liver *qi* stagnation, *Xiao Yao San* (Rambling Powder), consists primarily of nourishing herbs including *dang gui*, *bai shao*, *bai zhu*, *fu ling*, and *gan cao* and contains only two herbs to move stagnant liver *qi*: *chai hu* and *bo he*. It is primarily a *qi*- and blood-nourishing formula. This reinforces the thesis that the real concern regarding liver function is *qi-yang* deficiency.
If liver *qi* is deficient it cannot store the blood or supply it to the other organs, perhaps most importantly the heart, which depends more on the liver for this aspect of its function than the other organs. The kidney makes its own blood through the marrow; the lung's blood function is to aerate it and depends on lung and kidney *qi* to "grasp" the oxygen; the spleen creates blood through its digestive function.
The process of moving blood out of the uterus in the premenstrual phase of the cycle supersedes all other liver functions at that time and depends on the integrity of liver *qi*. If that *qi* is deficient, blood does not move sufficiently out of the uterus as well as to all of the other areas that depend on liver blood.
This is especially true for the head, since the liver and heart must overcome gravity. The headache is dull and generally around the entire head. Bursting headaches are associated with heat in the blood and expanding vessels.

Headache from an Old Injury

Pin Yin	Latin	English	Dosage
Dang gui	Angelica Sinensis Radix	Chinese angelica root, *tang-kuei*	6 g
Chuan xiong	Chuangxiong Rhizoma	Chuanxiong root, Szechuan lovage root, cnidium	4.5 g
Bai zhi	Angelicae Dahuricae Radix	Angelica root	6 g
Sang ji sheng	Taxilli Herba	Mulberry mistletoe stems, loranthus, taxillus, mistletoe	9 g
San qi	Notoginseng Radix	Noto ginseng root, root of pseudo-ginseng	3 g
Dan shen	Salviae Miltiorrhiziae Radix	Salvia root	6 g
Xiang fu	Cyperi Rotundi Rhizoma	Nut grass rhizoma, cyperus	4.5 g

Hamilton Rotte   Headaches that arise from trauma result from the blood stasis incurred during the trauma. These headaches are at a fixed location, have a stabbing nature, and can be traced back to the traumatic event.

Blood-moving and or pain-relieving herbs are the primary means of addressing the local conditions in the head at the site of the pain. The following herbs have a blood-moving effect: *dang gui, chuan xiong, san qi,* and *dan shen. San qi* is especially indicated for the treatment of trauma. The following herbs have pain-relieving effects: *chuan xiong, san qi,* and *bai zhi. Chuan xiong* and *bai zhi* target the head. *Xiang fu* is included as a *qi* regulator, which aids in the movement of blood. When administering herbs that move the blood, blood tonics should be included so as not to damage the blood. In this formula, *dang gui* and *sang ji sheng* serve this purpose.

Leon Hammer   Dr Shen stressed the importance of trauma to the head as the source of most intractable headaches. He advised palpating the scalp for tender spots and especially ones that are slightly swollen. He associated these spots in girls and women with obesity, the origin being unresolved trauma. He asserted that without needling these local tender spots (*ashi* points) the headaches would never resolve. I have found this to be accurate and have been amazed by the large number of women who love horses who have received repeated blows to the head from falls or being kicked who do not associate these injuries to their head with "trauma" when questioned.

Headache, Migraine from Anemia

FROM DR. SHEN: There are four causes of migraine. Either the nerves have been injured without receiving effective treatment; it is the sequelae of a slight cerebral concussion; it is caused by anemia; or it is due to nervous tension. Migraines may persist from adolescence until old age. For anemia, in addition to the formula take two pills of *Yunnan Baiyao* a day for 7 days.

Leon Hammer   As mentioned elsewhere, Dr. Shen placed great emphasis on trauma as a cause of headache. He recommended treating the *ashi* points on the head as a prerequisite for the treatment of intractable headaches, which I found to be accurate.

Whereas I have a different concept of the cause of "migraine" headaches, I have found his emphasis on head trauma absolutely valid.

FROM DR. SHEN: In Chinese medicine anemia refers to blood that is too weak to supply sufficient energy to the body. This condition can result in weakened circulation to the head, which manifests as migraines. Anemia is usually caused by a weak constitution and overwork. An injury that is not properly treated can also cause migraines by weakening the circulatory system. If migraines are caused by a weak constitution, they will have occurred before 14 years of age. The pulse in this condition will be weak and the tongue will be pale.

Pin Yin	Latin	English	Dosage
Dang gui	Angelicae Sinensis Radix	Chinese angelica root, *tang-kuei*	9 g
Shu di huang	Rehmanniae Preparata Radix	Prepared Chinese foxglove root (cooked in red wine), cooked rehmannia rhizome	9 g
Bai shao	Paeoniae Alba Radix	White peony root	6 g
Chuan xiong	Chuanxiong Rhizoma	Chuanxiong root, Szechuan lovage root, cnidium	6 g

Pin Yin	Latin	English	Dosage
Man jing zi	Viticis Fructus	Vitex fruit	6 g
Bai zhi	Angelicae Dahuricae Radix	Angelica root	6 g
Shan zhu yu	Corni Officinalis Fructus	Asiatic Cornelian cherry fruit, cornus	9 g
Tu si zi	Cuscutae Chinensis Semen	Chinese dodder seeds, cuscuta	9 g
Long gu	Fossilia Ossis Mastodi	Dragon bone, fossilized vertebrae and bones of the extremities (usually of mammals)	9 g

Hamilton Rotte This formula contains herbs that tonify liver blood, relieve pain and target the head, tonify liver and kidneys, and subdue *yang*.

The herbs that tonify liver blood include *dang gui, shu di huang*, and *bai shao. Chuan xiong* is usually included with these, as in the standard formula *Si Wu Tang* (Four Substance Decoction). It is notable that the dosage of *chuan xiong*, a pain-relieving substance that targets the head, is relatively high.

The herbs that target the head directly and exhibit pain-relieving effects include *man jing zi, bai zhi*, and *chuan xiong*. These tend to be drying herbs, but are adequately balanced by the previously mentioned moistening ingredients.

Shan zhu yu and *tu si zi* are kidney tonics. Both are fairly mild tonics and considered to tonify both *yin* and *yang*. One of the most effective ways to treat blood deficiency is through tonifying the kidneys.

Long gu is included to downbear *yang*. Dr. Shen included downbearing herbs in all of his formulas to treat migraines.

Headache, Migraine from Internal Stress

FROM DR. SHEN: Too much thinking or worry can impair the circulation. In this condition, the migraine migrates.

Formula I for migraine from internal stress:

Pin Yin	Latin	English	Dosage
Tian ma	Gastrodiae Rhizoma	Gastrodia rhizome	9 g
Chuan xiong	Chuanxiong Rhizoma	Chuanxiong root, Szechuan lovage root, cnidium	4.5 g
Jing jie	Schizonepetae Herba	Schizonepeta	4.5 g
Bai ju hua	Chrysanthemi Flos	Wild chrysanthemum flower (white)	9 g
Xiang fu	Cyperi Rotundi Rhizoma	Nut grass rhizoma, cyperus	4.5 g
Bai shao	Paeoniae Alba Radix	White peony root	6 g
Chai hu	Bupleuri Radix	Hare's ear root, thorowax root, bupleurum	3 g
Yu jin	Curcumae Radix	Curcuma tuber	9 g
Yan hu suo	Corydalis Yanhusuo Rhizoma	Corydalis rhizome	9 g

Hamilton Rotte The TCM literature usually attributes migraines to blood stasis, liver *qi* stagnation, liver *yin* deficiency and *yang* rising, liver blood deficiency, or phlegm.

This formula addresses liver *qi* stagnation and blood stasis. Migraines almost always occur at least partially because of blood stasis (patients with migraines have a history of trauma to the head or neck), but other pathologies of the liver frequently complicate the condition.

In the treatment of migraines in general, it is beneficial to descend energy because of the tendency of the liver to send its energies upward. When liver *qi* stagnation is part of a migraine presentation, using the standard liver *qi*-regulating formulas with a large dose of *chai hu* can be problematic because of the ascending nature of *chai hu*. In this formula we can see that the dose of *chai hu* is minimal and therefore offers a viable alternative.

This formula contains medicinals that regulate the liver *qi* (*xiang fu*, *yu jin*, *chai hu*), medicinals that move the blood and relieve pain (*chuan xiong*, *yu jin*, *yan hu suo*), and medicinals that target the head (*chuan xiong*, *ju hua*, *jing jie*). Perhaps most importantly, we find that this formula has a descending tendency with larger dosages of descending herbs: *tian ma*, *yu jin*, and *bai shao*. *Tian ma* is especially important in this formula as well because of its strong pain-relieving effect and its ability to enter both the main channels and the collaterals.

Formula II for migraine from internal stress:

Pin Yin	Latin	English	Dosage
Tian ma	Gastrodiae Rhizoma	Gastrodia rhizome	9 g
Chuan xiong	Chuanxiong Rhizoma	Chuanxiong root, Szechuan lovage root, cnidium	4.5 g
Jing jie	Schizonepetae Herba	Schizonepeta	4.5 g
Bai shao	Paeoniae Alba Radix	White peony root	6 g
Fu shen	Poria Cocos Pararadicis Sclerotium	Poria fungus	9 g
Yuan zhi	Polygalae Radix	Chinese senega root, polygala root	4.5 g
Duan long chi	Fossilia Dentis Mastodi	Calcined dragon teeth, fossilized teeth	15 g
Zhen zhu mu	Margarita	Mother-of-pearl	15 g[a]
Chao huang qin	Scutellariae Baicalensis Radix	Fried baical skullcap root, scutellaria, scute	4.5 g

[a] Cools liver.

Headache, Migraine from an Old Injury

FROM DR. SHEN: This type of migraine will tend to be on either the left or right side of the head. Over time, however, it can spread. Shock and injury cause poor circulation and weakened *qi*. When the body's energy is low, the migraine will manifest. To check for an old injury, look at the eyes—there will be a red line under the eyelid on the side of the injury. The pain from this type of migraine weakens the body's energy, and can therefore bring about more frequent occurrences. The pulse will be a little tight.

Pin Yin	Latin	English	Dosage
Dang gui	Angelicae Sinensis Radix	Chinese angelica root, *tang-kuei*	9 g
Chuan xiong	Chuanxiong Rhizoma	Chuanxiong root, Szechuan lovage root, cnidium	4.5 g
Bai zhi	Angelicae Dahuricae Radix	Angelica root	6 g
San qi	Notoginseng Radix	Noto ginseng root, root of pseudo-ginseng	0.6 g
Fang feng	Saposhnikoviae Radix	Ledebouriella root, saposhnikoviae root, siler	6 g
Dan shen	Salviae Miltiorrhizae Radix	Salvia root	6 g

Pin Yin	Latin	English	Dosage
Sang ji sheng	Taxilli Herba	Mulberry mistletoe stems, loranthus, taxillus, mistletoe	9 g
Hong hua	Carthami Tinctorii Flos	Safflower flower, carthamus	4.5 g
Niu xi or huai niu xi	Achyranthis Bidentatae Radix	Ox-knee root from Huai	9 g

Hamilton Rotte Migraines and headaches in general frequently arise from trauma to the head, which causes blood stasis. This formula primarily moves blood and targets the head, but contains other ingredients that exhibit pain-relieving effects in the head. Also, we find herbs that are markedly descending in order to bring energy down.

Herbs that move blood include *dang gui*, *chuan xiong*, *san qi*, *dan shen*, *hong hua*, and *niu xi*. Clearly, this is the main focus of the formula. *Dang gui*, *san qi*, *chuan xiong*, *hong hua*, and *niu xi* are especially indicated for treating pain. Among the blood-moving ingredients, *chuan xiong* and *hong hua* focus their actions on the head and upper body.

Bai zhi and *fang feng* both target the head and exhibit pain-relieving effects, usually attributed to their ability to expel wind.

This formula contains some herbs that nourish blood and *yin*, notably *dang gui*, *sang ji sheng*, and *niu xi*. These offset drying tendencies of blood-moving and wind-expelling herbs.

Sang ji sheng and *niu xi* both tend to exhibit their effects on the lower body and are therefore descending in nature, a method of treatment utilized in all of Dr. Shen's formulas for migraines.

Leon Hammer Again, Dr. Shen placed special emphasis on trauma as a prerequisite cause of intractable headache. He searched the skull for tender *ashi* points and pointed out to me swelling at some of these points that he associated in young women with trauma, which he said also caused obesity. While I observed the women we examined to indeed be obese, he never explained the connection.

My own extensive experience has supported his view, particularly with regard to women who ride horseback. On questioning, these equestrian women's history of considerable trauma to the head by horses is deeply repressed. From my perspective the affinity of women for horses is a mixed blessing since the kicks in the head, the endless trauma is as nothing to them. They suffer, but make no connection between their pain and their love in this unequal relationship. The horses have won and the women celebrate their triumph.

Headache, Migraine from Weakness

Pin Yin	Latin	English	Dosage
Dang gui tou	Angelica Sinensis Radix	Angelica root head	9 g
Chuan xiong	Chuanxiong Rhizoma	Chuanxiong root, Szechuan lovage root, cnidium	6 g
Shu di huang	Rehmanniae Preparata Radix	Prepared Chinese foxglove root (cooked in red wine), cooked rehmannia rhizome	12 g
Bai shao	Paeoniae Alba Radix	White peony root	6 g
Fu ling	Poria Cocos Sclerotium	Sclerotium of tuckahoe, poria, China root, hoelen, Indian bread	9 g
Yuan zhi	Polygalae Radix	Chinese senega root, polygala root	6 g

Pin Yin	Latin	English	Dosage
Shan yao	Dioscoreae Oppositae Rhizoma	Chinese yam root, dioscorea rhizome	12 g
Man jing zi	Viticis Fructus	Vitex fruit	6 g

Hamilton Rotte Here is another formula from Dr. Shen aimed at treating migraines in a deficient individual. The deficiencies addressed, like the previous formula, are blood deficiency and kidney deficiency. This formula also contains an herb that targets the head and relieves pain.

Blood tonics in this formula include *dang gui tou* (*dang gui* root head), *shu di huang*, and *bai shao*. *Chuan xiong* is included to move blood in order to balance the tonics, as in *Si Wu Tang* (Four Substance Decoction). *Dang gui tou* also has a blood-moving, pain-relieving effect.

Kidney tonics include *shan yao* and possibly *yuan zhi*. *Shan yao* is a highly regarded tonic for both the *yin* and *yang* of the kidneys and some sources indicate that *yuan zhi* is a kidney tonic, including a text from Ding Gan Ren.

Fu ling, which exhibits a descending tendency, is possibly included to prevent cloying effects from moistening blood tonics. Also, it is possibly included because dampness and phlegm often contribute to headaches. *Man jing zi*, utilized in many other of Dr. Shen's formulas for headaches and migraines, targets the head and exhibits pain-relieving effects.

Melancholia

FROM DR. SHEN: This kind of patient is lost in depressed meditation all day long, even when there is no particular reason for this. It comes mainly from mental vexation because so much burdens the mind. This causes the *qi* to stagnate, leading to disorders of the entire *qi* mechanism in the chest. There is a distaste for food and this type of melancholia leads to sleeplessness. It is of great significance to revive the individual psychologically, as well as with herbal treatments.

Formula for treating melancholia:

Pin Yin	Latin	English	Dosage
Dang shen	Codonopsis Pilosulae Radix	Codonopsis root	10 g
Bai zhu	Atractylodis Macrocephalae Rhizoma	White atractylodes rhizome	10 g
Fu ling	Poria Cocos Sclerotium	Sclerotium of tuckahoe, poria, China root, hoelen, Indian bread	10 g
Yuan zhi	Polygalae Radix	Chinese senega root, polygala root	6 g
Suan zao ren	Ziziphi Spinosae Semen	Spiny zizyphus seeds, sour jujube seeds, zizyphus	12 g
Sheng gan cao	Glycyrrhizae Radix	Fresh licorice root	6 g
Guang mu xiang	Saussureae Lappae Radix or Aucklandia Lappae Radix	Costus root, saussurea, aucklandia from Guangdong Province	6 g
Ju jin	Curcumae Radix	Curcuma tuber	10 g
Xiang fu	Cyperi Rotunda Rhizoma	Nutgrass rhizome, cyperus	10 g

Boil the medicines into tea and drink.

Hamilton Rotte   Depression can arise from pathology of any of the five *zang* organs. The most severe type of depression comes from kidney *yang* deficiency. This is a severe, endogenous depression. Stagnation of liver *qi* causes an agitated depression (depression with feelings of irritability and frustration or anger). The lung-type depression is marked by prolonged, intractable grief (melancholy). Heart-type depression is marked by lack of joy. Spleen-type depression is marked by lethargy and foggy mentation. This view of depression is specific to Dr. Shen and Dr. Hammer's viewpoint (Contemporary Oriental Medicine).

This formula primarily focuses on the middle burner, notably the spleen and liver. Frequently it is advisable to address pathologies in the middle burner before transitioning to treatment of other organs as the middle burner responds more quickly to treatment. The treatment principles for this formula are to tonify the spleen, expel dampness and phlegm, and regulate the liver *qi*. Herbs that tonify the spleen include *dang shen*, *bai zhu*, and *fu ling* and *gan cao*. This constitutes the famous *Si Jun Zi Tang* (Four Gentlemen Decoction). *Dang shen* is utilized instead of *ren shen* (ginseng, which has a greater tendency to make people agitated). *Mu xiang* is partially included to treat damp excess of the spleen.

Herbs that regulate the liver *qi* include *mu xiang*, *yu jin*, and *xiang fu*. *Xiang fu* and *yu jin*, in particular, are especially effective in treating mental-emotional aspects of liver *qi* stagnation.

Yuan zhi, one of Dr. Shen's favorite herbs, is included here to resolve "phlegm misting the orifices." "Phlegm misting the orifices" by itself causes dull, foggy mental function and has the ability to make mental-emotional conditions chronic. *Yuan zhi* also moves *qi* in the chest, thereby addressing lung and heart *qi* stagnation, prominent contributors to depression.

Suan zao ren may be included as a moistening agent to balance the drying tendencies of moving herbs. It is also sour and consolidating, highly beneficial to balancing a formula of acrid, moving herbs. It is also noteworthy that most cases of depression include an element of anxiety, for which *suan zao ren* is extremely effective.

Leon Hammer   Postpartum depression afflicts a large percentage of women in urbanized Western-style societies, especially after the second and subsequent children. This was largely unknown by people closer to their traditional roots but who even in China when I was there in 1981 routinely supplemented women's diet with blood- and *qi*-nourishing herbs from menarche to menopause.

From the viewpoint of Chinese medicine, postpartum depression is due to deficiency of both *qi* and blood. Proper nourishment is the remedy. It is most important that the young mother relaxes as much as possible and avoids anxieties.

Multiple Sclerosis

FROM DR. SHEN: In the case of a "true" MS condition still in the early stage, use 7-star needle, bleed a little for minor curve of the spine. Use a moxa roll, make warm. Bleeding the spine moves blood.

Pin Yin	Latin	English	Dosage
Chao dang gui	Angelicae Sinensis Radix	Fried Chinese angelica root, *tang-kuei*	9 g
Qiang huo	Notopterygii Rhizoma et Radix	Notopterygium root and rhizome, *chiang-huo*	9 g
Du huo	Angelicae Pubescentis Radix	Pubescent angelica root	9 g
Wei ling xian	Clematidis Radix	Chinese clematis root	9 g
Hong hua	Carthami Tinctorii Flos	Safflower flower, carthamus	6 g
Dan shen	Salviae Miltiorrhiziae Radix	Salvia root	6 g
Xu duan	Dipsaci Asperi Radix	Japanese teasel root, dipsacus	9 g
San qi	Notoginseng Radix	Noto ginseng root, root of pseudo-ginseng	4.5 g

Pin Yin	Latin	English	Dosage
Gou ji	Cibotii Rhizoma	Cibotium rhizome, chain fern	12 g
Fang feng	Saposhnikoviae Radix	Ledebouriella root, saposhnikoviae root, siler	4.5 g
Sang zhi	Ramulus Mori Albae	Mulberry twig, morus twig	12 g

Add as needed:

Pin Yin	Latin	English	Dosage
Nan sha shen	Adenophorae seu Glehniae Radix	Adenophora root or glehnia root, ladybell root	9–15 g
Yuan zhi	Polygalae Radix	Chinese senega root, polygala	6–15 g

Hamilton Rotte In the literature, MS is attributed to phlegm-heat, blood deficiency, qi deficiency, and kidney yin or yang deficiency.

In this formula, the focus is on expelling wind-dampness (as in a bi syndrome), moving blood, strengthening sinews and bones, and tonifying the kidneys.

Dr. Shen emphasized the effects of trauma in the development of MS. In Chinese medicine it known that wind-damp pathogens lodge in areas where there has been a trauma. In the later stages of trauma, herbs that strengthen sinews and bones (and tonify the liver and kidneys) have a special relevance. Here, Dr. Shen is treating MS as a trauma.

Herbs that expel wind-dampness include qiang huo, du huo, wei ling xiang, gou ji, fang feng, and sang zhi. This is the primary focus of the formula. Herbs that target the upper body include qiang huo, sang zhi, and fang feng. Herbs that target the lower body include du huo and wei ling xian.

Herbs that move blood include dang gui, dan shen, hong hua, and san qi. These directly address the trauma.

Herbs that strengthen the sinews and bones include xu duan and gou ji. These are also kidney yang tonics, which Dr. Shen indicated was an underlying condition that predisposed an individual to MS.

Herbs that were indicated as optional include nan sha shen (for yin deficiency) and yuan zhi, which may be included as a tonic for the kidneys.

Dang gui may have been included to offset the drying tendencies of the wind-damp-expelling herbs, and as means of tonifying blood. Blood deficiency has been documented as a contributing factor in MS.

Leon Hammer Dr. Shen's comments to me about the etiology of MS primarily involved trauma to the spine, especially at a young age, with perhaps a vulnerable "marrow" due to an inherent kidney essence deficiency.

This formula suggests a wind-cold invasion that is discussed in detail under "Allergies, Internal" and "Allergy and Chronic Fatigue" and was in Dr. Shen's opinion the source, if unresolved, of many chronic debilitating diseases.

Nervous System Tense, Original Formula

Pin Yin	Latin	English	Dosage
Chuan xiong	Chuanxiong Rhizoma	Chuanxiong root, Szechuan lovage root, cnidium	5 g
Yu jin	Curcumae Radix	Curcuma tuber	6 g
Lu lu tong	Liquidambaris Fructus	Sweetgum fruit, liquidambar fruit	12 g
Jing jie	Schizonepetae Herba	Schizonepeta	2 g

Pin Yin	Latin	English	Dosage
Bai shao	Paeoniae Alba Radix	White peony root	6 g
Yin chai hu	Stellariae Radix	Stellaria root	3 g
Xiang fu	Cyperi Rotundi Rhizoma	Nut grass rhizoma, cyperus	2 g
Yan hu suo	Corydalis Yanhusuo Rhizoma	Corydalis rhizome	10 g
Huang qin	Scutellariae Baicalensis Radix	Baical skullcap root, scutellaria, scute	2 g

Hamilton Rotte   Dr. Shen's concept of the nervous system seemed to be that it was the system that affected all other systems and tissues in the body. Nervous tension should be addressed by utilizing moving herbs for each tissue.

Chuan xiong may be included because of its well-known effect on the central nervous system. Yu jin exerts its effects on the liver and heart. Lu lu tong moves the channels. Jing jie works on the skin. Bai shao works on the smooth muscle. Yin chai hu works at the level of the bones.

Xiang fu operates on the triple burner, therefore affecting energy flow in the whole organism, and works on the liver and treats the reproductive organs. Xiang fu is also highly effective for mental-emotional constraint.

Yan hu suo and huang qin affect the organs of the digestive system. The two of them together move qi and blood in the digestive organs and reduce heat that occurs in these organs.

Nervous System Tense

FROM DR. SHEN: This is the basic nervous system formula from February 2000, used for "Nervous System Tense." Western doctors don't detect nervous system problems by testing; they are caused by a person's lifestyle.

Pin Yin	Latin	English	Dosage
Shi chang pu	Acori Tatarinowii Rhizoma	Grass-leaved sweetflag rhizome, acorus	2.4 g

For heart nerves:

Pin Yin	Latin	English	Dosage
Chuan xiong	Chuanxiong Rhizoma	Chuangxiong rhizome	4.5 g

Relaxes nerves (not move blood):

Pin Yin	Latin	English	Dosage
Jing jie	Schizonepetae Herba	Schizonepeta	3 g

Relaxes skin nerves:

Pin Yin	Latin	English	Dosage
Bai shao	Paeoniae Alba Radix	White peony root	6 g

Inside nerves:

Pin Yin	Latin	English	Dosage
Xiang fu	Cyperi Rotunda Rhizoma	Nutgrass rhizome, cyperus	4.5 g

Organ nerves:

Pin Yin	Latin	English	Dosage
Ge gen	Puerariae Radix	Kudzu root, pueraria	4.5 g
Gua lou pi	Trichosanthis Pericarpium	Peel of Mongolian snakegourd	9 g

Muscle nerves:

Pin Yin	Latin	English	Dosage
Yu jin	Curcumae Radix	Curcuma tuber	6 g

Nervous System Tense and *Yin*-deficient Heat

Formula from February 2000:

Pin Yin	Latin	English	Dosage
Zhi bie jia	Carapax Amydae Sinensis	Honey-fried Chinese soft-shelled turtle shell	12 g
Chai hu	Bupleuri Radix	Hare's ear root, thorowax root, bupleurum	3 g
Qing hao	Artemisiae Annuae Herba	Wormwood, *ching-hao*	9 g
Di gu pi	Lycii Radicis Cortex	Cortex of wolfberry root, lycium bark	9 g
Fu ling	Poria Cocos Sclerotium	Sclerotium of tuckahoe, poria, China root, hoelen, Indian bread	9 g
Yuan zhi	Polygalae Radix	Chinese senega root, polygala root	4.5 g
Long chi	Fossilia Dentis Mastodi	Dragon teeth, fossilized teeth	18 g
Mu li	Ostreae Concha	Oyster shell	12 g
Yu jin	Curcumae Radix	Curcuma tuber	9 g
Chao bai shao	Paeoniae Alba Radix	Dry-fried white peony root	9 g
Lu lu tong	Liquidambaris Fructus	Sweetgum fruit, liquidambar fruit	12 g

Hamilton Rotte This formula contains herbs that clear deficient heat, regulate *qi*, and calm the spirit. Herbs that clear deficient heat include *bie jia*, *qing hao*, and *di gu pi*. Herbs that regulate *qi* include *chai hu*, *yu jin*, and *lu lu tong*. *Bai shao* "softens the liver" and by nourishing liver blood aids in the smooth flow of *qi*.
Spirit-calming herbs include *fu ling*, *yuan zhi*, *long chi*, and *mu li*.

Leon Hammer When tension is found uniformly over the entire pulse, I refer to it as the "vigilance" pulse because it appears constitutionally in ethnic groups whose survival through the centuries has required extraordinary vigilance. A similar pulse quality can be found today in almost anyone living in a large city, or living constantly with the need to be vigilant. Therefore, a differential diagnosis is required be- tween a constitutional "nervous system tense" and one that is due to ongoing chronic stress. Making this distinction is important since individuals whose tension is related to their current life situation can alter their lifestyle as part of the solution. That is less true for those for whom the etiology is constitutional.
The principal symptom is an ongoing tension that may or may not be related to a particular life stress. The

tension can be in the family over several generations. Accompanying symptoms depend on the vulnerability of other organ systems that are affected by the stasis and especially excess heat that can be a consequence of this condition when it persists over a long period of time.

Nervous System Weak, Original Formula

Pin Yin	Latin	English	Dosage
Chuan xiong	Chuanxiong Rhizoma	Chuanxiong root, Szechuan lovage root, cnidium	4.5 g
Yu jin	Curcumae Radix	Curcuma tuber	4.5 g
Jing jie	Schizonepetae Herba	Schizonepeta	3 g
Bai shao	Paeoniae Alba Radix	White peony root	6 g
Xiang fu	Cyperi Rotundi Rhizoma	Nut grass rhizoma, cyperus	4.5 g
Yan hu suo	Corydalis Yanhusuo Rhizoma	Corydalis rhizome	9 g
Bai zhu	Atractylodis Macrocephalae Rhizoma	White atractylodes rhizome	6 g
Huang qi	Astragali Radix	Milk vetch root, astragalus root	9 g
Shan yao	Dioscoreae Oppositae Rhizoma	Chinese yam root, dioscorea rhizome	9 g
Gan cao	Glycyrrhizae Radix	Licorice root	4.5 g

Hamilton Rotte   This formula regulates *qi*, in particular the liver, and tonifies the *qi*, particularly the spleen *qi*. Liver *qi*-regulating herbs include *yu jin* and *xiang fu*. *Yan hu suo* moves liver blood. *Bai shao* is included to tonify liver blood, which aids in regulating the liver *qi*.

Chuan xiong and *jing jie* are ingredients that are both included in Dr. Shen's "Nervous System Tense" basic formula, implying that he utilized these in an unusual manner to relieve nervous tension.

Qi tonics in this formula especially target the spleen including *bai zhu*, *huang qi*, and *shan yao*.

Nervous System Weak, Recent Formula

Pin Yin	Latin	English	Dosage
Ren shen	Ginseng Radix	Ginseng root	4.5 g
Fu ling	Poria Cocos Sclerotium	Sclerotium of tuckahoe, poria, China root, hoelen, Indian bread	9 g
Da zao	Zizyphi Jujubae Fructus	Chinese date, jujube	9 g
Bie jia	Carapax Amydae Sinensis	Chinese soft-shelled turtle shell	12 g
Yuan zhi	Polygalae Radix	Chinese senega root, polygala root	6 g
Bai shao	Paeoniae Alba Radix	White peony root	6 g
Nuo dao gen xu	Oryzae Glutinosae Radix	Glutinous rice root	30 g
Chai hu	Bupleuri Radix	Hare's ear root, thorowax root, bupleurum	3 g
Di gu pi	Lycii Radicis Cortex	Cortex of wolfberry root, lycium bark	9 g

Nervous System Weak

From February 2000, this was mentioned as a modification of the "Nervous System Tense" formula when the organs are weak.

> **FROM DR. SHEN:**
> *Pulse:*
> Both sides same, tight and a little fast.

Pin Yin	Latin	English	Dosage
Shi chang pu	Acori Tatarinowii Rhizoma	Grass-leaved sweetflag rhizome, acorus	2.4 g

For heart nerves:

Pin Yin	Latin	English	Dosage
Chuan xiong	Chuanxiong Rhizoma	Chuangxiong rhizome	4.5 g

Relaxes nerves (not move blood):

Pin Yin	Latin	English	Dosage
Jing jie	Schizonepetae Herba	Schizonepeta	3 g

Relaxes skin nerves:

Pin Yin	Latin	English	Dosage
Bai shao	Paeoniae Alba Radix	White peony root	6 g

Inside nerves:

Pin Yin	Latin	English	Dosage
Xiang fu	Cyperi Rotunda Rhizoma	Nutgrass rhizome, cyperus	4.5 g

Organ nerves:

Pin Yin	Latin	English	Dosage
Ge gen	Puerariae Radix	Kudzu root, pueraria	4.5 g
Gua lou pi	Trichosanthis Pericarpium	Peel of Mongolian snakegourd	9 g

Muscle nerves:

Pin Yin	Latin	English	Dosage
Yu jin	Curcumae Radix	Curcuma tuber	6 g

Tonic herbs:

Pin Yin	Latin	English	Dosage
Dang gui	Angelicae Sinensis Radix	Chinese angelica root, *tang-kuei*	No dose mentioned
Huang qi	Astragali Radix	Milk vetch root, astragalus root	No dose mentioned

Leon Hammer   Another condition described by Dr. Shen is "nervous system weak." Again, this is a constitutional condition, and Dr. Shen describes a progression of pulse qualities over time not found in my own experience (Hammer, 2001, p. 577). While I have not found any predictable pulse picture with this condition, often there is a smooth vibration at all positions and all depths, a left side that is deep with reduced substance, especially the left proximal (kidney), both progressing over a long time to a "*qi* wild" pulse and emotionally chaotic condition. With a concomitant *yin*-deficient condition the pulse can be changing back and forth from reduced substance to tight at the left proximal position.

This condition is often found in a person who has a life-long history of "neurasthenia," one whose symptoms are always changing without identifiable biomedical disease. They are highly vulnerable, unstable, and easily disturbed or stressed, and also subject to constantly fluctuating allergies. The disorder doesn't represent illness as much as physical and mental instability and vulnerability to illness. However, due to this vulnerability they are like the "canary in the mine," experiencing reactions to toxic environmental stimuli before other more robust people and more likely to avoid them and survive longer.

Hammer formula for "nervous system weak" (altered lycium formula [Bensky 2009, p. 404]):

Pin Yin	Latin	English	Dosage
Shu di huang	Rehmanniae Preparata Radix	Prepared Chinese foxglove root (cooked in red wine), cooked rehmannia rhizome	9–30 g
Gou qi zi	Lycii Fructus	Chinese wolfberry, matrimony vine fruit, lycium fruit	6–15 g
Shan yao	Dioscoreae Oppositae Rhizoma	Chinese yam root, dioscorea rhizome	9–30 g
Fu shen	Poria Cocos Pararadicis Sclerotium	Poria fungus	9–15 g
Rou cong rong	Cistanches Herba	Cistanche, fleshy stem of the broomrape	3–18 g
Xiao hui xiang	Foeniculi Fructus	Fennel seed	3–9 g
Ba ji tian	Morinda Officinalis Radix	Morinda root	6–15 g
Du zhong	Eucommiae Cortex	Eucommia bark	6–15 g
Niu xi or *huai niu xi*	Achyranthis Bidentatae Radix	Ox-knee root from Huai	9–15 g
Wu wei zi	Schisandrae Chinensis Fructus	Schisandra fruit	6–9 g
Yuan zhi	Polygalae Radix	Chinese senega root, polygala root	3–9 g
Shi chang pu	Acori Tatarinowii Rhizoma	Grass-leaved sweetflag rhizome, acorus	3–9 g
Da zao	Ziziphi Jujubae Fructus	Chinese date, jujube	4 g
Chu shi zi	Broussonetia	Paper mulberry fruit	6–9 g
Shan zhu yu	Corni Officinalis Fructus	Asiatic Cornelian cherry fruit, cornus	6–12 g
Yin yang huo	Epimedii Herba	Aerial parts of epimedium	3–12 g
For heart fire:			
Lian zi	Nelumbinis Semen	Lotus seed	8 g

Nervous System: Diarrhea from Nervous System

FROM DR. SHEN: Diarrhea from nervous system comes from emotions; watery, comes out quickly, without pain.

Pin Yin	Latin	English	Dosage
Mu xiang	Saussureae Lappae Radix or Aucklandia Lappae Radix	Costus root, saussurea, aucklandia	6 g
Chuan lian zi	Meliae Toosendan Fructus	Szechuan pagoda tree fruit, Szechuan chinaberry, melia	4.5 g
Yan hu suo	Corydalis Yanhusuo Rhizoma	Corydalis rhizome	9 g
Bai shao	Paeoniae Alba Radix	White peony root	6 g

Hamilton Rotte Nervous tension causes stagnation of qi and blood and this affects the most vulnerable area of the body. If this is the intestines, urgent, watery, and possibly explosive diarrhea results. Dr. Shen's concept of nervous tension is roughly equivalent to stagnation of liver qi. In this formula the herbs that regulate the liver qi include mu xiang, chuan lian zi, and bai shao.

Herbs that especially regulate qi and blood in the intestines include mu xiang, yan hu suo, and bai shao. Because of the pain-relieving effects of all of the ingredients, this formula would also be indicated if diarrhea caused by emotional distress was also accompanied by the symptom of pain.

Muscle Nerve Pain, Herb Bath

Pin Yin	Latin	English	
Ma huang	Ephedrae Herba	Ephedra stem	As needed
Ma qian zi	Strychni Semen	Nux-vomica seeds	As needed
Ge gen	Puerariae Radix	Kudzu root, pueraria	As needed
Fang feng	Saposhnikoviae Radix	Ledebouriella root, saposhnikoviae root, siler	As needed
Ru xiang	Gummi Olibanum	Frankincense, mastic	As needed
Mo yao	Myrrha	Myrrh	As needed
Qiang huo	Notopterygii Rhizoma et Radix	Notopterygium root and rhizome, chiang-huo	As needed
Dang gui	Angelicae Sinensis Radix	Chinese angelica root, tang-kuei	As needed
Dan shen	Salviae Miltiorrhiziae Radix	Salvia root	As needed
Hong hua	Carthami Tinctorii Flos	Safflower flower, carthamus	As needed
Wang bu liu xing	Vaccariae Segetalis Semen	Vaccaria seed	As needed

Hamilton Rotte This formula is moving to both qi and blood (and pain relieving), it targets the muscles, and contains many surface-releasing ingredients. The surface-releasing ingredients may be included as a means to resolve stagnation through the exterior. The ingredients that move qi and especially blood include ru xiang, mo yao, dang gui, dan shen, hong hua, and wang bu liu xing. Many of these, notably ru xiang and mo yao, are the strongest pain-relieving ingredients in Chinese medicine. Ma qian zi, considered obsolete because of toxicity, exerts its moving effects on the channels and collaterals.

Herbs that target the muscles include *ge gen* and *qiang huo*.

Herbs that release the exterior include *ma huang*, *ge gen*, and *fang feng*, clearly indicating that Dr. Shen viewed this treatment principle as an important aspect of addressing this condition.

Leon Hammer
Ginger bath:
During the years when I was with Dr. Shen he prescribed the ginger bath for pain. The results from the ginger bath have been extraordinary. See page 92 above for instructions.
Pulse:
- Chronic severe pain on the pulse is represented with an extreme tight quality on the entire pulse and especially in the position as one rotates one's finger laterally or radially as follows, already mentioned on page 114:
  - Neck–head–shoulder pain: rolling radially from the distal positions
  - Hip–lower back pain: rolling radially from the middle positions
  - Knee–ankle: rolling radially from the proximal position

Organ Nerves Tight (Pain)

Pin Yin	Latin	English	Dosage
Xie bai	Albi Bulbus	Bulb of Chinese chive, macrostem onion, bakeri	4.5 g
Gua lou pi	Trichosanthis Pericarpium	Peel of trichosanthes fruit	9 g
Wu yao	Linderae Radix	Lindera root	3 g
Yu jin	Curcumae Radix	Curcuma tuber	4.5 g
E zhu	Curcumae Rhizoma	Zedoary rhizoma, zedoaria	1.8 g
Yan hu suo	Corydalis Yanhusuo Rhizoma	Corydalis rhizome	9 g
Lu lu tong	Liquidambaris Fructus	Sweetgum fruit, liquidambar fruit	9 g
Zhi ke	Citri Aurantii Fructus	Mature fruit of the bitter orange	4.5 g
Hou po	Magnoliae Officinalis Cortex	Magnolia bark	1.8 g
Ru xiang	Gummi Olibanumi	Frankincense, mastic	4.5 g
Mo yao	Myrrha	Myrrh	4.5 g
Shi chang pu	Acori Tatarinowii Rhizoma	Grass-leaved sweetflag rhizome, acorus	2.4 g
Ding xiang	Caryophilli Flos	Clove flower bud	3 g
Chuan xiong	Chuanxiong Rhizoma	Chuanxiong root, Szechuan lovage root, cnidium	2.4 g

Hamilton Rotte This formula contains *qi*- and blood-invigorating ingredients that relieve pain. *Shi chang pu*, *xie bai*, and *gua lou pi* target the chest. *Wu yao*, *yu jin*, *e zhu*, *chuan xiong* and *yan hu suo* target the liver. *Lu lu tong*, *zhi ke*, *ding xiang*, and *hou po* target the spleen and stomach.

Skin Nerves (Pain)

Pin Yin	Latin	English	Dosage
Jing jie	Schizonepetae Herba	Schizonepeta	3 g
Ge gen	Puerariae Radix	Kudzu root, pueraria	3 g
Fang feng	Saposhnikoviae Radix	Ledebouriella root, saposhnikoviae root, siler	3 g
Chan tui	Periostracum Cicadae	Cicada moultings	3 g
Chuan xiong	Chuanxiong Rhizoma	Chuanxiong root, Szechuan lovage root, cnidium	4.5 g
Gui zhi	Ramulus Cinnamomi Cassiae	Cinnamon twig, cassia twig	4.5 g
Chai hu	Bupleuri Radix	Hare's ear root, thorowax root, bupleurum	4.5 g

Hamilton Rotte This formula releases the exterior and moves blood to relieve pain. Herbs that release the exterior include *jing ji, ge gen, fang feng, chan tui, chuan xiong, gui zhi*, and *chai hu* (all of the ingredients). Herbs that are moving include *fang feng, gui zhi, chai hu*, and *chuan xiong*.

Leon Hammer The ginger bath is useful here as well (see above, p. 92).

Schizophrenia

Leon Hammer The terms "mental derangement" and "insanity" are not distinguishable in allopathic psychiatry. According to the texts, what is perhaps meant is that "mental derangement" may be what is commonly alluded to in Chinese medicine as "phlegm-cold" and associated with depression or the depressed aspect of bipolar disease and "phlegm-fire" and associated with the manic phase of bipolar disease.

The confusion between schizophrenia and bipolar disease has existed in allopathic psychiatry until recently. With the concept of "phlegm-misting the orifices" accounting for mental (neurosis to psychosis) to neurological conditions (epilepsy) the subject is even more confused in Chinese medicine than allopathically.

I have found the bipolar condition rooted in a triple burner defect in which the control of the wood feeding the fire goes out of control. The manic phase is one in which the wood is being consumed at a greatly increased rate, causing a heart fire condition. The balance of heart fire by kidney *yin* is strained to the extreme and ultimately lost.

When the wood is depleted and little is supplied to the heart the depressive phase begins, exacerbated by the kidney *yin* that is still being sent to the heart that is no longer on fire.

I find that there is a continuity between neurosis and psychosis including schizophrenia in the degree of the "phlegm misting the orifices" of the heart. The greater the "misting" the greater the loss of awareness and the more serious the loss of touch with reality and boundaries between the inner psyche of one's own thoughts and feelings, and the thoughts and feelings of others (Hammer, 2007).

FROM DR. SHEN: In Chinese medicine this disease is subdivided into two kinds: mental derangement and insanity.

A deranged person may at first be very much distressed by an unrealized ambition or astonished so much beyond his or her bounds of tolerance that his "*qi*" goes in conflict with the blood. This stagnant "*qi*" coagulates with fluids into phlegm. The phlegm enfolds the heart and its ingenuity and the patient loses his or her normal senses. A deranged person speaks incoherently, goes from sudden rapture to utter misery, is rarely found hungry or thirsty and has a thin tongue with a curdy coating. The pulses are stringy and slippery.

An insane person is always lost in delirium. They engage in violent actions or activities, attacking, singing, laughing or weeping, swearing, from one extreme to another, causing disturbances or even injury. The tongue coat is curdy and yellow and the pulses are stringy and slippery. This disease also comes from enormously frustrated emotions in their heart of hearts. They are so bewildered that the "*qi*" of their liver and gallbladder is transformed into fire that scorches the fluids into phlegm. The phlegm-fire shrouds the heart and its alertness. For the treatment of such a disease, we have to set the "*qi*" free, restoring it to its normal activity and releasing it from long-term pent-up depression so it can liquidate the clouded phlegm for the recovery of the lost wisdom. Only by cleaning the liver and the gallbladder can we hope to dispel phlegm and curtail the fire, the causes of all the trouble.

Formula for derangement:

Pin Yin	Latin	English	Dosage
Sheng zhi shi	Fructus Immaturus Citri Aurantii	Fresh immature bitter orange	10 g
Zhu ru	Bambussae in Taeniis Caulis	Bamboo shavings	10 g
Zhi ban xia	Pinelliae Preparatum Rhizoma	Dried processed pinellia rhizome	6 g
Chen pi	Citri Reticulatae Pericarpium	Tangerine peel	6 g
Fu ling	Poria Cocos Sclerotium	Sclerotium of tuckahoe, poria, China root, hoelen, Indian bread	12 g
Sheng gan cao	Glycyrrhizae Radix	Fresh licorice root	6 g
Yuan zhi	Polygalae Radix	Chinese senega root, polygala root	6 g
Shi chang pu	Acori Tatarinowii Rhizoma	Grass-leaved sweetflag rhizome, acorus	10 g
Yu jin	Curcumae Radix	Curcuma tuber	15 g
Tian zhi huang	Concretio Silicea Bambusae Textillis	Tabasheer or siliceous secretions of bamboo	10 g

Boil the medicines into tea.

Hamilton Rotte This formula, which is a modification of *Wen Dan Tang* (Warm the Gallbladder Decoction), clears heat, resolves "phlegm misting the orifices," and regulates liver *qi*.

The herbs that clear heat (with a focus on the heart) are *tian zhi huang* and *zhu ru*. The herbs the resolve "phlegm misting the orifices" include *zhu ru*, *tian zhi huang*, *shi chang pu*, *yuan zhi*, and to a mild degree *yu jin*. This is the major focus of the formula. It has been well documented how "phlegm misting the orifices" contributes to mental disorders. *Zhi shi*, *zhi ban xia*, and *chen pi* resolve dampness in the spleen and stomach, which frequently contribute to "phlegm misting the orifices" of the heart.

Yu jin is included to regulate the liver *qi*.

Leon Hammer See the text following the next formula for a commentary about both the formulas concerned with mental illness (see also Hammer, 2007).

Formula for insanity:

Pin Yin	Latin	English	Dosage
Long dan cao	Gentianae Longdancao Radix	Chinese gentian root, gentiana	5 g
Hei shan zhi zi	Gardeniae Jasminoidis Fructus	Charred cape jasmine fruit, gardenia fruit	10 g
Chai hu	Bupleuri Radix	Hare's ear root, thorowax root, bupleurum	5 g
Sheng di huang	Rehmannia Radix	Fresh Chinese foxglove root, rehmannia root	15 g
Bai shao	Paeoniae Alba Radix	White peony root	12 g
Sheng gan cao	Glycyrrhizae Radix	Fresh licorice root	6 g
Huang lian	Coptidis Rhizoma	Coptis rhizome	4 g
Da huang	Rhei Rhizoma et Radix	Rhubarb root and rhizome	6 g
Yuan zhi	Polygalae Radix	Chinese senega root, polygala root	6 g
Dan nan xing	Arisaematis Praeparatum Rhizoma cum Felle Bovis	Arisaema pulvis, Jack in the pulpit rhizome with cow bile	5 g

Hamilton Rotte   This formula, which is a modification of *Long Dan Xie Gan Tang* (Gentiana Decoction to Drain the Liver), is designed to clear heat in the liver and heart and resolve "phlegm misting the orifices." Heat in the liver and heart cause agitation and irritability and "phlegm misting the orifices" causes a distortion of reality.
The herbs that cool the liver include *long dan cao, zhi zi, chai hu, huang lian, bai shao, sheng di huang,* and *da huang. Chai hu* is also utilized as a guide to the liver. The herbs that cool the heart include *zhi zi* and *huang lian.*
Herbs that resolve "phlegm misting the orifices" include *yuan zhi* and *dan nan xing.*
Dang gui and *bai shao,* included in *Long Dan Xie Gan Tang* provide nourishment to *yin* and blood to offset the drying tendencies of the other herbs.

Leon Hammer   Regarding "phlegm misting the orifices" please see Hammer (2007). For further comments about mental illness I recommend Chapter 14 of *Dragon Rises Red Bird Flies,* which is a discussion of Dr. Shen's concept of the "nervous system" (Hammer, 2005).
The formulas listed above under "mental derangement" and "insanity" are ones familiar to me with a gallbladder–heart disharmony. The first formula seems to emphasize the phlegm aspect and the second the heat aspect of "phlegm misting the orifices." From Dr. Shen's descriptions of the conditions, the second formula I associate with more manic-depressive (bipolar) illness in the manic phase and the first with schizophrenia.

Trigeminal Neuralgia

FROM DR. SHEN: Pain at the trigeminal nerves falls into the realm of unilateral severe headache according to Chinese medicine. It is mainly caused by internal emotional injury that causes liver *qi* stagnation to transform into rising fire as described above and occludes the "upper aperture of wisdom" (cranial nerve V). Other possible causes are dental problems or tooth extractions that have hurt the facial nerves. The pain may come and go for a dozen years, afflicting the patient for a long time and not responding to treatment. The Chinese way of treatment is dispersion of the aching nerves through activation of the blood and clearing the channels.

Formula I for trigeminal pain:

Pin Yin	Latin	English	Dosage
Bai shao	Paeoniae Alba Radix	White peony root	30 g
Bai zhi	Angelicae Dahuricae Radix	Angelica root	10 g
Chuan xiong	Chuanxiong Rhizoma	Chuanxiong root, Szechuan lovage root, cnidium	30 g
Dan shen	Salviae Miltiorrhiziae Radix	Salvia root	15 g
Gan cao	Glycyrrhizae Radix	Licorice root	10 g
Di long	Lumbricus	Earthworm, lumbricus	10 g
Quan xie	Buthus Martensi	Scorpion, buthus	10 g
Gou teng	Ramulus cum Uncis Uncariae	Stems and thorns of the gambir vine, uncaria	15 g
Mu li	Ostreae Concha	Oyster shell	30 g
Xi xin	Asari Herba cum Radice	Chinese wild ginger, asarum	3 g

Boil the medicines into tea. Supplement the treatment by employing acupuncture and moxibustion to obtain better effects.

Hamilton Rotte   This formula contains herbs that move *qi* and blood to relieve pain, herbs that target the head, herbs that open the channels, herbs that extinguish wind (addressing neurological conditions), herbs that nourish the liver (which nourishes the nerves), and herbs that expel cold.

Herbs that move *qi* and blood include *dan shen*, *chuan xiong*, *xi xin*, and *di long*. Herbs that target the head include *bai zhi* and *chuan xiong*. Herbs that open the channels and collaterals include *di long*, *quan xie*, and *xi xin*. Herbs that extinguish wind include *gou teng* and *mu li*.

Bai shao is included to nourish the liver *yin* (and therefore the nerves).

Formula II for trigeminal pain:

FROM DR. SHEN: No spicy food, alcohol, or sex. If problem is severe, rest in bed for 2 weeks. Not resting causes nerve problems. Take this formula internally (in two doses daily), then apply as a compress.

Pin Yin	Latin	English	Dosage
Chuan xiong	Chuanxiong Rhizoma	Chuanxiong root, Szechuan lovage root, cnidium	4.5 g
Bai zhi	Angelicae Dahuricae Radix	Angelica root	4.5 g
Jing jie	Schizonepetae Herba	Schizonepeta	4.5 g
Ge gen	Puerariae Radix	Kudzu root, pueraria	4.5 g
Gan cao	Glycyrrhizae Radix	Licorice root	3 g
Qiang huo	Notopterygii Rhizoma et Radix	Notopterygium root and rhizome, *chiang-huo*	4.5 g
Xiang fu	Cyperi Rotundi Rhizoma	Nut grass rhizoma, cyperus	4.5 g

Oncologic Diseases

Leon Hammer
Generic signs of cancer:
Pulse:
- Fl: muffled (3+–5)
- Left middle position: muffled (5) to dead (late) depending on stage
- Engorged positions all present

- Proximal positions: choppy and muffled
- Pelvic lower body: choppy and muffled
Tongue:
- Entire tongue loses shape
- Amorphous and milky
- Sides shriveled and/or loss of color in specific areas

FROM DR. SHEN: Three stages of cancer:
1. Beginning stage
2. Middle stage—people who have strong minds may survive
3. End stage—no hope for survival
Take care of life (style).
If energy goes down then the disease goes up, and vice versa. Don't make the patient nervous or they will die early. Help the patient to relax. Use herbs and a prepared medicine named Snake Venom capsules, #787, following dosage as listed on packaging. Cancer is a blood problem—snake poison clears the blood and helps the immune system. Two to 3 weeks will start to show results. Very early cancer can be cleared up in 6 months to 1 year.
If the doctor's energy is strong the patient's energy becomes strong. Dress well, sleep well, keep your *shen* strong; speak slowly and strongly.

Cancer, Early or Pre-cancer

FROM DR. SHEN: Can be used for lymph, breast, uterus, or prostate problems. This formula can also be used in breast infection (postpartum mastitis). "In two days it will go away. I promise." Strong people should take every day. *Wu gong* is very moving and can tax the energy. The patient must rest.
Cysts may become malignant if the body condition is weak. If a cyst moves on palpation it is not serious. If it does not move the problem comes from the organs and is serious.

Pin Yin	Latin	English	Dosage
Wu gong[a]	Scolopendra Subspinipes	Centipede, scolopendra	10 pieces
Jin yin hua	Lonicerae Flos	Honeysuckle flower, lonicera	30 g

[a] Toxic

Add these for deficient conditions:

Pin Yin	Latin	English	Dosage
Dang gui	Angelicae Sinensis Radix	Chinese angelica root, *tang-kuei*	4.5–15 g
Duang qi	Astragali Radix	Fried milk vetch root, fried astragalus root	9–15 g

Hamilton Rotte   This formula utilizes *wu gong*, one of the strongest collateral-invigorating substances used in TCM to address early stages of cancer or masses that have the possibility of becoming cancerous. In the treatment of cancer, heat toxin-clearing substances are also frequently used and *wu gong* also "attacks toxins and dissipates nodules," slightly paradoxically because of its own inherent toxicity.

Jin yin hua is included here in a large dose to clear heat and toxicity and mitigate the toxicity of *wu gong* and render it more tolerable to the patient.

This two-herb formula is very draining because of the strong moving effects of *wu gong* and the cold nature of *jin yin hua*. Naturally, it requires a significant expenditure of the body's energy to support a very moving herb like *wu gong*. For deficient individuals *qi* and blood tonic herbs (*huang qi* and *dang gui*) are administered along with the formula in order to prevent it from becoming too draining. Regardless, Dr. Shen indicates that the patient must rest while taking this formula because of its draining tendency.

Cancer of the Bladder, Prostate, Ovaries

Pin Yin	Latin	English	Dosage
Niu xi or *huai niu xi*	Achyranthis Bidentatae Radix	Ox-knee root from Huai	6–15 g
Xiang fu	Cyperi Rotundi Rhizoma	Nut grass rhizoma, cyperus	6–12 g
Chuan xiong	Chuanxiong Rhizoma	Chuanxiong root, Szechuan lovage root, cnidium	3–9 g
Shan dou gen	Menispermi Rhizoma/Sophorae Tonkinensis Radix	Root and rhizome of sophora	3–9 g

San Miao San (Three Marvel Powder):

Pin Yin	Latin	English	Dosage
Cang zhu	Atractylodis Rhizoma	Black atractylodes rhizome	3–9 g
Huang bai	Phellodendri Cortex	Amur corktree bark, phellodendron bark	3–12 g
Yi yi ren	Coicis Semen	Seeds of Job's tears, coix seeds	9–30 g

Hamilton Rotte   This is not a formula, but a list of ingredients that can be applied to cancer of the bladder, prostate, and ovaries. Herbs from this list should be selected according to the specifics of the situation. Cancer is usually attributed to dampness and phlegm, stagnation of *qi* and blood and heat toxicity. Certainly herbs that target the effected area are indicated.

Herbs that resolve dampness include *cang zhu*, *huang bai*, and *yi yi ren*. These make up the additional formula called *San Miao San* (Three Marvel Powder), treating dampness in the lower burner.

Blood-invigorating ingredients include *niu xi* and *chuan xiong*. Of these, *niu xi* especially targets the lower burner. *Xiang fu* is a *qi*-regulating ingredient that especially targets the liver. The liver is responsible for regulating *qi* in the reproductive organs, and is therefore especially applicable in this case.

Cancer of the Bones

Pin Yin	Latin	English	Dosage
Gou qi zi	Lycii Fructus	Chinese wolfberry, matrimony vine fruit, lycium fruit	18 g
Xu duan	Dipsaci Asperi Radix	Japanese teasel root, dipsacus	18 g
Bu gu zhi	Psoraleae Corylifoliae Fructus	Psoralea fruit	18 g
Xi xin	Asari Herba cum Radice	Chinese wild ginger, asarum	4.5 g

Hamilton Rotte   This formula contains ingredients to tonify the kidney essence, warm the kidney *yang* and move blood. Bone cancer is marked by pain and weakening of the bones. Herbs that tonify the kidneys include *gou qi zi, xu duan,* and *bu gu zhi* (literally meaning "tonify bone resin"). *Xu duan* and *bu gu zhi* are used specifically to strengthen the bones. *Xu duan* moves blood and has strong pain-relieving effects. *Xi xin* and *bu gu zhi* both warm the interior and expel cold; *xi xin* exhibits particularly strong pain-relieving effects.

Cancer of the Breasts

Formula I for cancer of the breasts:

Pin Yin	Latin	English	Dosage
Jie geng	Platycodi Radix	Root of balloonflower, platycodon root	3–9 g
Chai hu	Bupleuri Radix	Hare's ear root, thorowax root, bupleurum	3–9 g
Pu gong ying	Taraxaci Herba	Dandelion, taraxacum	9–30 g
Chuan shan jia [a]	Mantis Pentadactylae Squama	Pangolin scales	3–9 g
Quan gua lou	Trichosanthis Fructus	Trichosanthes fruit	9–21 g
Qing pi	Citri Reticulatae Pericarpium Viride	Unripe tangerine peel, green tangerine peel, blue citrus	3–9 g
Wang bu liu xing	Vaccariae Segetalis Semen	Vaccaria seeds	4.5–9 g

[a] Obsolete

Add to soften hardness:

Pin Yin	Latin	English	Dosage
Hai zao	Sargassum	Sargassum, seaweed	15 g
Mu li	Ostreae Concha	Oyster shell	15 g

Hamilton Rotte   This is a not intended to be a formula, but it is rather a list of herbs that Dr. Shen suggested would be beneficial for breast cancer. Herbs from this list should be selected according to the specifics of the situation.

Cancer is usually attributed to dampness and phlegm, stagnation of *qi* and blood, and heat toxicity. Herbs that target the effected area are indicated.

Herbs that move blood include *chuan shan jia* and *wang bu liu xing*. Both of these substances target the breasts. *Chuan shan jia* is unavailable because it is a protected species.

Qi regulators in this formula include *jie geng, chai hu, quan gua lou,* and *qing pi. Jie geng* and *quan gua lou* regulate *qi* in the chest in general (more directly affecting the lungs) and *chai hu* and *qing pi* regulate *qi* in the liver. Energy movement in the breasts is mostly related to movement in the lungs and liver.

Pu gong ying is an herb that clears heat and toxicity and directly targets the breasts (i.e., it is indicated for breast abscesses).

Hai zao and *mu li* are salty substances that soften hardness. Masses readily develop in the breasts, and the salty and softening substances are an important means of addressing this condition.

Formula II for cancer of the breasts: use "Leukemia" formula below and add:

Pin Yin	Latin	English	Dosage
Wu gong[a]	Scolopendra Subspinipes	Centipede, scolopendra	10 pieces
Jin yin hua	Lonicerae Flos	Honeysuckle flower, lonicera	30 g

[a] Toxic

Formula for early-stage breast cancer:

Pin Yin	Latin	English	Dosage
Chai hu	Bupleuri Radix	Hare's ear root, thorowax root, bupleurum	10 g
Dang gui	Angelicae Sinensis Radix	Chinese angelica root, *tang-kuei*	10 g
Yu jin	Curcumae Radix	Curcuma tuber	10 g
Gua lui pi	Trichosanthis Pericarpium	Husk of trichosanthes fruit	30 g
Qing pi	Citri Reticulatae Pericarpium Viride	Unripe tangerine peel, green tangerine peel, blue citrus	6 g
San leng	Sparganii Stoloniferi Rhizoma	Bur-reed rhizoma, scirpus	10 g
E zhu	Curcumae Rhizoma	Zedoary rhizoma, zedoaria	10 g
Bai shao	Paeoniae Alba Radix	White peony root	10 g
Chi shao	Paeoniae Rubra Radix	Red peony root	10 g
Chuan bei mu	Fritillaria Cirrhosae Bulbus	Szechuan fritillaria bulb, tendrilled fritillary bulb, fritillaria	10 g
Bai ji li	Tribuli Terrestris Fructus	Caltrop fruit, puncture-vine fruit, tribulus	15 g

Boil the medicine into tea for daily drinking over an extended period of time.

Hamilton Rotte This is a formula designed to treat early-stage breast cancer. It contains ingredients that move *qi* and blood, nourish blood, resolve phlegm, and reduce masses.

Herbs that move *qi* include *chai hu, yu jin, gua lou pi, qing pi*, and *bai ji li. Chai hu, yu jin, qing pi*, and *bai ji li* move *qi* in the liver channel and therefore affect the breasts. *Gua lou pi* moves *qi* in the chest (especially targeting the lungs), therefore affecting the breasts.

Blood movers include *dang gui, yu jin, san leng, e zhu*, and *chi shao. San leng* and *e zhu*, strong blood movers, also reduce masses.

Chuan bei mu resolves phlegm and is indicated for abscesses, particularly in the breasts.

Blood tonics in this formula include *dang gui* and *bai shao*. It is important to tonify blood in order to protect the blood when using strong moving ingredients.

Formula for later-stage breast cancer:

Pin Yin	Latin	English	Dosage
Nu zhen zi	Ligustri Lucidi Fructus	Privet fruit, ligustrum	30 g
Han lian cao	Ecliptae Prostratae Herba	Eclipta	10 g
Dang gui	Angelicae Sinensis Radix	Chinese angelica root, tang-kuei	10 g
Xuan shen	Scrophulariae Radix	Ningpo figwort root, scrophularia	12 g
Shan zhu yu	Corni Officinalis Fructus	Asiatic Cornelian cherry fruit, cornus	10 g
Chuan bei mu	Fritillaria Cirrhosae Bulbus	Szechuan fritillaria bulb, tendrilled fritillary bulb, fritillaria	10 g
Lu jiao shuang	Cornu Cervi Degelatinatium	Leftover dregs after boiling deer antler glue	15 g
Ji xue teng	Jixueteng Radix et Caulis	Spatholobus or milettia root and vine	30 g
Dan shen	Salviae Miltiorrhiziae Radix	Salvia root	15 g
Ban zhi lian	Scutellariae Barbatae Herba	Barbat skullcap, scutellaria	30 g
Si gua luo	Fasciculus Vascularis Luffae	Dried skeleton of vegetable sponge	10 g
Gua lou pi	Trichosanthis Pericarpium	Peel of trichosanthes fruit	30 g

FROM DR. SHEN: Boil the medicines into tea for daily drinking with some addition or deduction of medicines to suit different cases.

Hamilton Rotte This formula is designed to treat kidney yin and yang deficiency, move qi and blood, resolve phlegm, soften hardness, and clear heat and toxicity. Compared to the formula for early-stage breast cancer, this formula addresses deficiency to a much greater degree, suggesting that long-term stagnation and heat in cancer consumes the body's resources.

Kidney yin tonics in this formula include nu zhen zi, han lian cao, shan zhu yu, and xuan shen. Kidney yang tonics include lu jiao shuang. All of these are mild, well tolerated, and do not tend to create stagnation to the degree that many other kidney tonics do.

Herbs that soften hardness include xuan shen and chuan bei mu. Chuan bei mu also treats phlegm. Herbs that move blood include ji xue teng, dan shen, dang gui, and si gua luo. Among these, ji xue teng and si gua luo open the collaterals. Herbs that open the collaterals are especially indicated for long-term stagnation. Si gua luo especially targets the breasts.

Gua lou pi, a qi regulator, especially targets the chest. Ban zhi lian clears heat and toxicity and targets the liver channel (which supplies the breasts). Herbs that clear heat and toxicity are widely used to treat cancer.

Cancer of the Colon

Pin Yin	Latin	English	Dosage
Di yu	Sanguisorbae Radix	Sanguisorba, burnet-bloodwort root	9–15 g
Huai jiao	Sophorae Fructus[a]	Sophora seeds	3–6 g
Huai hua	Sophorae Flos	Sophora flower	4.5–9 g
Di long	Lumbricus	Earthworm, lumbricus	4.5–15 g
Niu xi or huai niu xi	Achyranthis Bidentatae Radix	Ox-knee root from Huai	6–15 g

[a] For hemorrhoids.

To soften hardness and scatter toxins add:

Pin Yin	Latin	English	Dosage
Tian kui zi	Semiaquilegiae Radix	Semiaquilegia tuber/root	15–30 g
Ban zhi lian	Scutellariae Barbatae Herba	Barbat skullcap, scutellaria	9–30 g
Hai zao	Sargassum	Sargassum, seaweed	6–15 g
Mu li	Ostreae Concha	Oyster shell	9–30 g
Zao jiao	Gleditsiae Sinensis Fructus	Chinese honey locust fruit, gleditsia	1–1.5 g

Hamilton Rotte   This is not a formula, but a list of herbs that Dr. Shen considered useful in the treatment of colon cancer. These herbs clear heat, stop bleeding, and move blood. Herbs that clear heat and toxicity and soften hardness may also be applicable. Dr. Shen suggested these herbs to clear heat and stop bleeding: *di yu*, *huai jiao*, and *huai hua*. Because rectal bleeding is a prominent symptom of colon cancer, these herbs are especially applicable. *Di long*, *niu xi*, and *zao jiao* are included to move blood. *Niu xi*, in particular, targets the lower burner.

To clear heat and toxicity we have *tian kui zi*, *ban zhi lian*, and *zao jiao*. *Tian kui zi* and *ban zhi lian* are modern favorites for the treatment of cancer.

Hai zao and *mu li* soften hardness and treat masses.

Cancer of the Esophagus

Pin Yin	Latin	English	Dosage
Huang yao zi	Dioscoreae Bulbiferae Rhizoma	Airpotato yam rhizome	6–15 g
Yuan zhi	Polygalae Radix	Chinese senega root, polygala root	6–15 g[a]
Chuan shan jia	Mantis Pentadactylae Squama	Pangolin scales	3–9 g[b]
Wei ling xian	Clematidis Radix	Chinese clematis root	6–9 g
Zhu ru	Bambussae in Taeniis Caulis	Bamboo shavings	4.5–9 g
Hai piao xiao	Sepiae Endoconcha	Cuttlefish bone	6–12 g
Pi pa ye	Eriobotryae Folium	Loquat leaf, dried leaf of *Eriobotrya japonica*	6–15 g

[a] Protects stomach and esophagus membrane.
[b] Obsolete.

Hamilton Rotte   This is not a formula, but a list of herbs that Dr Shen suggested would be useful for the treatment of esophagus cancer. The treatment principles are to move blood, clear heat and toxicity, descend stomach *qi*, and generate flesh.

Huang yao zi resolves toxicity and dissipates nodules. *Wei ling xian* also softens hardness and targets the middle burner. *Yuan zhi* dissipates swellings, especially applicable for cancer. *Chuan shan jia* is used to move blood. *Zhu ru* and *pi pa ye* clear heat and descend stomach *qi*. *Hai piao xiao* is used to absorb acidity and generate flesh.

Cancer of the Kidneys

Pin Yin	Latin	English	Dosage
Sha yuan zi	Astragali Complanati Semen	Astragalus seed	9–18 g
Xu duan	Dipsaci Asperi Radix	Japanese teasel root, dipsacus	9–18 g
Du zhong	Eucommiae Cortex	Eucommia bark	9–15 g
Bu gu zhi	Psoraleae Corylifoliae Fructus	Psoralea fruit	4.5–9 g
Mu hu die	Oroxyli Semen	Oroxylum seeds	1.5–3 g

Hamilton Rotte   This is not a formula, but a list of herbs that Dr. Shen recommended for the treatment of cancer. They should be selected according to the needs of the patient. *Xu duan*, *du zhong*, and *bu gu* *zhi* all tonify kidney *yang*. *Xu duan* and *du zhong* are both invigorating to the blood. *Sha yuan zi* and *bu gu zhi* are both stabilizing to the kidneys.

Cancer of the Liver

Formula I for cancer of the liver:

Pin Yin	Latin	English	Dosage
Chai hu	Bupleuri Radix	Hare's ear root, thorowax root, bupleurum	3–9 g
Chuan lian zi	Meliae Toosendan Fructus	Szechuan pagoda tree fruit, Szechuan chinaberry, melia	4.5–9 g
Xiang fu	Cyperi Rotunda Rhizoma	Nut-grass rhizome, cyperus	6–12 g
Chuan shan jia[a]	Mantis Pentadactylae Squama	Pangolin scales	3–9 g
Yin chen	Artemisiae Scopariae Herba	Virgate wormwood	9–30 g

[a] Obsolete

Hamilton Rotte   This is not intended to be a formula, but is rather a list of herbs that Dr. Shen suggested would be beneficial for liver cancer. Herbs from this list should be selected according to the specifics of the situation.
Cancer is usually attributed to dampness and phlegm, stagnation of *qi* and blood, and heat toxi-city. Herbs that target the effected area are indicated. *Chai hu*, *chuan lian zi*, and *xiang fu* regulate *qi* in the liver. *Chuan shan jia*, deemed obsolete because of its endangered status, moves blood and targets the liver channel.
Yin chen is used to clear heat from the liver.

Formula II for cancer of the liver:

Pin Yin	Latin	English	Dosage
Chai hu	Bupleuri Radix	Hare's ear root, thorowax root, bupleurum	9 g
Chuan xiong	Chuanxiong Rhizoma	Chuanxiong root, Szechuan lovage root, cnidium	12 g
Bai shao	Paeoniae Alba Radix	White peony root	8 g
Huang lian	Coptidis Rhizoma	Coptis rhizome	15 g
Mu xiang	Saussureae Lappae Radix or Aucklandia Lappae Radix	Costus root, saussurea, aucklandia	12 g
Fu ling	Poria Cocos Sclerotium	Sclerotium of tuckahoe, poria, China root, hoelen, Indian bread	15 g
Zhi ke	Citri Aurantii Fructus	Mature fruit of the bitter orange	9 g
Yu jin	Curcumae Radix	Curcuma tuber	18 g
Bai hua she she cao	Heydyotis Diffusae Herba	Heydyotis, oldenlandia	15 g
Ban zhi lian	Scutellariae Barbatae Herba	Barbat skullcap, scutellaria	15 g
Gan cao	Glycyrrhizae Radix	Licorice root	6 g
Yuan hu suo	Corydalis Rhizoma	Corydalis rhizome	18 g

Pin Yin	Latin	English	Dosage
Nan sha shen	Adenophorae seu Glehniae Radix	Adenophora root or glehnia root, ladybell root	18 g
Lu lu tong	Liquidambaris Fructus	Sweetgum fruit, liquidambar fruit	8 g
Mai men dong	Ophiopogonis Radix	Ophiopogon tuber/root	18 g
Zhe bie mu	Fritillariae Thunbergii Bulbus	Zhejiang fritillaria, Thunberg fritillaria bulb, fritillaria	18 g
Yu zhu	Polygonati Odorati Rhizoma	Solomon's seal rhizome, polygonatum	18 g
Long gu	Fossilia Ossis Mastodi	Dragon bone, fossilized vertebrae and bones of the extremities (usually of mammals)	24 g

Decoction is sipped all day

Three together if added to the above soften liver, or any hard mass in the lower burner:

Pin Yin	Latin	English	Dosage
Mu li	Ostreae Concha	Oyster shell	18–24 g
Long gu	Fossilia Ossis Mastodi	Dragon bone, fossilized vertebrae and bones of the extremities (usually of mammals)	24 g
Mai men dong	Ophiopogonis Radix	Ophiopogon tuber/root	9 g

Hamilton Rotte   Cancer is treated as stagnation of *qi* and blood, phlegm and heat toxicity.

Herbs in this formula that move *qi* in the liver include *chai hu*, *mu xiang*, and *yu jin*. *Lu lu tong*, which regulates the *qi* and blood, enters the liver channel. Herbs that move blood in the liver include *chuan xiong*, *yu jin*, and *yan hu suo*. Herbs that resolve heat toxicity include *ban zhi lian*, *huang lian*, and *bai hua she she cao*. Among these, *ban zhi lian* particularly targets the liver.

This formula contains many *yin* tonics. *Bai shao* tonifies the liver *yin* and blood. Other *yin* tonics include *nan sha shen*, *mai men dong*, and *yu zhu*. *Nan sha shen*, *mai men dong*, and *yu zhu* affect the lungs and stomach. It is not clear why Dr. Shen chose these herbs for a condition that affects the liver.

Fu ling and *zhi ke* enter the spleen and stomach. Stagnation and excess of the liver commonly cause problems in these organs and these herbs probably are included for this reason.

Long gu is included because of its ability to treat masses. Consuming a decoction of herbs with high dosages slowly all day yields a stronger effect and is indicated for severe pathology such as cancer.

Leon Hammer   Regarding the use of *yin*-nourishing herbs in this formula Dr. Shen regarded cancer as a condition that was due to the "separation of *yin* and *yang*" in the organ or area involved.

The "separation of *yin* and *yang*" is usually the result of severe deficiency of either *yin* or *yang* or both. Unless one is absolutely certain which is the most deficient, it is safer to nourish both. In this formula Dr. Shen clearly leaned toward *yin* deficiency.

The stagnation that is addressed in all of the cancer conditions and herbs herein prescribed is a secondary condition due to deficiency, to physiologic chaos that precludes orderly movement of *qi*, blood, and phlegm.

What is interesting to me is the shift over the last 40 years from *yin* deficiency that predominated in Dr. Shen's time to *yang* deficiency in our time. I account for this change for increased drain on liver *qi-yang* in dealing with the enormous and ubiquitous increase during this time span in environmental toxicity (by the order of millions) and the likewise concomitant use of cold substances, especially marijuana, and also including LSD and heroin. Of interest in this regard is the extensive presence of anti-toxic herbs in many current formulas treating cancer.

Cancer of the Lungs

Pin Yin	Latin	English	Dosage
Bai hua she she cao	Heydyotis Diffusae Herba	Heydyotis, oldenlandia	6–15 g
Bai mao gen	Imperatae Cylindricae Rhizoma	Rhizome of woolly grass, imperata, white grass	9–30 g
Xing ren	Armeniacae Semen	Apricot seed or kernel	3–9 g
Bai bu	Stemonae Radix	Stemona root	3–9 g
Jie geng	Platycodi Radix	Root of balloonflower, platycodon root	3–9 g
Pi pa ye	Eriobotryae Folium	Loquat leaf, dried leaf of *Eriobotrya japonica*	6–15 g

Hamilton Rotte This is a not intended to be a formula, but is rather a list of herbs that Dr. Shen suggested would be beneficial for lung cancer. Herbs from this list should be selected according to the specifics of the situation.

Cancer is usually attributed to dampness and phlegm, stagnation of *qi* and blood, and heat toxicity. Herbs that target the affected area are indicated.

Herbs that clear heat from the lungs include *bai mao gen* and *pi pa ye*. *Bai hua she she cao* is a modern favorite for cancer. *Xing ren* is slightly moistening and is utilized to move *qi* in the lungs. *Bai bu* nourishes lung *yin* and moves lung *qi*.

Cancer of the Lymphatic System

Pin Yin	Latin	English	Dosage
Qiang huo	Notopterygii Rhizoma et Radix	Notopterygium root and rhizome, chiang-huo	18 g
Chuan xiong	Chuanxiong Rhizoma	Chuanxiong root, Szechuan lovage root, cnidium	12 g
Sang ji sheng	Taxilli Herba	Mulberry mistletoe stems, loranthus, taxillus, mistletoe	18 g
Mu gua	Chaenomelis Fructus	Chinese quince fruit, chaenomeles	18 g
Fang feng	Saposhnikoviae Radix	Ledebouriella root, saposhnikoviae root, siler	12 g
Chi shao	Paeoniae Rubra Radix	Red peony root	18 g
Mu dan pi	Moutan Radicis Cortex	Tree peony root bark, moutan root bark	1 g
Chuan shan jia	*Mantis* Pentadactylae *Squama*	Pangolin scales	18 g

Hamilton Rotte Lymph cancer is marked by swollen lymph nodes in the neck, underarm or groin. Dr. Shen apparently viewed this as stagnation and heat in the channels and collaterals.

This formula contains herbs that open *qi* and blood circulation in the channels and collaterals including *qiang huo*, *sang ji sheng*, *mu gua*, *fang feng*, and *chuan sha jia*. *Chuan shan jia* is not available and suitable substitutes include *wang bu liu xing* (vaccaria seeds) or *zao jiao ci* (spine of honeylocust plant).

Herbs that move blood include *chuan xiong*, *chi shao*, and *mu dan pi*. Of these, *chi shao* and *mu dan pi* also clear heat.

This formula contains many ingredients that target the liver channel (and therefore the inguinal region). These include *chuan xiong*, *mu gua*, *chi shao*, and *mu dan pi*.

Cancer of the Prostate

Pin Yin	Latin	English	Dosage
Chao sheng di huang	Rehmanniae Radix	Dry-fried fresh Chinese foxglove root, rehmannia root	18 g
Zhi mu	Anemarrhenae Asphodeloidis Rhizoma	Anemarrhena rhizome	18 g
Huang bai	Phellodendri Cortex	Amur corktree bark, phellodendron bark	15 g
Ze xie	Alismatis Rhizoma	Water plantain rhizome, alisma rhizome	18 g
Long dan cao	Gentianae Longdancao Radix	Chinese gentian root, gentiana	12 g

Hamilton Rotte   For prostate cancer, Dr. Shen suggested this in addition to *wu gong* and *pu gong ying*. It contains ingredients to clear damp-heat in the lower burner, including *zhi mu*, *huang bai*, *ze xie* and *long dan cao*. *Ze xie* clears damp-heat in the lower burner by promoting urination. *Long dan cao* clears damp-heat in the lower burner because it especially targets the liver channel, which supplies the reproductive organs.

This formula can also be used by itself, without the *wu gong* or *jin yin hua*, for an enlarged prostate in the absence of cancer. Dr. Shen suggested that this formula should be taken daily for periods of 1 to 2 months, followed by a break, and then resumed.

Leon Hammer   Whereas the insect- and snake-derived herbs were among Dr. Shen's favorites, in the raw forms in which they were dispensed during the years I was with him, they were not tolerated well by American recipients and compliance was very low.

Cancer of the Stomach

Pin Yin	Latin	English	Dosage
Huang yao zi	Dioscoreae Bulbiferae Rhizoma	Airpotato yam rhizome	6–15 g
Bi ba	Piperis Longi Fructus	Long pepper	1.5–4.5 g
Gao liang jiang	Alpiniae Officinari Rhizoma	Lesser galangal rhizome	3–9 g
Hai piao xiao	Sepiae Endoconcha	Cuttlefish bone, cuttlebone	6–12 g
Sha ren	Amomi Fructus	Cardamom	3–6 g
Zhi ban xia	Pinelliae Preparatum Rhizoma	Dried processed pinellia rhizome	3–9 g

Hamilton Rotte   This is not a formula, but a list of herbs that Dr. Shen suggested for the treatment of stomach cancer. All of these enter the middle burner. *Huang yao zi* clears heat and toxicity and is used for many types of cancers, including those that involve the esophagus and stomach. *Bi ba* and *gao liang jiang* are warming to the middle burner. *Hai piao xiao* absorbs acidity and is especially indicated when reflux is a prominent symptom. *Sha ren* warms the middle burner and excels at regulating *qi*. *Zhi ban xia* excels at descending stomach *qi* and is especially indicated when nausea and vomiting are prominent symptoms.

Chemotherapy

FROM DR. SHEN: Also good for low appetite after catching a cold. Symptoms: nausea, low appetite, vomiting.

Pin Yin	Latin	English	Dosage
Shan yao	Dioscoreae Oppositae Rhizoma	Chinese yam, dioscorea rhizome	15 g
Mu xiang	Saussureae Lappae Radix or Aucklandia Lappae Radix	Costus root, saussurea, aucklandia	9 g
Shan zha	Crataegi Fructus	Hawthorn fruit, crataegus fruit	No dose mentioned
Shen qu	Massa Medicata Fermentata	Medicated leaven (dough)	No dose mentioned
Mai ya	Hordei Germinatus Fructus	Barley sprout, malt	No dose mentioned
Zhu ru	Bambussae in Taeniis Caulis	Bamboo shavings	9 g
Xiang fu	Cyperi Rotundi Rhizoma	Nut grass rhizoma, cyperus	9 g
Chen pi	Citri Reticulatae Pericarpium	Tangerine peel	9 g
Wu zhu yu	Evodiae Fructus	Evodia fruit	6 g
Chao huang lian	Coptidis	Dry-fried coptis rhizome	6 g
Hou po	Magnoliae Officinalis Cortex	Magnolia bark	9 g
Ban xia	Rhizoma Pinelliae	Pinellia rhizome	9 g
Xha ren	Amomi Fructus	Cardamom	6 g

Hamilton Rotte   This formula focuses on regulating and descending stomach *qi* and contains a few tonics for the middle burner.

Herbs that regulate the stomach *qi* include *mu xiang*, *xiang fu*, *chen pi*, *wu zhu yu*, *hou po*, and *sha ren*. Herbs that are particularly descending to the stomach *qi* include *zhu ru*, *wu zhu yu*, *huang lian*, *hou po*, and *zhi ban xia*.

Shan yao is the only true tonic in this formula, a mild food-level substance that does not exacerbate stagnation or improper ascent of stomach *qi*. A favorite method of Dr. Shen to indirectly benefit the spleen and stomach is to utilize herbs that resolve food stagnation, as food stagnation burdens the spleen. Herbs that resolve food stagnation in this formula include *mu xiang*, *shan zha*, *shen qu*, *mai ya*, and *hou po*.

Chemotherapy with Diarrhea

Pin Yin	Latin	English	Dosage
Shan yao	Dioscoreae Oppositae Rhizoma	Chinese yam, dioscorea rhizome	60 g
Fu ling	Poria Cocos Sclerotium	Sclerotium of tuckahoe, poria, China root, hoelen, Indian bread	30 g
Duan mu li	Ostreae Concha	Calcined oyster shell	30 g
Duan long gu	Fossilia Ossis Mastodi	Calcined fossilized dragon bone, fossilized vertebrae and bones of the extremities (usually of mammals)	30 g

Pin Yin	Latin	English	Dosage
Lian zi	Nelumbinis Semen	Lotus seed	30 g
Qian shi	Euryales Ferocis Semen	Euryale seeds	30 g
Bai shao	Paeoniae Alba Radix	White peony root	30 g
Bai zhu	Atractylodis Macrocephalae Rhizoma	White atractylodes rhizome	15 g
Sha ren	Amomi Fructus	Cardamom	6 g

Hamilton Rotte   This formula tonifies the spleen, regulates *qi* of the spleen, and stabilizes the intestines. Spleen *qi* tonics include *shan yao, fu ling, lian zi,* *qian shi,* and *bai zhu. Qi* regulators include *sha ren.* Stabilizing ingredients include *mu li, long gu, lian zi, qian shi,* and *bai shao.*

With cold add:

Pin Yin	Latin	English	Dosage
Gan jiang	Zingiberis Rhizoma	Dried ginger	15 g
Rou gui	Cinnamomi Cassiae Cortex	Inner bark of Saigon cinnamon	15 g
Fu zi	Aconiti Lateralis Praeparata Radix	Aconite	12 g
Long yan rou	Longan Arillus	Flesh of the longan fruit, longan	30 g

With heat add:

Pin Yin	Latin	English	Dosage
Huang lian	Coptidis Rhizoma	Coptis rhizome	6–9 g

Leukemia

FROM DR. SHEN: Put herbs in a big pan and add enough water to cover with 1 inch of water, then boil for 45 minutes. The same batch of herbs should be cooked two to three times, and will last 5 days to 1 week. Drink a little all day, each day.

Pin Yin	Latin	English	Dosage
Xi yang shen	Panacis Quinquefolii Radix	American ginseng root	18 g
Chao huang qi	Astragali Radix	Fried milk vetch root, fried astragalus root	18 g
Dang gui	Angelicae Sinensis Radix	Chinese angelica root, *tang-kuei*	15 g
Shu di huang	Rehmanniae Preparata Radix	Prepared Chinese foxglove root (cooked in red wine), cooked rehmannia rhizome	18 g
Sheng di huang	Rehmannia Radix	Fresh Chinese foxglove root, rehmannia root	18 g
Du zhong	Eucommiae Cortex	Eucommia bark	18 g
Gou ji	Cibotii Rhizoma	Cibotium rhizome, chain fern	18 g
Shan yao	Dioscoreae Oppositae Rhizoma	Chinese yam, dioscorea rhizome	18 g
Qiang huo	Notopterygii Rhizoma et Radix	Notopterygium root and rhizome, *chiang-huo*	12 g
Xi xin	Asari Herba cum Radice	Chinese wild ginger, asarum	9 g

Pin Yin	Latin	English	Dosage
Fu ling	Poria Cocos Sclerotium	Sclerotium of tuckahoe, poria, China root, hoelen, Indian bread	18 g
Yuan zhi	Polygalae Radix	Chinese senega root, polygala root	12 g
Da zao	Zizyphi Jujubae Fructus	Chinese date, jujube	18 g
Mu gua	Chaenomelis Fructus	Chinese quince fruit, chaenomeles	18 g
He shou wu	Radix Polygoni Multiflori	Fleece-flower root, polygonum hosuwu	18 g

Hamilton Rotte Dr. Shen considered leukemia to involve deficiency of *qi*, blood, and kidney *yang*. Qi tonics in this formula include *xi yang shen, huang qi, shan yao, fu ling,* and *da zao*. In this formula more emphasis is placed on the tonification of blood with the inclusion of *dang gui, shu di huang, sheng di huang, da zao,* and *he shou wu*. Kidney *yang* tonics include *du zhong* and *gou ji*. Dr. Shen also frequently used *yuan zhi* in kidney tonic formulas. *Xi xin* is included to warm the kidney *yang* and it is also known to reach the level of the bones, where the pathology of leukemia occurs. This formula contains ingredients that "strengthen sinews and bones," as leukemia is a disorder of the bones.

Uterine Tumor

FROM DR. SHEN: Uterine tumors are not limited to only one etiology. There are three causes for their formation. They are made up either of blood or water or *qi*. These factors may intermingle in different compositions to be subdivided into still more forms. So the prerequisite for effective treatment is to first discern the etiology of the tumor.

When the tumor is made of blood, the swellings in the uterus feel hard and remain constant in size. If the tumor is made up of water, it may feel hard or soft, while the size seems sometimes large and sometimes small. If the tumors are made up of *qi*, some are soft. Upon palpation they sometimes feel large but disappear altogether at other times.

Formation of uterine tumors is the bitter aftermath of inappropriate ways of life. Tumors made up of blood have their root in deficiency of the womb (*qi* deficiency in the lower burner), which is too weak to expel all the menstrual blood freely so some is retained inside. If the patient's defective ways of life are not improved in time, clumps of blood will grow in size and number and become tumors.

Qi and water are gradually stockpiled in the womb from repressed emotion that is too weak to expel them. They will gradually grow into tumors. When the patient is stronger, her womb will expel the remnant stagnant blood or *qi*-fluid. So the lumps are sometimes large and sometimes small.

Pin Yin	Latin	English	Dosage
Dan shen	Salviae Miltiorrhizae Radix	Salvia root	15 g
Mu dan pi	Moutan Radicis Cortex	Tree peony root bark, moutan root bark	15 g
Yi mu cao	Leonuri Herba	Chinese motherwort, leonurus	15 g
Tu si zi	Cuscutae Chinensis Semen	Chinese dodder seeds, cuscuta	18 g
Duan long gu	Fossilia Ossis Mastodi	Calcined fossilized dragon bone, fossilized vertebrae and bones of the extremities (usually of mammals)	24 g
Yan hu suo	Corydalis Yanhusuo Rhizoma	Corydalis rhizome	18 g

Hamilton Rotte   This formula moves blood, clears heat, softens hardness, and mildly tonifies and stabilizes the kidneys. Blood-invigorating ingredients include *dan shen*, *mu dan pi*, *yi mu cao* and *yan hu suo*. *Dan shen*, *mu dan pi* and *yi mu cao* clear heat.
Duan long gu was a favorite herb of Dr. Shen to soften hardness and treat masses. Dr. Shen widely used *tu si*

zi for kidney-deficient conditions affecting the uterus. Its presence here implies that Dr. Shen considered uterine cancer to involve an underlying deficiency (as kidney energies supply energy to maintain movement of the organs in the lower burner). *Tu si zi* and *Duan long gu* stabilize the kidneys and offset moving tendencies of other herbs in the formula.

Leon Hammer

Pulse:
• Pelvis lower body: choppy; slippery
• Proximal position: choppy

Tongue:
Swollen with purple spots

FROM DR. SHEN: The most important approach to treating uterine tumors is to overcome the defective ways of life and choose different formulas to suit different patients.

Formula for uterine tumors arising from blood stagnation:

Pin Yin	Latin	English	Dosage
Dang gui	Angelicae Sinensis Radix	Chinese angelica root, *tang-kuei*	6 g
Chuan xiong	Chuanxiong Rhizoma	Chuanxiong root, Szechuan lovage root, cnidium	6 g
Chi shao	Paeoniae Rubra Radix	Red peony root	9 g
Bai shao	Paeoniae Alba Radix	White peony root	6 g
Dan shen	Salviae Miltiorrhiziae Radix	Salvia root	6 g
Yi mu cao	Herba Leonuri	Chinese motherwort, leonurus	6 g
E zhu	Curcumae Rhizoma	Zedoary rhizoma, zedoaria	2.4 g
Xiang fu	Cyperi Rotundi Rhizoma	Nut grass rhizoma, cyperus	4.5 g
Chuan lian zi	Meliae Toosendan Fructus	Szechuan pagoda tree fruit, Szechuan chinaberry, melia	9 g
Huai niu xi	Achyranthis Bidentatae Radix	Ox-knee root, achyranthes root	9 g

Hamilton Rotte   This formula focuses on moving blood in the uterus. Blood movers include *dang gui*, *chuan xiong*, *chi shao*, *dan shen*, *yi mu cao*, *e zhu*, and *huai niu xi*. *Yi mu cao* and *huai niu xi* particularly focus on the uterus. *E zhu*, a strong blood mover, also dissolves masses.
We also find herbs that move *qi* in the formula, to aid in movement of blood. *Xiang fu* and *chuan lian zi* serve this purpose, both targeting the liver organ.

This formula contains blood tonic ingredients to protect the blood from damage caused by *qi*- and blood-moving ingredients. These include *dang gui* and *bai shao*.

Formula for uterine tumors arising from water accumulation:

Pin Yin	Latin	English	Dosage
Dang gui	Angelicae Sinensis Radix	Chinese angelica root, *tang-kuei*	6 g
Cang zhu	Atractylodis Rhizoma	Black atractylodes rhizome	4.5 g
Bi xie	Dioscoreae Rhizoma Hypoglaucae	Fish poison yam rhizome, tokoro	4.5 g
Xiang fu	Cyperi Rotundi Rhizoma	Nut grass rhizoma, cyperus	4.5 g
Chi fu ling	Sclerotium Poria Cocos Rubrae	Red sclerotium of tuckahoe, china root, poria, hoelen	9 g
Lu lu tong	Liquidambaris Fructus	Sweetgum fruit, liquidambar fruit	12 g
Yan hu suo	Corydalis Yanhusuo Rhizoma	Corydalis rhizome	9 g
Yu jin	Curcumae Radix	Curcuma tuber	6 g
Ze xie	Alismatis Rhizoma	Water plantain rhizome, alisma rhizome	9 g
Sheng yi yi ren	Coicis Semen	Fresh seeds of Job's tears, fresh coix seeds	12 g
Shu yi yi ren	Coicis Semen	Prepared seeds of Job's tears, coix seeds	12 g

Hamilton Rotte   This formula focuses on damp excess in the lower burner. The herbs that treat dampness include *cang zhu, bi xie, fu ling, ze xie,* and two preparations of *shu yi yi ren. Bi xie, fu ling, ze xie,* and *shu yi yi ren* promote urination.

A mass also implies stagnation of *qi* and blood. This formula also contains ingredients that move *qi* and blood. *Qi* movers include *xiang fu, lu lu tong,* and *yu jin.* Blood-moving ingredients include *dang gui, yu jin, lu lu tong,* and *yan hu suo. Dang gui* is also included to protect the blood from damage that could be caused by moving ingredients.

Formula for uterine tumors arising from *qi stagnation:*

Pin Yin	Latin	English	Dosage
Dang gui	Angelicae Sinensis Radix	Chinese angelica root, *tang-kuei*	6 g
Chuan xiong	Chuanxiong Rhizoma	Chuanxiong root, Szechuan lovage root, cnidium	6 g
Chai hu	Bupleuri Radix	Hare's ear root, thorowax root, bupleurum	3 g
Bai shao	Paeoniae Radix Alba	White peony root	9 g
Fu ling	Poria Cocos Sclerotium	Sclerotium of tuckahoe, poria, China root, hoelen, Indian bread	9 g
Yan hu suo	Corydalis Yanhusuo Rhizoma	Corydalis rhizome	9 g
E zhu	Curcumae Rhizoma	Zedoary rhizoma, zedoaria	3 g
Da fu pi	Arecae Catechu Pericarpium	Betel husk, areca peel	9 g
Huang qin	Scutellariae Baicalensis Radix	Baical skullcap root, scutellaria, scute	4.5 g
Huai nui xi	Achyranthis Bidentatae Radix	Ox-knee root, achyranthes root	12 g

Boil the above medicines into tea and drink twice a day until the tumors disappear.

Hamilton Rotte   This formula is indicated for uterine tumors due to *qi* stagnation. Herbs that move *qi* include *chai hu* and *da fu pi*. *Da fu pi* is also especially indicated for stagnant fluid. *Chai hu* combines with *bai shao* to regulate the liver *qi*.

This formula also contains many ingredients that regulate the blood, suggesting that a uterine tumor also includes stagnation of blood. Blood movers in this formula include *dang gui*, *chuan xiong*, *yan hu suo*, *e zhu*, and *huai niu xi*. *E zhu* is especially indicated for masses.

Dang gui and *bai shao* are blood tonics that are included to protect the blood from potential damage caused by *qi* and blood movers.

Huang qin is included to treat the heat that develops because of stagnation of *qi* and blood.

Ophthalmologic Conditions

FROM DR. SHEN: In a robust individual eye problems come from overuse (**Fig.13**). This causes heat and the heat causes wind. These problems occur on the right side. Weakness causes left-sided problems.

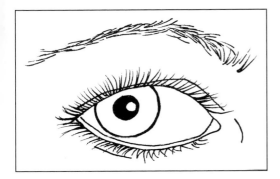

Fig.13 Ophthalmology: the eye.

Left Eye

Pin Yin	Latin	English	Dosage
Chao jing jie	Schizonepetae Herba	Dry-fried schizonepeta	4.5 g
Chan tui	Periostracum Cicadae	Cicada moultings	4.5 g
Ju hua	Chrysanthemi Flos	Chrysanthemum flower	9 g
Gu jing cao	Eriocauli Flos	Pipewort scapus and inflorescence	3 g
Gan cao	Glycyrrhizae Radix	Licorice root	3 g
Mu dan pi	Moutan Radicis Cortex	Tree peony root bark, moutan root bark	6 g
Bai mao gen	Imperatae Cylindricae Rhizoma	Rhizome of woolly grass, imperata, white grass	9 g
Ze xie	Alismatis Rhizoma	Water plantain rhizome, alisma rhizome	9 g
Sheng di huang	Rehmannia Radix	Fresh Chinese foxglove root, rehmannia root	9 g

Hamilton Rotte This formula is for left eye problems, which according to Dr. Shen is due to weakness of the blood. This formula also contains herbs that remove heat from the eyes. The suggestion is that there is also excess heat in addition to deficiency. This could be because a vulnerability of the eyes forces them to overwork in daily activities. As indicated in the previous commentary, the herbs that remove heat from the eyes include *chan tui*, *mu dan pi*, and *bai mao gen*. *Gu jing cao* is an additional herb in the formula for clearing heat and targeting the eyes.

Tonic herbs in this formula include *ju hua* and *sheng di huang*. *Sheng di huang* can be used as a milder and easier to digest substitute for *shu di huang* in tonifying liver blood.

This formula would be appropriate in instances where there is a combination of excess heat and underlying blood deficiency. In severe deficiency, an appropriate formula to strengthen the eyes would be *Qi Ju Di Huang Wan* (Lycium Fruit, Chrysanthemum and Rehmannia Pill). *Gou qi zi* in particular is considered the premier substance in Chinese medicine for tonifying the eyes from liver and kidney deficiency.

Formula for left eye weak:

Pin Yin	Latin	English	Dosage
Chao dang gui	Angelicae Sinensis Radix	Fried Chinese angelica root, *tang-kuei*	6 g
E jiao	Corii Colla Asini	Donkey hide gelatin	12 g
Chao bai shao	Paeoniae Alba Radix	Dry-fried white peony root	9 g
Duan mu li	Ostreae Concha	Calcined oyster shell	12 g
Gou qi zi	Lycii Fructus	Chinese wolfberry, matrimony vine fruit, lycium fruit	9 g
Gu jing cao	Eriocauli Flos	Pipewort scapus and inflorescence	9 g

Hamilton Rotte This formula, gleaned from Dr. Shen's clinical records, is a formula that treated weakness of the left eye. It contains many blood tonics, including *dang gui, e jiao, bai shao,* and *gou qi zi. Mu li* is also considered a tonic herb for the liver. *Gou qi zi,* in particular, is prized for treating vision problems from deficiency.

Right Eye

Pin Yin	Latin	English	Dosage
Chan tui	Periostracum Cicadae	Cicada moultings	4.5 g
Chao jing jie	Schizonepetae Herba	Dry-fried schizonepeta	4.5 g
Mu zei	Equiseti Hiemalis Herba	Equisetum, scouring rush, shave grass, Dutch rushes, rough horsetail	9 g
Gan cao	Glycyrrhizae Radix	Licorice root	3 g
Long dan cao	Gentianae Longdancao Radix	Chinese gentian root, gentiana	2.4 g
Mu dan pi	Moutan Radicis Cortex	Tree peony root bark, moutan root bark	6 g
Ze xie	Alismatis Rhizoma	Water plantain rhizome, alisma rhizome	9 g
Bai mao gen	Imperatae Cylindricae Rhizoma	Rhizome of woolly grass, imperata, white grass	9 g

Hamilton Rotte This formula is designed to remove heat in the eyes that arises from overuse. The herbs that target the eyes tend to be either surface-releasing herbs (which tend to go to the upper body) or herbs that target the liver channel. The herbs that release the surface are all cooling and include *chan tui, jing jie,* and *mu zei.* Of these, *chan tui* and *mu zei* in particular focus on the eyes. *Long dan cao* and *mu dan pi* both remove heat from the liver channel. *Long dan cao* is used at a particularly light dose and this focuses it on the eyes. As a general rule, lighter dosage of herbs tends to affect the upper body or the surface. In this case, the light dose of *long dan cao* affects the eyes rather than the liver organ itself.

Ze xie may be included to provide balance to the formula that has the tendency to target the upper burner. *Ze xie* settles ministerial fire and has a marked descending effect. *Ze xie* targets the kidneys. Dr. Shen emphasized that both the liver and kidneys influence the eyes, which bears out in practical experience if one examines herbs that influence the eyes (i.e., *gou qi zi, shi hu,* and *tu si zi* are all very important herbs for the eyes and affect the kidneys). *Ze xie* may have been included here because of its influence on the kidneys. *Bai mao gen* may be included because it influences the bladder channel, which supplies the eyes.

Formula for right eye heat:

Pin Yin	Latin	English	Dosage
Chao huang bai	Phellodendri Cortex	Fried amur corktree bark, phellodendron bark	6 g
Zhi mu	Anemarrhenae Asphodeloidis Rhizoma	Anemarrhena rhizome	9 g
Sheng gan cao	Glycyrrhizae Radix	Fresh licorice root	3 g
Ze xie	Alismatis Rhizoma	Water plantain rhizome, alisma rhizome	9 g

Hamilton Rotte This formula, gleaned from Dr. Shen's clinical records, is a formula that treated heat in the right eye. *Huang bai* and *zhi mu* are a two-herb combination that clears deficient heat. These two are both strongly descending. *Sheng gan cao* slows the pathogenic progression of heat with a sweet flavor and harmonizing effect. *Ze xie* clears heat with its cooling and descending nature.

Pediatric Conditions

San Huang Tang (Three Yellow Decoction) for discharging the meconium:

Pin Yin	Latin	English	Dosage
Huang bai	Phellodendri Cortex	Amur corktree bark, phellodendron bark	3 g
Huang lian	Coptidis Rhizoma	Coptis rhizome	3 g
Da huang	Rhei Radix et Rhizoma	Rhubarb root and rhizome	3 g

FROM DR. SHEN: Mother should not feed a baby before its first bowel movement. Give *San Huang Tang* to baby before feeding.

Hamilton Rotte Dr. Shen emphasized the importance of discharging the meconium before feeding a newborn.

The meconium is an accumulation of amniotic fluid on the inside of the intestines of a fetus. If a newborn is fed, it will begin to absorb it, which is toxic.

This formula contains three herbs that resolve heat and toxicity: *huang bai*, *huang lian*, and *da huang*.
Da huang is a purgative, which helps to discharge the meconium.

Leon Hammer MEDLINE at the US National Library of Medicine defines meconium as: "The thick green-to-black mucilaginous material found in the intestines of a full-term fetus. It consists of secretions of intestinal glands, bile pigments, fatty acids, amniotic fluid, and intrauterine debris. It constitutes the first stools passed by the newborn" (MEDLINE).

Due to the fact that infants are pure *yang*, the strong cooling substance used in small amounts in this formula for treating infants to eliminate meconium is not too strong.

Dr. Shen said only that the meconium should pass before the baby is fed anything. The contention by Dr. Shen is that if the baby is fed before it passes meconium, the digestive tract is engaged and re-absorption of toxins occurs. The problems that can arise are jaundice, digestive problems, colic, skin problems, baby acne, psoriasis, and difficult allergies as a child.

A common sign of birth trauma used today is meconium present in the amniotic fluid during labor, which may be more along the lines of fetal diarrhea. The meconium is absorbed through the gut into the blood that attempts to excrete it through the skin since it does not seem to be excreted through the stool.

Toxicity will always affect the liver since the liver stores the blood and the liver is the principal detoxifier from a chemical point of view. It will also affect the most vulnerable organ (the skin is an organ).

Theoretically, it can be also be diverted to the joints, muscles, ligaments, fascia through the divergent and muscular-sinew channels and remain a silent retained pathogen until the body becomes too weak to hold it. I say "theoretically" because I do not know at what age these channels reach maturity and operate as described.

The meconium can be drained at any time in life along with other toxicities by employing the extraordinary channel, the *dai mai*, which is a "depository for postnatal junk" and "absorption of excess from the postnatal environment" (Jacob, 1996).

Respiratory Conditions

Allergies, Internal

> **FROM DR. SHEN:** Sinus problems and allergies are usually caused by weakened *qi* in the body. Often, a cold not treated properly is the original source of these problems. The problems caused by colds are underestimated. When a cold is not treated properly, it stays in the organs and weakens the body. If, in this condition, a cold is caught again, chronic sinus conditions and allergies can result.
>
> If an allergy is brought on by smell, it usually means that the lungs are both weak and cold. The stomach may also be weak, and eating habits may be wrong. If the allergies are brought on by eating, the function of the large intestine may be impaired. These conditions are treated by an internal formula, and a formula that is inhaled with steam.

Formula for internal allergies:

Pin Yin	Latin	English	Dosage
Bai zhi	Angelicae Dahuricae Radix	Angelica root	9 g
Cang er zi	Xanthii Sibirici Fructus	Cocklebur fruit, xanthium fruit	9 g
Chuan xiong	Chuanxiong Rhizoma	Chuanxiong root, Szechuan lovage root, cnidium	3 g
Xin yi hua	Magnoliae Flos	Magnolia flower	6 g
Zhe bie mu	Fritillariae Thunbergii Bulbus	Zhejiang fritillaria, Thunberg fritillaria bulb, fritillaria	9 g
Jiang can	Bombyx Batryticatus	Silkworm, body of sick silkworm	9 g
Ge gen	Puerariae Radix	Kudzu root, pueraria	6 g
Qiang huo	Notopterygii Rhizoma et Radix	Notopterygium root and rhizome, chiang-huo	3 g
Fang feng	Saposhnikoviae Radix	Ledebouriella root, saposhnikoviae root, siler	3 g

Hamilton Rotte Dr. Shen discovered that allergies and certain forms of asthma were due to exterior cold pathogens lodged in the lungs. The pathogen lodged in the lungs creates a chronic problem. He indicated that a deficiency of the lungs predisposed an individual to this condition, yet the first priority in treatment was to remove the cold pathogen. This is achieved by utilizing surfacing-relieving herbs.

All of the ingredients in this formula release the exterior except *zhe bie mu*. All of the ingredients are warm or neutral except *zhe bie mu* and *ge gen*. These ingredients increase fluids to offset any potential drying effects from warming diaphoretic herbs.

Allergies, Steam

Pin Yin	Latin	English	Dosage
Ge gen	Puerariae Radix	Kudzu root, pueraria	9 g
Fang feng	Saposhnikoviae Radix	Ledebouriella root, saposhnikoviae root, siler	9 g
Bai zhi	Angelicae Dahuricae Radix	Angelica root	9 g
Xin yi hua	Magnoliae Flos	Magnolia flower	9 g
Bo he	Menthae Haplocalycis Herba	Field mint, mentha, peppermint leaves	3 g
Cang er zi	Xanthii Sibirici Fructus	Cocklebur fruit, xanthium fruit	9 g

Hamilton Rotte   This is a modification of *Cang Er Zi San* (Xanthium Powder). Additions include *ge gen* and *fang feng*, also surface-releasing ingredients. Overall, this formula is slightly warm and contains surface-releasing ingredients that focus on opening the sinuses such as *bai zhi*, *xin yi hua*, and *cang er zi*.

Allergy and Chronic Fatigue

FROM DR. SHEN: *Qi* is weak—person catches cold, cold goes in. Chronic fatigue is caused by deep cold. The body gradually becomes weaker. Gradually take cold out from the body.
If smelling aggravates allergies—the lungs are weak and cold.

Basic formula:

Pin Yin	Latin	English	Dosage
Gui zhi	Ramulus Cinnamomi Cassiae	Cinnamon twig, cassia twig	1.5 g
Ge gen	Puerariae Radix	Kudzu root, pueraria	4.5 g
Chao jing jie	Schizonepetae Herba	Dry-fried schizonepeta	4.5 g
Chao fang feng	Saposhnikoviae Radix	Fried ledebouriella root, saposhnikoviae root, siler	4.5 g
Yuan zhi	Polygalae Radix	Chinese senega root, polygala root	4.5 g
Zhe bie mu	Fritillariae Thunbergii Bulbus	Zhejiang fritillaria, Thunberg fritillaria bulb, fritillaria	9 g

Use only a little—takes out deep cold, helps the heart.

Modifications of basic "Allergy and Chronic Fatigue" formula:

Lung:

Pin Yin	Latin	English	Dosage
Ma huang	Ephedrae Herba	Ephedra stem	2–9 g
Jiang can	Bombyx Batryticatus	Silkworm, body of sick silkworm	3–9 g

Food allergies:

Pin Yin	Latin	English	Dosage
Shan yao	Dioscoreae Oppositae Rhizoma	Chinese yam root	9–30 g
Bai zhu	Atractylodis Macrocephalae Rhizoma	White atractylodes rhizome	6–15 g

Kidneys weak:

Pin Yin	Latin	English	Dosage
Du zhong	Eucommiae Cortex	Eucommia bark	9–15 g
Rou cong rong	Cistanches Herba	Cistanche, fleshy stem of the broomrape	9–21 g

Energy:

Pin Yin	Latin	English	Dosage
Da zao	Zizyphi Jujubae Fructus	Chinese date, jujube	10–30 g
Shan zhu yu	Corni Officinalis Fructus	Asiatic Cornelian cherry fruit, cornus	6–12 g

Eyes red:

Pin Yin	Latin	English	Dosage
Bai ji li	Tribuli Terrestris Fructus	Caltrop fruit, puncture-vine fruit, tribulus	6–15 g
Ju hua	Chrysanthemi Flos	Chrysanthemum flower	4.5–15 g

Muscles:

Pin Yin	Latin	English	Dosage
Mu gua	Chaenomelis Fructus	Chinese quince fruit, chaenomeles	6–12 g
Wei ling xian	Clematidis Radix	Chinese clematis root	6–12 g

Memory:

Pin Yin	Latin	English	Dosage
Hu tao ren	Juglandis Regiae Semen	English walnut seed	9–15 g
Hei zhi ma	Sesami Nigrum Semen	Black sesame seed	9–30 g

Helps the heart:

Pin Yin	Latin	English	Dosage
Gui zhi	Ramulus Cinnamomi Cassiae	Cinnamon twig, cassia twig	1.5 g
Bai fu zi	Typhonii seu Radix Aconiti Rhizoma	Typhonium root	3 g
Yuan zhi	Polygalae Radix	Chinese senega root, polygala root	4.5 g

Leon Hammer
Etiology:
Complaint:
- Chronic fatigue syndrome
- Fibromyalgia

Pathogenesis of root:
- Severe "flu" that persists for months
- Recurs every year at the same time over a number of years
- True *qi* (*wei qi*) deficiency allows the cold to penetrate deeply and not be expelled.
- Organism attempts to eliminate exterior cold by bringing heat (*yang*) to move it out.
- Exterior cold continues to cause *qi* stagnation over the years while (floating slippery pulse with pounding).
- Futile attempt by body to eliminate internal heat adds to true *qi* deficiency experienced as chronic fatigue syndrome.
- Exterior cold gradually fatigues circulation:
  - Body attempts to bring the heat, causing stagnation.
  - An artificial blood deficiency occurs from poor blood circulation to nerve endings in the skin.
  - Resulting condition: fibromyalgia.

Etiology of the root and the individual:
- Terrain (pulse) shows heart and kidney most deficient.

- History:
  - Heart shock during pregnancy: mother psychotic during unplanned pregnancy
  - Nutrition poor
  - Mother's emotional state affects circulation in fetus (placenta)
- Root condition: heart-kidney *yang* deficiency
- Adaptation—the individual: mental-emotional:
  - Obsessive personality (mind)—controlling
  - Underlying anxiety—worrier
  - Drains heart and kidney *yin*
  - Obsessive work habits: drains heart and kidney *qi*

Signs:
Pulse:
- Proximal positions:
  - Reduce substance—diffuse
  - Feeble-absent progressing to "separation of *yin* and *yang*" (empty and change in qualities) and extreme physiological chaos

Tongue:
- Same as above, plus:
  - Body pale
  - Slightly swollen
  - Root: depressed, very pale

Asthma, Elderly Heart Condition

FROM DR. SHEN: Asthma is caused by:
- Deep cold
- Heart problems
- Liver problems
- Weakness of kidneys
- Emotions
- Poor eating habits and a weak digestive system

In asthma stop sex, until condition is resolved.

"Not true one"—moving a little causes asthma; heart problem. Not moving—no asthma:

Pin Yin	Latin	English	Dosage
Xi yang shen	Panacis Quinquefolii Radix	American ginseng root	4.5 g
Ge jie	Gekko Gecko Linnaeus	Gecko	1 tail
Su zi	Perillae Fructus	Perilla fruit	6 g
Wu wei zi	Schisandrae Chinensis Fructus	Schisandra fruit	4.5 g

Hamilton Rotte   Heart conditions frequently affect the lungs, especially deficiencies of the heart. In this case a deficiency of the heart *qi* causes asthma. Conditions that are worse on exertion are related to *qi* deficiency.

Xi yang shen is the *qi* tonic that directly targets the heart in this formula. It was one of Dr. Shen's favorite herbs to tonify heart *qi*. *Ge jie* is included to tonify the lungs. It also tonifies kidney *yang*, which Dr. Shen evidently considered part of this condition, and heart and kidney *qi-yang* deficiencies frequently co-exist. Asthma that is worse on exertion is frequently from kidney *yang* deficiency (kidneys not grasping *qi*).

Wu wei zi is a stabilizing herb that targets the lung and heart, among other organs. Stabilizing herbs are very effective to treat shortness of breath caused by deficiency.

Su zi, one of Dr. Shen's favorite herbs in the treatment of asthma, regulates and descends lung *qi*. Even in deficiency conditions he considered moving herbs to be important. Moving herbs can be contraindicated in deficiency, but in this formula it is balanced by the stabilizing and tonifying effects of the other herbs.

Leon Hammer
Etiology:
Since this formula primarily affects the lungs, this is one form of cardiopulmonary disease in which the lungs cannot oxygenate the blood, depriving the heart of oxygen.

Signs:
Pulse and tongue:
• See above for signs under "Allergies, Internal" (p. 156).

Asthma, Heart

"True one"—heart weak, worse on exertion:

Pin Yin	Latin	English	Dosage
Su zi	Perillae Fructus	Perilla fruit	6 g
Tian ting li zi	Descurainiae Semen	Sweet descurainia seeds, lepidium seeds	6 g
Wu wei zi	Schisandrae Chinensis Fructus	Schisandra fruit	4.5 g
Yuan zhi	Polygalae Radix	Chinese senega root, polygala root	4.5 g
Bai shao	Paeoniae Alba Radix	White peony root	6 g
Duan long gu	Fossilia Ossis Mastodi	Calcined fossilized dragon bone, fossilized vertebrae and bones of the extremities (usually of mammals)	12 g[a]
Mai men dong	Ophiopogonis Radix	Ophiopogon tuber/root	9 g

[a] Opens chest.

Hamilton Rotte   This formula is indicated for deficiency conditions (which are worse on exertion), and it contains a combination of moving and tonic herbs. *Su zi* is a strong herb for moving *qi* in the lungs. The type of *ting li zi* indicated here is the sweet variety (*tian ting li zi*). Ding Gan Ren indicated that it is important to distinguish between the sweet and bitter types of *ting li zi*. *Wu wei zi* stabilizes the lung *qi*:

• *Yuan zhi* is a moving and phlegm-resolving substance.
• According to Ding Gan Ren, *bai shao* treats rebellious lung *qi*, coughing, and asthma
• According to Ding Gan Ren, *long gu* enters the heart and dispels stasis.
• *Mai men dong* nourishes heart *yin*.

Leon Hammer

Etiology:

Here the asthma is a cardiopulmonary deficit due to heart *qi* deficiency in which the heart *qi* cannot move the blood circulation through *qi* and fluid obstruction in the lungs.

The rationale for this formula is the combined improvement of heart function and lung function by clearing lung phlegm-heat stagnation that will relieve asthma through the increased flow of blood and *qi* through the lungs. *Qi* moves the blood, which is perhaps why there is a liver-nourishing herb (*bai shao*). Except for *yuan zi* that resolves "phlegm misting the orifices," facilitates the flow of *qi* in the heart and calms the spirit, and *long gu* that calms the spirit, the other herbs serve to contain lung *qi* (*wu wei zi*) and clear heat.

Signs:

Pulse:

- LDP:
  - Deep to absent
  - Thin
  - Tight
  - Slippery
- Rate on exertion is less than 12 beats more than the resting rate
- RDP:
  - Deep
  - Feeble-absent
- SLP:
  - Slippery
  - Robust pounding
  - Muffled
  - Tense
  - Inflated
  - Rough vibration
  - Narrow
  - Restricted

Asthma, Herbal Inhaler

Pin Yin	Latin	English	Dosage
Ma huang	Ephedrae Herba	Ephedra stem	6 g[a]
Su zi	Perillae Fructus	Perilla fruit	6 g
Mi zhi zi wan	Asteris Radix	Honey-cooked purple aster, aster root	6 g
Jie geng	Platycodi Radix	Root of balloonflower, platycodon root	6 g
Bai zhi	Angelicae Dahuricae Radix	Angelica root	6 g
Zhe bie mu	Fritillariae Thunbergii Bulbus	Zhejiang fritillaria, Thunberg fritillaria bulb, fritillaria	6 g

[a] Does not have stimulating effect when inhaled.

Hamilton Rotte   This is a formula that should be decocted in a wide pan. The patient should hold their head about 30–60 cm over the decoction and inhale the steam as the herbs cook. This is an especially suitable treatment for an acute asthma episode.

This formula contains mostly herbs that move and descend lung *qi*. These include *ma huang*, *su zi*, *zi wan*, and *jie geng*. *Ma huang* does not have the stimulating effect when it is inhaled. *Zhe bie mu* is moistening and cooling and offsets the drying and warming tendencies of other herbs.

Asthma, Kidney

Pin Yin	Latin	English	Dosage
Su zi	Perillae Fructus	Perilla fruit	4.5 g
Bai zhu	Atractylodis Macrocephalae Rhizoma	White atractylodes rhizome	6 g
Bai shao	Paeoniae Alba Radix	White peony root	6 g
Mi zhi zi wan	Asteris Radix	Honey-cooked purple aster root	6 g
Zhe bie mu	Fritillariae Thunbergii Bulbus	Zhejiang fritillaria, Thunberg fritillaria bulb, fritillaria	9 g
Chuan bei mu	Fritillariae Cirrhosae Bulbus	Szechuan fritillaria bulb, tendrilled fritillary bulb, fritillaria	9 g
Tu si zi	Cuscutae Chinensis Semen	Chinese dodder seeds, cuscuta	9 g
Chao sheng di huang	Rehmanniae Radix	Dry-fried fresh Chinese foxglove root, rehmannia root	9 g[a]
Nan sha shen	Adenophorae seu Glehniae Radix	Adenophora root or glehnia root, ladybell root	9 g
Bu gu zhi	Psoraleae Corylifoliae Fructus	Psoralea fruit	6 g
Nu zhen zi	Ligustri Lucidi Fructus	Privet fruit, ligustrum	9 g

[a] Fried: more to blood, kidneys.

Hamilton Rotte This formula contains herbs that regulate and descend lung *qi*, resolve damp excess of the spleen and lungs, nourish lung *yin*, and tonify kidney *yin* and *yang*.

The herbs that regulate and descend lung *qi*, two of Dr. Shen's favorites for the treatment of asthma, include *su zi* and *mi zhi zi wan*. *Bai zhu* is included to resolve damp excess of the spleen.

Lung *yin* tonics include *chuan bei mu* and *nan sha shen*. Herbs that resolve phlegm in the lungs include *zhe bie mu*, *chuan bei mu*, *su zi*, and *mi zhi zi wan*.

Kidney *qi-yang* tonics in this formula include *tu si zi* and *bu gu zhi*. Kidney *yin* tonics include *sheng di huang* and *nu zhen zi*.

The inclusion of *bai shao* in many of Dr. Shen's formulas for asthma is difficult to explain, as it is usually used as a blood tonic for the liver.

Leon Hammer

Etiology:

Kidney *jing* is the energetic source of lung *qi* and is involved with all lung problems in childhood.

Signs:

Pulse:

- Proximal positions: any of the following with increasing amounts of deficiency:
  - Mild deficiency: *qi* depth, yielding, diminished, absent
  - Moderate deficiency: diffuse, reduced substance and reduced pounding
  - Severe deficiency: deep (*qi* and blood depths absent)
  - Chaotic *qi* ("separation of *yin* and *yang*"): empty, changing qualities

Tongue:

- Same as above, plus:
  - Body pale
  - Slightly swollen
  - Root: depressed, very pale

Comment:

This formula is frequently described in literature. Refer to "Allergies" section above (p. 156).

Asthma, Liver

FROM DR. SHEN: During the day no problem, problem at night; liver asthma, related to emotions.

Add to "Asthma, True" formula on page 165:

Pin Yin	Latin	English	Dosage
Xuan fu hua	Inulae Flos	Inula flower	6 g
Bai shao	Paeoniae Alba Radix	White peony root	6 g

Hamilton Rotte *Bai shao* is well known for its ability to "soften and comfort the liver." *Xuan fu hua* descends lung and liver *qi*. It is listed as entering the liver channel in standard texts, even though it is not commonly used for this purpose.

Leon Hammer I have found that the liver controls the peripheral nervous system, which includes the autonomic nervous system, sympathetic and parasympathetic. It is the relaxation and constriction of bronchi and bronchioles by the autonomic nervous system and its relationship to the effects of stress that concern us here. When the liver is functioning normally it regulates this relaxation and constriction according to the needs of the body to aerate the lungs.

Repression of emotions creates liver *qi* stagnation due to the responsibility of the liver to contain *qi* as well as move *qi*. There are two scenarios involving the consequences of liver *qi* stagnation that affect the sympathetic nervous system and the constriction and relaxation of bronchi and bronchioles, and therefore asthma. In either instance liver *qi* is no longer functioning normally and able to respond appropriately to the needs of the body to aerate the lungs.

One situation is usually more acute and occurs when the stagnant liver *qi* cannot be contained due to either a very great deal of stagnant liver or if liver *qi* is too deficient to contain even a moderate or small amount of *qi*. In either case the *qi* escapes from the liver and is diverted to the most vulnerable organ or area, as a retained pathogen in the case of asthma, to the lungs. This escaped liver *qi* is not functional and disrupts the sympathetic control of the bronchi and bronchioles so that when the need is for relaxation (sympathetic) the result might be constriction (parasympathetic).

The second instance when repression of liver *qi* and consequent stagnation affects the liver's normal control of the sympathetic nervous system is more gradual, therefore a chronic condition. This involves the well-known "liver *yang* rising" condition, which is primarily a deficient state of either *yin* or *yang* in which "metabolic heat" is required to relieve chronic liver *qi* stagnation. If it fails to overcome the stagnation "excess heat" accumulates.

The liver mobilizes its *yin* to balance the "excess heat" and over time, possibly years, the *yin* is depleted. Eventually the depleted *yin* cannot hold onto *yang*, "*yin* and *yang* separate" and *yang*, without the centripetal force of the *yin*, becomes out of control and dysfunctional. *Yang* is a lighter energy and rises, becoming the condition, "liver *yang* rising."

Again, this dysfunctional liver *yang* is diverted to the most vulnerable organ or area, and if it is the lungs, disrupts the normal sympathetic control of the bronchioles and bronchi, creating a deficient chronic asthmatic condition. "Separation of liver *yin* and *yang*" and "*yang* rising" can also occur with the increasingly common liver *yang* deficiency associated with the cold substances (marijuana, LSD and heroin).

This may be more of a problem at night when the containing function of the liver is relatively more relaxed and less vigilant.

Bai shao goes to the liver (and spleen) and nourishes blood that is stored in the liver. Blood is more *yin* than *yang*. That moistens, allows for softening; softness is blood. The blood is that part of *qi* that allows for receptivity and response to what is there; an acknowledgment of what has happened. Hence it is likened to memory. Blood is related to accessing memory, self-awareness. Being comfortable in the moment is more a blood phenomenon than a *qi* phenomenon. *Qi* is more about going places, dynamic and engaging; blood is about being places. If heaven is equated with *qi*, then earth is related to blood (see chapters and

hexagrams in *I Ching* [*Book of Changes*]—'The Creative,' 'The Receptive'; personal communication, Ted Kapchuck, LAc ca. 1983/84).
Therefore, with regard to the stagnation of *qi* either due to excess or deficiency *bai shao*'s enhancing of blood in the liver will soften the struggle between the *qi* that moves and the *qi* that contains and the consequences of that struggle described above.

Asthma, Spleen and Stomach

FROM DR. SHEN: Poor nutrition, problem goes to lung—a lot of mucus.

Pin Yin	Latin	English	Dosage
Su zi	Perillae Fructus	Perilla fruit	4.5 g
Bai zhu	Atractylodis Macrocephalae Rhizoma	White atractylodes rhizome	6 g
Bai shao	Paeoniae Alba Radix	White peony root	6 g
Fu hai shi	Costaziae Os	Constaziae skeleton	12 g
Mi zhi zi wan	Asteris Radix	Honey-cooked purple aster, aster root	6 g
Nan sha shen	Adenophorae seu Glehniae Radix	Adenophora root or glehnia root, ladybell root	9 g
Zhe bie mu	Fritillariae Thunbergii Bulbus	Zhejiang fritillaria, Thunberg fritillaria bulb, fritillaria	9 g
Chuan bei mu	Fritillariae Cirrhosae Bulbus	Szechuan fritillaria bulb, tendrilled fritillary bulb, fritillaria	9 g
Dan nan xing	Arisaematis Praeparatum Rhizoma cum Felle Bovis	Arisaema pulvis, Jack in the pulpit rhizome with cow bile	4.5 g[a]
Lai fu zi	Raphani Semen	Radish seed, raphanus	2.4 g

[a] Do not use if tongue is dry—substitute *tian zhi huang* (tabasheer or siliceous secretions of bamboo) 2 g.

Hamilton Rotte Damp excess produced by the spleen frequently affects the lungs. Phlegm in the lungs is sticky and cloying and disruptive to the orderly descent of lung *qi*. In this situation the treatment is to dry dampness in the spleen, expel phlegm in the lungs, and descend lung *qi*.
The herb that dries dampness in the spleen is *bai zhu*. *Lai fu zi* reduces food stagnation, thereby aiding in the separation of pure and impure in the middle burner.

Herbs that expel phlegm from the lungs include *su zi, mi zhi zi wan, zhe bie mu, chuan bei mu, dan nan xing,* and *lai fu zi*. All of these also descend lung *qi*. *Fu hai shi* is salty and softens viscous phlegm.
Nan sha shen descends lung *qi* and is moistening, offsetting the drying tendencies of the phlegm-resolving herbs.
Bai shao is included here because it descends lung *qi* and tonifies the middle (as described by Ding Gan Ren).

Leon Hammer
Etiology:
According to the "internal duct of the triple burner," pure (*gu*) *qi* from food goes to the spleen, which separates it into the "concentrated essence" that forms the "five tastes" distributed by the spleen to each solid organ. "Impure *qi*" is condensed to form "fluids" via the lungs to the kidneys (kidney *yin*) (in accor-

dance with the philosophy of the earth–metal–water *sheng* cycle).
If lung *qi* is deficient it does not descend fluids to the kidneys and accumulates in the lungs. If a person drinks excessive amounts of fluid, which seems to be the prevalent practice, even normal lung *qi* will have trouble descending the fluid that will accumulate in the lung. Metabolic heat is brought to the lung to

move the stagnant fluid and accumulates if it fails, combining with the fluid to form phlegm-heat that obstructs the bronchioles and bronchi.

Signs:

Pulse:

• Right distal position and special lung position:
  – Slippery with robust pounding feeble or even changing to absent.

Tongue:

• A thick yellow coat is found especially in the lung area that might be sunken
• Mucus threads are common lengthwise between the center and edge of the tongue

Asthma, True

> **FROM DR. SHEN:** Affected by changes in weather, deep cold, pathogenic factor, hypo-function. Bronchitis becomes asthma. True asthma changes with the weather—this shows that it is related to the lung.

Pin Yin	Latin	English	Dosage
Ma huang	Ephedrae Herba	Ephedra stem	2.4 g
Su zi	Perillae Fructus	Perilla fruit	6 g
Niu bang zi	Arctii Lappae Fructus	Great burdock fruit, arctium	6 g
Mi zhi zi wan	Asteris Radix	Honey-cooked purple aster, aster root	6 g
Zhe bie mu	Fritillariae Thunbergii Bulbus	Zhejiang fritillaria, Thunberg fritillaria bulb, fritillaria	9 g
Bai jie zi	Sinapis Albae Semen	White mustard seed	9 g
Ting li zi	Descurainiae seu Lepidii Semen	Descurainia seeds, lepidium seeds	6 g
Pi pa ye	Eriobotryae Folium	Loquat leaf, dried leaf of *Eriobotrya Japonica*	9 g
Chan tui	Periostracum Cicadae	Cicada moultings	4.5 g

Hamilton Rotte This formula addresses a situation described by Dr. Shen that can also cause allergies and chronic fatigue, where a cold pathogen enters the lungs amidst a background of lung deficiency. As with the allergies and chronic fatigue protocols, emphasis is first placed on eliminating the pathogen. This formula contains the following ingredients to release the exterior: *ma huang*, *niu bang zi*, and *chan tui*.

Although it is a cold pathogen that has lodged in the lungs, internal heat is produced as the body tries to deal with the pathogen. Therefore, both warming and cooling herbs are included in this formula to address both aspects of the situation. The cooling herbs include *niu bang zi*, *zhe bie mu*, *ting li zi*, *pi pa ye*, and *chan tui*. The warming herbs include *ma huang*, *su zi*, *mi zhi zi wan*, and *bai jie zi*.

The single unifying treatment principle of this formula is to regulate lung *qi*. All of the herbs in this formula with the possible exception of *chan tui* descend lung *qi*.

After the pathogen has been cleared and symptoms improve, tonic therapy is indicated, but experience has shown that patients with this condition do not respond to tonics if they are introduced too early.

In the TCM literature, asthma is related to exterior conditions, phlegm in the lungs, and deficiencies of the lung and the kidneys. Dr. Shen emphasized the importance of exterior conditions in asthma.

This formula is designed to address an exterior pathogen that has lodged in the lungs, a cause of chronic asthma. Even though the presence of a pathogen that has moved into the interior implies a vulnerability of the lungs, this formula first addresses the pathogen. This formula contains the following to release the exterior: *ma huang*, *pi pa ye*, and *chan tui*. Every ingredient except for *niu bang zi* and *chan tui* has the function of downbearing lung *qi*. Most of the ingredients resolve phlegm, and we find that the formula is balanced between hot and cold herbs.

In our experience, this formula is especially useful when allergy and asthma symptoms are present, but once they subside, tonic therapy that address the lungs and kidneys is indicated.

Leon Hammer The reason that heat-clearing herbs are used in cold conditions is that the organism abhors stagnation. Wherever there is stagnation the organism will attempt to overcome it to restore the normal flow of *qi*, blood, and other body fluids. It does this in all cases by bringing metabolic heat to move the stagnation.

The invasion of cold creates stagnation of all of the above substances. If the metabolic heat that is focused on moving that stagnation does not succeed, it accumulates and itself becomes a pathogen. Therefore, a formula that attempts to release a cold pathogen must include heat-clearing herbs to remove this secondary heat pathogen.

Chronic Fatigue

FROM DR. SHEN: Worse than allergies; deep-level cold; weak organs.

First treatment: cupping on back (especially BL-12, *feng men*)

Second treatment:

Pin Yin	Latin	English	Dosage
Ge gen	Puerariae Radix	Kudzu root, pueraria	6 g
Cang er zi	Xanthii Sibirici Fructus	Cocklebur fruit, xanthium fruit	9 g
Xin yi hua	Magnolia Flos	Magnolia flower	4.5 g
Jie geng	Platycodi Radix	Root of balloonflower, platycodon root	6 g
Jiang can	Bombyx Batryticatus	Silkworm, body of sick silkworm	9 g
Fang feng	Saposhnikoviae Radix	Ledebouriella root, saposhnikoviae root, siler	6 g
Dang shen	Codonopsis Pilosulae Radix	Codonopsis root	6 g
Qiang huo	Notopterygii Rhizoma et Radix	Notopterygium root and rhizome, chiang-huo	6 q

Hamilton Rotte Dr. Shen described a retained cold pathogen as a primary cause of allergies, asthma, and chronic fatigue.

Conventional methods within TCM for addressing fatigue utilize tonic therapy, utilizing *qi*, blood or *yang* tonics. Here Dr. Shen is utilizing surface-releasing herbs to dredge a retained cold pathogen to address fatigue. The following herbs "release the exterior": *ge gen*, *cang er zi*, *xin yi hua*, *jiang can*, *fang feng*, and *qiang huo*. *Jie geng* is a guide herb for the lungs, descends lung *qi*, and aids in releasing the exterior. Most of the exterior-releasing herbs in this formula are warm, though *ge gen* is cooling and fluid nourishing, which offsets the drying tendencies of the other herbs. *Dang shen* is a *qi* tonic, the one tonic in the formula. It is commonly utilized to tonify *qi* in the presence of pathogens because of its ability to tonify without retaining excess conditions, as stronger tonics often do.

Third treatment—inhale only, don't drink:

Pin Yin	Latin	English	Dosage
Ma qian zi	Strychni Semen	Nux-vomica seeds	6 g[a]
Qiang huo	Notopterygii Rhizoma et Radix	Notopterygium root and rhizome, chiang-huo	6 g
Fang feng	Saposhnikoviae Radix	Ledebouriella root, saposhnikoviae root, siler	6 g
Ge gen	Puerariae Radix	Kudzu root, pueraria	6 g
Xin yi hua	Magnolia Flos	Magnolia flower	6 g
Cang er zi	Xanthii Sibirici Fructus	Cocklebur fruit, xanthium fruit	6 g
Bo he	Menthae Haplocalycis Herba	Field mint, mentha, peppermint leaves	3 g

[a] Strychnine—illegal; removes nasal polyps. Toxic and obsolete.

FROM DR. SHEN: Make sure to cover chest, upper back, and neck when getting out of bed. This area is delicate at this time—the *wei qi* is not ready to protect. Exposure to cold at this time can cause allergies and sinus problems.

Leon Hammer While Dr. Shen did attribute the chronic fatigue syndrome to the invasion of a cold pathogen, which has been confirmed on more than one occasion, it is clear to me and others that there are many causes.

A very common scenario in my clinical practice was a woman with a deadbeat husband who supported her family by working as a nurse from 11 p.m. to 7 a.m., returning home to get her children ready for school, including breakfast and dressing. She then cleaned the house, took care of all the business aspects of family life (bills etc.), made appointments for her family health care, and tried to get a few hours sleep. She was there for her children when they returned from school, fed them supper, helped with the homework and put them to bed before she set off for another night as a nurse. After 30 years of this, chronic fatigue set in.

Another condition that I associate with all chronic disease is the "separation of *yin* and *yang*" of many organ systems that we call the "*qi* wild" syndrome (Hammer, 1998, p. 15). In particular, this condition is associated with autoimmune diseases in which the *yin* cannot hold onto the *yang* that once separated from the grounding *yin* becomes an erratic source of heat that disturbs the function of all aspects of physiology, especially the most vulnerable.

Lungs Weak

Pin Yin	Latin	English	Dosage
Chuan bei mu	Fritillariae Cirrhosae Bulbus	Szechuan fritillaria bulb, tendrilled fritillary bulb, fritillaria	9 g
Dong chong xia cao	Cordyceps Sinensis	Chinese caterpillar fungus	9 g

Hamilton Rotte This elegant formula combines two of the most useful tonic herbs in Chinese medicine for the lungs. *Chuan bei mu* is used for lung *yin* deficiency (and phlegm) and does not have the cloy- ing effects of many richer lung *yin* tonics. *Dong chong xia cao* is a *qi* and *yin* tonic for the lungs and also lacks the cloying or excessively warming effects of other tonic herbs.

Sores of the Mouth, Temporary

FROM DR. SHEN: Sores in the mouth can occur with varying frequency. Sores that appear infrequently can be brought on by a cold or a slightly weak body condition. Sores that appear more frequently, and are accompanied by a sensation of heat, are caused by a weaker body condition and heat in the lung.

Pin Yin	Latin	English	Dosage
Jing jie	Schizonepetae Herba	Schizonepeta	4.5 g
Fang feng	Saposhnikoviae Radix	Ledebouriella root, saposhnikoviae root, siler	4.5 g
She gan	Belamcandae Rhizoma	Belamcanda rhizome	3 g
Ting li zi	Descurainiae seu Lepidii Semen	Descurainia seeds, lepidium seeds	6 g
Chan tui	Periostracum Cicadae	Cicada moultings	4.5 g
Jie geng	Platycodi Radix	Root of balloonflower, platycodon root	6 g
Xuan shen	Scrophulariae Radix	Ningpo figwort root, scrophularia	9 g
Chi shao	Paeoniae Rubra Radix	Red peony root	9 g
Zhe bie mu	Fritillariae Thunbergii Bulbus	Zhejiang fritillaria, Thunberg fritillaria bulb, fritillaria	9 g
Ma bo	Fructificatio Lasiosphaera seu Calvatia	Fruiting body of puff-ball	3 g

Hamilton Rotte   Sores of the mouth can arise from digestive problems (notably heat in the stomach or spleen deficiency), and they can also occur in respiratory conditions. This formula is indicated for an exterior invasion of wind-heat lodging in the lungs, creating a heat toxin condition.

Herbs that release the exterior include *jing jie*, *fang feng*, *chan tui*, and *jie geng*.

Herbs that clear heat from the lungs include *ting li zi*, *xuan shen*, and *zhe bie mu*. Both of these are also moistening, offsetting drying effects of other herbs.

Herbs that resolve heat toxicity in the lungs include *she gan* and *ma bo*. *Chi shao*, while not strictly considered an herb for heat toxicity is indicated for the early stages of abscesses and boils. Dr. Shen probably chose the herb for this reason.

Sores of the Mouth, Constant

Pin Yin	Latin	English	Dosage
Chan tui	Periostracum Cicadae	Cicada moultings	4.5 g
Jing jie	Schizonepetae Herba	Schizonepeta	4.5 g
Fang feng	Saposhnikoviae Radix	Ledebouriella root, saposhnikoviae root, siler	4.5 g
Mu dan pi	Moutan Radicis Cortex	Tree peony root bark, moutan root bark	9 g
Ma bo	Fructificatio Lasiosphaera seu Calvatia	Fruiting body of puff-ball	3 g
Gan cao	Glycyrrhizae Radix	Licorice root	4.5 g
Zhe bie mu	Fritillariae Thunbergii Bulbus	Zhejiang fritillaria, Thunberg fritillaria bulb, fritillaria	9 g
Jiang can	Bombyx Batryticatus	Silkworm, body of sick silkworm	9 g
Huang qin	Scutellariae Baicalensis Radix	Baical skullcap root, scutellaria, scute	6 g
Hei shan zhi zi	Gardeniae Jasminoidis Fructus	Charred cape jasmine fruit, gardenia fruit	9 g

Hamilton Rotte   This formula, like the previous formula, releases the exterior, cools heat in the lungs, and resolves toxicity. Herbs that release the exterior include *chan tui, jing jie, fang feng*, and *jiang can*. Herbs that cool the lungs include *zhe bie mu* and *huang qin. Ma bo* clears heat and toxicity.

Dr. Shen must have viewed the heat as being deeper in the body in the case of constant sores, because we find herbs that cool the blood. These include *mu dan pi, huang qin*, and *shan zhi zi*.

Sores of the Mouth, Virus/Canker Sores

FROM DR. SHEN: In Chinese medicine, the concept of viruses is less important than understanding why one person gets sick and another does not, or why different parts of the body become dysfunctional in different people. These sores are therefore seen to be caused by digestive problems and a very weak body condition. Digestive sores are considered "strong" and can develop from consuming spicy foods or alcohol, which make the stomach too hot. These sores can be aggravated by lack of sleep. Another type of sore appears more frequently and is considered "weak." These are caused by a poor body condition, and can be a precursor to more serious disease.

Pin Yin	Latin	English	Dosage
Fang feng	Saposhnikoviae Radix	Ledebouriella root, saposhnikoviae root, siler	6 g
Xuan shen	Scrophulariae Radix	Ningpo figwort root, scrophularia	9 g
Huang bai	Phellodendri Cortex	Amur corktree bark, phellodendron bark	9 g
Gan cao	Glycyrrhizae Radix	Licorice root	4.5 g
Long dan cao	Gentianae Longdancao Radix	Chinese gentian root, gentiana	4.5 g
Mai men dong	Ophiopogonis Radix	Ophiopogon tuber/root	9 g
Shen qu	Massa Medicata Fermentata	Medicated leaven (dough)	9 g
Mu dan pi	Moutan Radicis Cortex	Tree peony root bark, moutan root bark	9 g
Lu gen	Phragmitis Communis Rhizoma	Reed rhizome	9 g

Hamilton Rotte   This formula is indicated for sores due to an excess condition. The focus is on taking heat out of the stomach and liver, though there are also herbs to treat the lungs.
Herbs that cool the liver include *long dan cao* and *mu dan pi*. Herbs that treat heat in the stomach include *xuan shen, mai men dong*, and *lu gen*.

Shen qu resolves food stagnation, suggesting the etiology of this condition includes improper eating. *Huang bai* clears heat in the intestines.
We also find an herb to release the exterior (*fang feng*), and herbs that cool the lungs including *xuan shen, mai men dong*, and *lu gen*.

Dr. Shen's Life Cycle Formulas

Formulas in this section that also have commentaries in the previous section are indicated by "See

Leon Hammer Dr. Shen's original comments make up the main text. The authors' comments are marked by a sidebar and their names.
Some of what follows is exactly in Dr Shen's own words and is obvious from his inexact English. Whereas I know that the ideas in each section are his since I was with him when they were spoken and did the first three edits, subsequently they were revised by English-speaking assistants in China with somewhat more, but still less than standard, sophisticated English.
While this was intended for a lay audience in an unpublished book called *Book of Life* and will be lacking in the conceptual depth expected of a master of Chinese medicine, it was one of his unique abilities to communicate the medicine and their conditions in the patient's own language.
We have retained the herbal formulas in this part of the book that accompanied the original of Dr. Shen's *Book of Life* and repeated those that are discussed and analyzed in detail in the previous section "Dr. Shen's Formulas in Systems."
The cognitive foundation of his approach is important in its own right. The format is his own plan for a book that would take the layperson through an entire life cycle from conception to death and is in everyday language. This is important because in communicating to his patients, Dr. Shen used similes familiar to everyone as we will see below.
This brings us to the central issue: lifestyle.
Lifestyle:
Lifestyle is the constant theme of Dr. Shen's clinical practice and consequently of this section of the book, and he stated frequently "Chinese medicine is in the life." What I have written here in the service of coherency is incrementally repeated in Dr. Shen's narratives accompanying each formula.
Dr. Shen expressed the medicine in tangible practical common sense terms of real life experience of the individual rather than just the pattern. He made it

also Dr. Shen's Formulas in Systems," with a page reference.

abundantly clear that without changes in lifestyle the prescribed treatments would not succeed.
A common admonishment to a patient who was not recovering was "Your fault, not mine. What you do?" meaning in which of the many ways was this person going beyond their energy and abusing themselves that rendered his considered treatment unworkable?
While this included emotional stress, his formula of "stop worrying" was somewhat infuriating to the psychologically sophisticated New York City clientele. He referred them to me. Yet, with some patients he devoted considerable time listening and responding to their problems and is well remembered by them for this.
Dr. Shen used everyday analogies to explain his concepts. Again, with regard to lifestyle he used one involving an object familiar to all of his clients: a car. He said that there were four kinds: one is good and well taken care of, one is good and over-used, one is poor and well taken care of, and the other is poor and poorly taken care of.
Obviously, the good car that is well taken care of will be the best. However, the point he was making was that the poor car that is well taken care of, a Model T Ford, will be better than the good car that is neglected, a Rolls Royce.
The quality of the car I refer to as the "terrain" and the care of the car as the "stress" (Hammer, 2010a). Diagnostically we can differentiate terrains and can advise our patients according to their terrain as to the limits of the stresses they can endure without developing symptoms. Therefore, a person with a good terrain can do 50 sit-ups without untoward depletion of their *qi*, while a person with a lesser terrain might be advised to do only 10.
Many people with lesser terrains, men included, break down in tears of relief when informed that they were never meant to operate three businesses at once and be healthy. Finally being free of the imperative to perform beyond their inherent endowment, I have seen

profound changes in people's lives with this liberating information. And with Dr. Shen's diagnostic system this "constitutional" information is available.

Dr. Shen, as we should all appreciate, was primarily concerned with prevention. Prevention depends on early detection of the disease process. Early detection depends upon a diagnosis sensitive to the earliest signs of that process that identifies the insults and abuses to physiology. While he had a multitude of diagnostic tools, for Dr. Shen the pulse was the principal diagnostic methodology.

This is discussed in detail in *Chinese Pulse Diagnosis: A Contemporary Approach* (Hammer, 2001). Deep, feeble, or empty proximal positions in a person under the age of 60 without a history of extraordinary stress such as childhood slave labor would indicate a kidney essence deficiency associated with a constitutional etiology. A history of childhood inability to keep up physically with peers, severe allergies and asthma, profound fear, learning disabilities (for example, ADHD), afternoon fevers and physical disabilities such as childhood hernias were other indicators of a constitutional, kidney essence deficiency ("nervous system weak").

"Lifestyle" abuses include overwork or over-exercise (also stopping either suddenly [Hammer, 2011]), lifting, swimming in very cold water (especially women), drinking very cold drinks (or chewing ice), eating excessively, irregularly, or rapidly, poor grade food, consuming over-spiced food, emotional instability (repression of feelings, thinking or worrying while eating), bulimia, and anorexia. Others include excessive sex or abstinence, substances of abuse, unnecessary medication and surgeries, poor sleep habits, dangerous activities, working conditions (unventilated room, poor posture, repetitive physical activity), exposure to toxins, pace of life, and lack of rest, among a few of the many.

All of the "overs" above are of course over and beyond one's innate capacity for such activity. We are not all created equal.

In passing, I wish to emphasize Dr. Shen's thesis illustrated in the following discussions of the concept of multiple etiology encapsulated in his repeating frequently that "you cannot make a sound with one *bao ding* ball" and which I expounded in the article "Science east and west" (Hammer, 2010b).

Cold:

Dr. Shen considered the invasion of and retained "cold" to be an extremely important factor in many diseases including those seemingly remote from our usual associations with it such as respiratory conditions. As far-fetched as it may seem and as skeptical as I was to begin with, I found, as he predicted, that some chronic fatigue syndromes, for example, could be traced to a "cold" invasion. Of course, these were *qi*-deficient people to begin with, which permitted the retention rather than elimination of the "cold." However, eliminating the cold was, in my experience, a necessary part of the management.

In Preparation for Conception

When a couple is ready to have a baby, they must take good care of themselves by nourishing themselves with herbal medicine and by cultivating a cordial and happy mood.

Some women become so weak that they lose too much blood during their menstrual flow, which exacerbates the weakness. If they overwork at the same time, dizziness and palpitations may be experienced. A simple treatment is to drink ginger tea made in the following way: cut three thin pieces of fresh ginger (approximately the thickness of a nickel) and boil them for 10 minutes. Sweeten with a little red rock sugar. The rock sugar should not be average brown sugar; it should be the kind of sugar bought at a Chinese grocery store in block form.

Sometimes, even if they don't lose too much blood with menstruation, stomach pain is sometimes felt, which may be caused by stagnant blood in the abdomen. In this case improvement may be made by drinking several cups of hot ginger tea. Put several slices of peeled fresh ginger in water and simmer, sweeten it with a small cube of white rock sugar (the thickness of a nickel), and drink before each period, one cup a day for several days.

Sexual Intercourse

Already alluded to above, when a couple is ready to have a baby, they must be aware of several important considerations. They should never have sex when drunken or exhausted. Any sort of irritation or tension, such as great anger, would constitute an unfavorable condition for conception.

Alcohol and other chemicals are harmful to the blood. These substances have an adverse effect on both the semen and the egg, and in turn on the fetus, which can lead to natal diseases. Exhaustion, especially due to intercourse, lowers one's immunity and harms the health of both partners. Any sort of drastic changes in emotion should be avoided as they will act unfavorably upon fetal development.

The gender of the child is decided upon at the instant of the climax. When the woman's climax comes first, the child will be a boy, when the man's climax comes before that of the woman it will be a girl. In my personal investigation of my clients' experience, this point has been proved quite accurate.

Female Infertility/Sterility

Infertility of a woman should not be assumed to be so based entirely on Western medical methods. Consider the following three cases:
- Infertility due to a cold womb
- Infertility due to a womb that is too warm
- Infertility due to deficiency in the womb

When sperm enters the womb, it arrives in much the same way that a stranger enters a new room. If the room temperature is too cold or warm, the stranger will feel uncomfortable. If the room is without ventilation, the stranger will also feel uneasy. In both cases the visitor will find the room inhospitable. Only with the use of these Chinese medical diagnostic considerations can one effectively treat a patient's particular fertility issues.

The typical features during periods of the above-mentioned cases of infertility are listed in the table below (see also "Dr. Shen's Formulas in Systems," p. 75):

Condition	Pain in Periods	Color	Quantity	Pulse	Other Symptoms
Cold womb	Pain in the belly	Pale, dark	Little	Deep	With clots in blood, dislikes tight clothing, prefers warm dress and drinks
Warm womb strong body	Slight pain 1–2 days before	Dark	Much	Fine	Dark clots in blood
Warm womb	No pain	Pale	A bit more	Fine	A longer period
Weak womb	Feeling pain	Pale red	Little	Very weak	Feeling cold, dizzy at the end of period, dim-sighted, short periods (3 days)

Treatment of a Cold Womb

Formula for a cold womb (see also "Dr Shen's Formulas in Systems, " p. 71):

Pin Yin	Latin	English	Dosage
Jiu dang gui	Angelicae Sinensis Radix	Chinese Angelica root, tang-kuei prepared with 1 tsp of wine	6 g
Ai ye	Artemisiae Argyi Folium	Mugwort leaf, artemesia	3 g
Gan jiang	Zingiberis Rhizoma	Dried ginger	3 g
Dan shen	Salviae Miltiorrhiziae Radix	Salvia root	9 g
Yi mu cao	Leonuri Herba	Chinese motherwort, leonurus	6 g
Lu lu tong	Liquidambaris Fructus	Sweetgum fruit, liquidambar fruit	12 g
Rou gui	Cinnamomi Cassiae Cortex	Inner bark of Saigon cinnamon	0.3 g

Treatment of a Warm Womb

Formula for an overly warm womb (see also "Dr. Shen's Formulas in Systems," p. 72):

Pin Yin	Latin	English	Dosage
Sheng di huang	Rehmannia Radix	Fresh Chinese foxglove root, rehmannia root	9 g
Dang gui	Angelicae Sinensis Radix	Chinese Angelica root, tang-kuei	6 g
Chuan xiong	Chuanxiong Rhizoma	Chuanxiong root, Szechuan lovage root, cnidium	4.5 g
Bai shao	Paeoniae Alba Radix	White peony root	6 g
Fu ling	Poria Cocos Sclerotium	Sclerotium of tuckahoe, poria, China root, hoelen, Indian bread	9 g
Dan shen	Salviae Miltiorrhiziae Radix	Salvia root	6 g
Mu dan pi	Moutan Radicis Cortex	Tree peony root bark, moutan root bark	6 g
Chi shao	Paeoniae Rubra Radix	Red peony root	9 g
Hei shan zhi zi	Gardeniae Jasminoidis Fructus	Charred cape jasmine fruit, gardenia fruit	9 g

Treatment for Infertility Due to Deficiency with Womb that is Slightly Too Warm

Formula for a deficient, slightly warm womb (see also "Dr. Shen's Formulas in Systems," p. 73):

Pin Yin	Latin	English	Dosage
Dang gui	Angelicae Sinensis Radix	Chinese Angelica root, tang-kuei	6 g
Dan shen	Salviae Miltiorrhiziae Radix	Salvia root	6 g
Hong hua	Carthami Tinctorii Flos	Safflower flower, carthamus	6 g
Chao sheng di huang	Rehmannia Radix	Fried root of rehmannia, fried Chinese foxglove root	9 g
Chao huang qi	Astragali Radix	Fried milk vetch root, fried astragalus root	4.5 g
Yu jin	Curcumae Radix	Curcuma tuber	9 g
Chuan xiong	Chuanxiong Rhizoma	Chuanxiong root, Szechuan lovage root, cnidium	4.5 g
Yan hu suo	Corydalis Yanhusuo Rhizoma	Corydalis rhizome	9 g
Xi yang shen	Panacis Quinquefolii Radix	American ginseng root	4.5 g
Di gu pi	Lycii Radicis Cortex	Cortex of wolfberry root, lycium bark	6 g

Deficiency in the Womb

Formula for deficiency of the womb (see also "Dr. Shen's Formulas in Systems," p. 74):

Pin Yin	Latin	English	Dosage
Huang qi	Astragali Radix	Milk vetch root, astragalus root	15 g
Dang shen	Codonopsis Pilosulae Radix	Codonopsis root	15 g
Dang gui	Angelicae Sinensis Radix	Chinese Angelica root, tang-kuei	15 g
Shu di huang	Rehmanniae Preparata Radix	Prepared Chinese foxglove root (cooked in red wine), cooked rehmannia rhizome	15 g
Da zao	Ziziphi Jujubae Fructus	Chinese date, jujube	7 dates
Tu si zi	Cuscutae Chinensis Semen	Chinese dodder seeds, cuscuta	12 g
Shu nu zhen zi	Ligustri Lucidi Fructus	Prepared fruit of glossy privet	12 g

Miscarriage

Formula for the prevention of miscarriage (see also "Dr. Shen's Formulas in Systems," p. 75):

Pin Yin	Latin	English	Dosage
Chao bai zhu	Atractylodis Macrocephalae Rhizoma	Dry-fried white atractylodes rhizome	6 g
Shan yao	Dioscoreae Oppositae Rhizoma	Chinese yam, dioscorea rhizome	12 g
Chao bai shao	Paeoniae Alba Radix	Fried root of white peony	6 g
Fu ling	Poria Cocos Sclerotium	Sclerotium of tuckahoe, poria, China root, hoelen, Indian bread	9 g

Pin Yin	Latin	English	Dosage
Yuan zhi	Polygalae Radix	Chinese senega root, polygala root	4.5 g
Tu si zi	Cuscutae Chinensis Semen	Chinese dodder seeds, cuscuta	9 g
Nu zhen zi	Ligustri Lucidi Fructus	Privet fruit, ligustrum	9 g
Zhu huang qi	Astragali Radix	Dried Milk vetch root, astragalus root	4.5 g

Anxiety

A childless woman over 35 is very anxious for a baby. Failure always makes her feel very troubled and nervous. When women with histories of miscarriage become pregnant again they are always afraid of its recurrence. The fact is, the more they worry, the farther away are they from their aspiration. When other factors are excluded, anxiety can be the single cause of infertility. The patient is advised to relax as much as possible and overcome anxiety, which is the only obstacle in her way.

Formula for anxiety:

Pin Yin	Latin	English	Dosage
Cu chai hu	Bupleuri Radix	Fried hare's ear root, thorowax root, bupleurum with vinegar	6 g
Chao dang gui	Angelicae Sinensis Radix	Fried Chinese Angelica root, tang-kuei	9 g
Bai shao	Paeoniae Alba Radix	White peony root	9 g
Sheng gan cao	Glycyrrhizae Radix	Fresh licorice root	6 g
Fu ling	Poria Cocos Sclerotium	Sclerotium of tuckahoe, poria, China root, hoelen, Indian bread	9 g
Sheng bai zhu	Atractylodis Macrocephalae Rhizoma	Fresh white atractylodes rhizome	6 g
Bo he	Menthae Haplocalycis Herba	Field mint, mentha, peppermint leaves	6 g
Mu dan pi	Moutan Radicis Cortex	Tree peony root bark, moutan root bark	9 g
Chao shan zhi zi	Gardeniae Jasminoidis Fructus	Fried cape jasmine fruit, gardenia fruit	9 g
Sheng jiang	Zingiberis Officinalis Recens Rhizoma	Fresh ginger rhizome	3 slices

Soak the herbal medicine in water before boiling for 20 minutes and drink the filtrate in two parts, twice a day. Continue the practice until the anxiety is relieved.

Male Infertility

Formula for male infertility (see also "Dr. Shen's Formulas in Systems," p. 66):

Pin Yin	Latin	English	Dosage
Wu wei zi	Schisandrae Chinensis Fructus	Schisandra fruit	20 g
Tu si zi	Cuscutae Chinensis Semen	Chinese dodder seeds, cuscuta	20 g
Che qian zi	Plantaginis Semen	Plantago seeds	20 g
She chuang zi	Cnidii Fructus	Cnidium seed	20 g
Fu pen zi	Rubi Fructus	Palm leaf raspberry fruit	20 g

Pin Yin	Latin	English	Dosage
Rou cong rong	Cistanches Herba	Cistanche, fleshy stem of the broomrape	20 g
Zhi yuan zhi	Polygalae Radix	Prepared Chinese senega root, polygala root	
			20 g
Zhong ru shi	Stalactitum	Stalactite	40 g
Lu rong	Cornu Cervi Parvum	Velvet of young deer antler, cervi	20 g

This formula should be taken in powder form, 3 g twice daily, to improve male sexual function.

Pregnancy and Childbirth

Thousands of years of medical history have shown that Chinese medicine is very effective in treating all the symptoms that appear in pregnancy and childbirth.

Diet

In her pregnancy, the expectant mother should avoid hot, chilly, or pungent foods. She should avoid drinking alcohol or consuming any food or beverage other than those absolutely free of chemicals. Diet has a direct effect on the blood of the mother, upon which the fetus depends for growth and nourishment. When the blood is contaminated, the mental and physical health, first of the mother herself then of the infant, will be unavoidably impaired. Strict control of diet must be exercised in pregnancy. Generally speaking, a pregnant mother will gain 9 to 13 kg of additional weight.

Sexual Intercourse

According to an old Chinese tradition, a wife should not share the same room with her husband after 3 months of pregnancy. At 5 months of pregnancy she must live separately in her "harem" to guard against male intrusion. The family should take good care of her and her diet. Nothing should happen to cause her worry or anger.

Too much or untimely sexual intercourse will irritate not only the womb but also the fetus. It can lead the mother to give birth to a weak and dull infant, with possible skin diseases to stain the unlucky newcomer.

Miscarriage often takes place in the early stages of pregnancy. Physical deficiency, too much sex, carrying heavy loads, or overwork of any kind should be avoided.

An infant may present with a variety of inexplicable infantile diseases. They can be traced back to either the chemicals or alcohol taken, and unrestricted sex or any other unfavorable influences upon the infant while residing in the womb. The material and spiritual environment around a pregnant woman will be reflected upon the baby throughout its life.

Blood Deficiency

The most frequent occurrences of miscarriage from blood deficiency occur between the third and fifth month of pregnancy. By observing the skin color of the inside lower eyelid we determine if the patient is blood deficient. If it appears colorless or pale white then blood deficiency is present. If it appears red, then either the patient or the blood is infected. If the color is in between the two, the blood isn't blood deficient. Usually a blood deficient patient has thin pulses.

Formula for blood deficiency (see also "Dr. Shen's Formulas in Systems," p. 94):

Pin Yin	Latin	English	Dosage
Huang qi	Astragali Radix	Milk vetch root, astragalus root	30 g
Dang gui	Angelicae Sinensis Radix	Chinese Angelica root, tang-kuei	15 g
Da zao	Zizyphi Jujubae Fructus	Chinese date, jujube	5 g
Ji xiong pu	Gallus	Skinless chicken breast	2 pieces

Put the herbal medicine into a Yunnan steam pot together with two skinned chicken legs. Boil the soup for 3 to 4 hours. Drink one or two bowls of the soup. Repeat two to three times a week until the inside of the eyelid shows a normal color.

The ingestion of the livers of chickens, ducks, and pigs treats blood deficiency. Soak 85 g of each type of liver in wine and onions for a while. Bring water to a boil. Put the livers in water for 1 second then eat the livers. Repeat the process for 3 months for effectiveness.

Reactions in Pregnancy

During the first 3 months of pregnancy the woman tends to vomit and can find taking food intolerable. Slippery and comparatively rapid pulses are felt in different degrees for different physiques. It is also possible that some women don't show these signs.

Formula for slight pregnancy reactions:

Pin Yin	Latin	English	Dosage
Bai dou kou	Amomi Kravanh Fructus	Cardamom fruit/round seed	3 g
Sheng jiang	Zingiberis Officinalis Recens Rhizoma	Fresh ginger rhizome	2 slices

Put the herbal medicines into just enough water and simmer heat for 10 minutes. Drink the tea one to two times a day. Continue the practice until the reactions subside.

If the above formula is not effective and the pregnant woman shows additional serious signs of reaction such as dizziness and palpitations then she is advised to take the following formula.

Formula for serious pregnancy reactions (see also "Dr. Shen's Formulas in Systems," p. 83):

Pin Yin	Latin	English	Dosage
Bai zhu	Atractylodis Macrocephalae Rhizoma	White atractylodes rhizome	4.5 g
Bai shao	Paeoniae Alba Radix	White peony root	4.5 g
Bai dou kou	Amomi Kravanh Fructus	Cardamom fruit/round seed	3 g
Chen pi	Citri Reticulatae Pericarpium	Tangerine peel	3 g
Zhu ru	Bambussae in Taeniis Caulis	Bamboo shavings	4.5 g
Gu ya	Oryzae Germinatus Fructus	Rice sprout	9 g
Ban xia	Rhizoma Pinelliae	Pinellia rhizome	4.5 g
Sheng jiang	Zingiberis Officinalis Recens Rhizoma	Fresh ginger rhizome	3 slices

If symptoms persist, see a doctor for treatment.

Preservation of the Fetus after Five Months of Pregnancy

After 5 months of pregnancy the expectant mother should be very careful of her dietary intake. She should abstain completely from sex in order to ensure the health and safety of both herself and her child. This will engender a smooth labor. If she doesn't take this precaution, she may have a long, difficult, and painful labor or possibly a premature birth or a malpositioned fetus. All these create suffering for both mother and child.

During this period the expectant mother must keep a correct posture when walking, sitting, and sleeping, all of which might influence the position of the child in the womb (**Fig. 14**).

She should vary the side on which she sleeps, changing from side to side so that the child will not always be in the same position.

During the fifth month, she may very well take some Chinese herbal medicine to "tranquilize" the fetus for a favorable smooth birth.

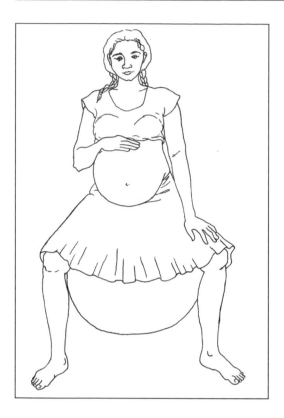

Fig. 14   Pregnant woman on a ball to maintain posture.

Formula for ensuring health and safety of both mother and child:

Pin Yin	Latin	English	Dosage
Dang gui	Angelicae Sinensis Radix	Prepared Chinese Angelica root, *tang-kuei*	4.5 g
Huang qin	Scutellariae Baicalensis Radix	Baical skullcap root, scutellaria, scute	3 g
Qiang huo	Notopterygii Rhizoma et Radix	Notopterygium root and rhizome, *chiang-huo*	3 g
Jing jie	Schizonepetae Herba	Schizonepeta	3 g
Chuan xiong	Chuanxiong Rhizoma	Chuanxiong root, Szechuan lovage root, cnidium	3 g
Bai shao	Paeoniae Alba Radix	White peony root	4.5 g
Gan jiang	Zingiberis Rhizoma	Dried ginger	2 g
Ai ye	Artemisiae Argyi Folium	Mugwort leaf, artemisia	0.24 g
Tu si zi	Cuscutae Chinensis Semen	Chinese dodder seeds, cuscuta	4.5 g
Hong hua	Carthami Tinctorii Flos	Safflower flower, carthamus	3 g
Bai zhu	Atractylodis Macrocephalae Rhizoma	White atractylodes rhizome	4.5 g
Hou po	Magnoliae Officinalis Cortex	Magnolia bark	0.15 g
Shan yao	Dioscoreae Oppositae Rhizoma	Chinese yam, dioscorea rhizome	6 g

In a normal case the medicine should be taken once a week beginning in the fifth month, twice a week from the sixth to the eighth months, and increased to three times a week in the ninth month.

For women over 30 years of age with a history of difficult breech birth, the medicine should be taken once a week in the fifth month, twice a week in the sixth month, three times a week in the seventh month, four times a week in the eighth month, and taken every day in the ninth month until a healthy birth is achieved.

Lower Back and Sciatic Pain

When a woman first becomes pregnant, she may find her lower back aches so much that it is difficult to either stand for extended periods of time or to walk long distances. Her condition can be subdivided into two cases. If it occurs after the seventh month of pregnancy, very probably the fetus is sitting in a position that is too low. If this is so, stimulate GV-26 *shui gou/ren zhong* to release her pain. If the pain occurs in the first 3 months, it is due to kidney deficiency and should be alleviated by nourishment.

Formula for lower back pain:

Pin Yin	Latin	English	Dosage
Du zhong	Eucommiae Cortex	Eucommia bark	12 g
Xi xin	Asari Herba cum Radice	Chinese wild ginger, asarum	2 g
Gou qi zi	Lycii Fructus	Chinese wolfberry, matrimony vine fruit, lycium fruit	12 g
Xu duan	Dipsaci Asperi Radix	Japanese teasel root, dipsacus	12 g
Qiang huo	Notopterygii Rhizoma et Radix	Notopterygium root and rhizome, chiang-huo	1 g
Tu si zi	Cuscutae Chinensis Semen	Chinese dodder seeds, cuscuta	12 g

The dose is to be taken twice a day until the symptoms disappear.

Other Symptoms That May Occur with Pregnancy

From the perspective of Chinese medicine, symptoms that may occur with pregnancy are by no means considered disease; rather they are seen as natural reactions to conception. They may include indigestion, varicosity, hemorrhoids, hypertension, edema, and so on. When the expectant mother can truly rest, the symptoms will naturally subside. If they persist, then she must see a doctor for advice. If there is a pre-existing condition of diabetes before pregnancy, she must pay special attention to her health after conception.

Hypertension

Leon Hammer Hypertension in a pregnant woman is a serious sign; if the inside of her lower eyelids are red, then the case is very serious. However, even if the lids are not red, she is still not out of danger. In addition to the herbs, she is required to have extended bed rest.

Formula for hypertension in pregnancy:

Pin Yin	Latin	English	Dosage
Gou teng	Ramulus cum Uncis Uncariae	Stems and thorns of the gambir vine, uncaria	18 g
Ju hua	Chrysanthemi Flos	Chrysanthemum flower	9 g
Sheng di huang	Rehmanniae Radix	Fresh Chinese foxglove root, fresh rehmannia root	12 g
Sang ji sheng	Taxilli Herba	Mulberry mistletoe stems, loranthus, taxillus, mistletoe	15 g
Mu li	Ostreae Concha	Oyster shell	30 g

Pin Yin	Latin	English	Dosage
Long chi	Fossilia Dentis Mastodi	Dragon teeth, fossilized teeth	15 g
Fu shen	Poria Cocos Pararadicis Sclerotium	Poria fungus	10 g
Dang gui	Angelicae Sinensis Radix	Chinese Angelica root, tang-kuei	10 g

Boil the medicine in water for 20 minutes and take it twice a day. Take one dose per day until the symptoms are alleviated.

Edema

While in the womb, the fetus often poses a heavy load upon the mother's kidneys, leading to edema. Other situations can also cause kidney-deficient edema. Too much water intake, tremendous emotional upheaval or hypertension can all result in edema. A pregnant woman must maintain an optimistic attitude and lead a normal way of life to guard against disease.

Formula for edema:

Pin Yin	Latin	English	Dosage
Chi xiao dou	Phaseoli Calcarati Semen	Aduki bean	50 g
Dan dou chi	Sojae Praeparatum Semen	Prepared soybean	15 g

Put the above two medicines into 500 mL of water and simmer for 30 minutes. Sweeten with sugar. Drink the fluid and eat the red beans, half in the morning and half in afternoon. Continue to take the herbs until the edema subsides.

Fetus in the Wrong Position

After 5 months of pregnancy, if the fetus is in the wrong position, "tranquilize" the fetus by applying moxa to BL-67 (*zhi yin*) (**Fig. 15**).

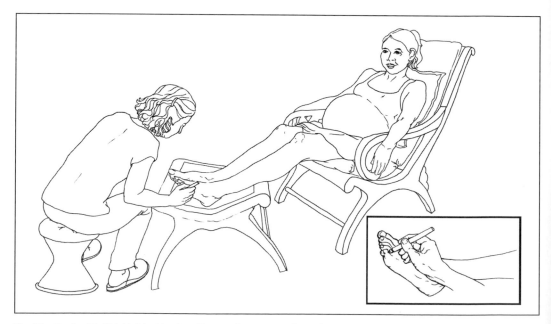

Fig. 15   Fuming BL-67 (*zhi yin*), side of small toe, with pure moxa (*ai tiao*).

Childbirth

Before giving birth, the pregnant mother should engage in moderation in all life activities, including exercise, resting, eating, food that is digestible, and sleeping in the correct position. She should walk up and down the room from time to time, stay relaxed, and maintain a clean environment. She should also take Chinese medicine to prepare herself for a smooth childbirth.

The throes of childbirth can be relieved by deep breathing. If conditions allow, acupuncture anesthesia can be introduced to alleviate the pain. Generally speaking, even if the woman suffers great pain, she should avoid chemical pain killers.

When a woman is too feeble to exert herself in childbirth, administer nourishment from Chinese medicine for strength and conviction to smooth the process.

Formula to help childbirth:

Pin Yin	Latin	English	Dosage
Xi yang shen	Panacis Quinquefolii Radix	American ginseng root	9 g
Gao li shen	Ginseng Coreensis Radix	Korean ginseng	9 g

Soak the ginseng in a container of water. Put the container in a pot of water and stew it for 3 to 4 hours, making it ready for use. The moment the fetus's head first shows itself, the mother should drink a full cup to fortify herself. Never do it before or after that very moment. This formula will not only help smooth the birth but also alleviate her pain and give her strength, thus avoiding the possibility of an operation.

Metroptosis or Prolapse of Uterus

Prolapse of the uterus in Chinese medicine is understood as "female piles, female prostration or female collapse." It is mostly caused by serious postpartum exhaustion or by overworking during periods, which results in *qi* deficiency. As a result

the *qi* is unable to hold the womb firmly. In this case nourish the body as a whole and the kidneys will be strong enough, thus preventing the *qi* from sinking. Such patients usually present with a thin tongue coating and deficient, slippery pulses.

Formula for uterine prolapse:

Pin Yin	Latin	English	Dosage
Dang shen	Codonopsis Pilosulae Radix	Codonopsis root	10 g
Huang qi	Astragali Radix	Milk vetch root, astragalus root	30 g
Bai zhu	Rhizoma Atractylodis Macrocephalae	White atractylodes rhizome	10 g
Sheng ma	Cimicifugae Rhizoma	Bugbane rhizome, black cohosh rhizome, cimicifuga	10 g
Chai hu	Bupleuri Radix	Hare's ear root, thorowax root, bupleurum	6 g
Jie geng	Platycodi Radix	Root of balloonflower, platycodon root	6 g
Dang gui	Angelicae Sinensis Radix	Chinese Angelica root, *tang-kuei*	10 g
Chen pi	Citri Reticulatae Pericarpium	Tangerine peel	6 g

Boil the medicines into tea and drink.

When the patient experiences low back and leg soreness, stomach sinking, frequent urination, tinnitus, a pale tongue body and thin white coating, and deep and feeble pulses, she is advised to take this formula:

Formula for prostration:

Pin Yin	Latin	English	Dosage
Dang shen	Codonopsis Pilosulae Radix	Codonopsis root	10 g
Shan yao	Dioscoreae Oppositae Rhizoma	Chinese yam, dioscorea rhizome	10 g
Shu di huang	Rehmanniae Preparata Radix	Prepared Chinese foxglove root (cooked in red wine), cooked rehmannia rhizome	12 g
Du zhong	Cortex Eucommiae	Eucommia bark	10 g
Dang gui	Angelicae Sinensis Radix	Chinese Angelica root, tang-kuei	10 g
Shan zhu yu	Corni Officinalis Fructus	Asiatic Cornelian cherry fruit, cornus	10 g
Gou qi zi	Lycii Fructus	Chinese wolfberry, matrimony vine fruit, lycium fruit	10 g
Zhi gan cao	Glycyrrhizae Radix	Processed licorice root[a]	6 g
Sheng ma	Cimicifugae Rhizoma	Bugbane rhizome, black cohosh rhizome, cimicifuga	6 g

[a] Often coated in honey and baked.

An external treatment is as follows:

Boil 60 g of *zhi ke* (mature fruit of the bitter orange) and 60 g of *wu mei* (mume fruit) in water. Allow the steam to warm up the affected area and even wash it, twice or three times a day.

Postnatal Care for Both the Mother and the Infant

Things a Young Mother Has to Observe

After having given birth, the young mother should rest for at least 2 weeks and if possible keep indoors for she is too feeble to resist the external pathogenic factors. Either hot and cold climate could retard her recovery. After that, she is advised to exercise lightly but by no means do any sort of hard physical labor. Sound sleep and sufficient rest will do her a lot of good. She has to keep herself clean but never wash with cold water. Neither is she allowed to have any cold drinks or she would run the risk of developing rheumatism. Resume sex no less than 30 days later.

According to Chinese custom she has to drink soup made of boiling motherwort. Boil a big pot of motherwort soup sweetened with some brown sugar; it will help the contraction of the womb and relieve the pain that is involved in the process. The metabolism will shift in favor of creating new flesh and in getting rid of the parts of the placenta that may still remain inside her.

Nourishment

Throughout giving birth a woman has lost so much blood and energy as to become too feeble to resist diseases. During the 2 weeks' rest after giving birth, she needs proper nourishment.

Formula I for nourishment:

Pin Yin	Latin	English	Dosage
Huang qi	Astragali Radix	Milk vetch root, astragalus root	12 g
Dang gui	Angelicae Sinensis Radix	Chinese Angelica root, tang-kuei	9 g
Shu di huang	Rehmanniae Preparata Radix	Prepared Chinese foxglove root (cooked in red wine), cooked rehmannia rhizome	12 g
Shan yao	Dioscoreae Oppositae Rhizoma	Chinese yam, dioscorea rhizome	12 g
Tu si zi	Cuscutae Chinensis Semen	Chinese dodder seeds, cuscuta	12 g
Dan shen	Salviae Miltiorrhiziae Radix	Salvia root	6 g
Bai zhu	Atractylodis Macrocephalae Rhizoma	White atractylodes rhizome	8 g
Shan zha	Crataegi Fructus	Hawthorn fruit, crataegus fruit	12 g
Huang qin	Scutellariae Baicalensis Radix	Baical skullcap root, scutellaria, scute	4.5 g

Boil the medicines in water and take twice a day. Continue for 2 weeks to a month according to the woman's physical condition until she has fully recovered her health. If the patient's digestive system is weak with loose stools, omit *shu di huang*.

Formula II for nourishment:

Pin Yin	Latin	English	Dosage
Huang qi	Astragali Radix	Milk vetch root, astragalus root	12 g
Dang gui	Angelicae Sinensis Radix	Chinese Angelica root, tang-kuei	9 g
Shan yao	Dioscoreae Oppositae Rhizoma	Chinese yam, dioscorea rhizome	12 g
Fu ling	Poria Cocos Sclerotium	Sclerotium of tuckahoe, poria, China root, hoelen, Indian bread	9 g
Yuan zhi	Polygalae Radix	Chinese senega root, polygala root	6 g
Shi chang pu	Acori Tatarinowii Rhizoma	Grass-leaved sweetflag rhizome, acorus	3 g
Gua lou pi	Trichosanthis Pericarpium	Peel of trichosanthes fruit	9 g
Yu jin	Curcumae Radix	Curcuma tuber	9 g
Shen qu	Massa Medicata Fermentata	Medicated leaven (dough)	12 g
Da zao	Zizyphi Jujubae Fructus	Chinese date, jujube	5 pieces

Follow the same directions.

Blood Deficiency

Formula for blood deficiency (see also "Dr. Shen's Formulas in Systems," p. 94):

Pin Yin	Latin	English	Dosage
Huang qi	Astragali Radix	Milk vetch root, astragalus root	30 g
Dang gui	Angelicae Sinensis Radix	Chinese Angelica root, tang-kuei	15 g
Da zao	Zizyphi Jujubae Fructus	Chinese date, jujube	5 g
San qi	Notoginseng Radix	Noto ginseng root, root of pseudo-ginseng	6 g
Ji xiong pu	Gallus	Skinless chicken breast	2 pieces

Put the medicines in a Yunnan steam pot and steam for 4 to 5 hours; eat one or two bowls of the soup a day two to three times a week to effectively promote the circulation of blood. If the case is serious consume each day. For gestational blood deficiency, add three kinds of livers to the soup.

Melancholia

From the viewpoint of Chinese medicine, postpartum depression is due to deficiency of both *qi* and blood. Proper nourishment is the remedy. It is most important that the young mother relaxes as much as possible and avoids anxieties.

Leon Hammer   Postpartum depression afflicts a large percentage of women in the urbanized Western-style societies especially after the second and subsequent children. This was largely unknown by people closer to their traditional roots who, even in China when I was there in 1981, routinely supplemented women's diet with blood- and *qi*-nourishing herbs from menarche to menopause and beyond.

Breast-feeding

Breast-feeding is the most natural way of feeding and it is favorable for both mother and child. However, we often find that some young mothers have insufficient lactation.

Formula I for stimulating the secretion of milk:

Pin Yin	Latin	English	Dosage
Bie jia	Carapax Amydae Sinensis	Soft-shelled turtle	1 whole turtle
Sheng jiang	Zingiberis Officinalis Recens Rhizoma	Fresh ginger rhizome	3 slices
Cong bai	Allii fistulosi bulbus	White part of scallion, spring onion	1 piece
Liao jiu		Cooking wine	3 tablespoons

Formula II for stimulating the secretion of milk:

Pin Yin	Latin	English	Dosage
Huang dou	Glycine	Soybeans	3 ounces
Zhu jiao	Suinae	Pig's feet	1–2 pieces
Sheng jiang	Zingiberis Officinalis Recens Rhizoma	Fresh ginger rhizome	3 pieces
Cong bai	Allii Fistulosi Bulbus Allium	Scallion	1 whole
Liao jiu	n. a.	Cooking wine	3 tablespoons

Put the herbal medicines into a pot of water and boil for 2 hours. If bie jia is to be included, first boil the other ingredients for an hour and then put the turtle into the fluid and go on boiling for another hour. When pig's feet and soybeans are to be included, then boil the soup until the pig's feet and the beans become soft. Take the soup twice a day until enough lactation is restored. Sometimes the mother's milk doesn't flow easily. The following formula can be adopted.

Formula to help the milk flow:

Pin Yin	Latin	English	Dosage
Lu lu tong	Liquidambaris Fructus	Sweetgum fruit, liquidambar fruit	1 g

Formula to stop breast-feeding:

Pin Yin	Latin	English	Dosage
Gu ya	Oryzae Germinatus Fructus	Rice sprout	50 g
Mai ya	Hordei Germinatus Fructus	Barley sprout, malt	50 g

Mastitis

When breast-feeding mothers find their breasts aching or infected with a fever, they require immediate treatment.

Formula for aching and infected breasts:

Pin Yin	Latin	English	Dosage
Wu gong[a]	Scolopendra Subspinipes	Centipede, scolopendra	10 pieces
Jin yin hua	Lonicerae Flos	Honeysuckle flower, lonicera	30 g

[a] Toxic

The simplest way to cure infected breasts is to buy nonpoisonous centipedes and honeysuckle from a herbal medicine store and put them into a pot with two to three cups of water. Boil until half of the water is left. The same mass can be boiled twice. Drink one cup of the liquid every day until the condition improves. The centipede invigorates the circulation of blood. When the body temperature drops, enfeebled mothers are advised to take other herbal medicine for nourishment.

Newborn Infants

Leon Hammer   My personal experience treating infants and very young children who resist the oral route for herbs is to administer the liquid rectally. This has proved to be a very successful practice with difficult conditions such as ADHD.

While still inside the mother's womb, the infant has already started its metabolic activity, especially when it approaches its birth. It is possibly for the neonate to take in an amount of amniotic fluid or even its own excrement and urine. If it is immediately fed with milk after it comes into the wide world, the dirt inside its digestive system is difficult to clean. Without that cleaning process, the child's health is vulnerable to diseases of the digestive system such as jaundice or skin diseases. For this purpose, let the infant go without food for some while until it has been given some medicine to rid its digestive system of its dirt.

Formula for cleaning the digestive system of meconium (*San Huang Tang* [Three Yellow Decoction], see also "Dr. Shen's Formulas in Systems," p. 55):

Leon Hammer   Colic and skin diseases due to the retention of meconium after the first feeding is discussed in "Dr. Shen's Formulas in Systems," (p. 55).

Pin Yin	Latin	English	Dosage
Huang bai	Phellodendri Cortex	Amur cork tree bark, phellodendron bark	3 g
Huang lian	Coptidis Rhizome	Coptis rhizome	3 g
Da huang	Rhei Rhizoma et Radix	Rhubarb root and rhizome	3 g

Boil the medicine for 20 minutes. Feed the baby several drops of the liquid two to three times a day, until its first excrement is expelled and its digestion channels have been cleaned. The whole process should take 10 to 24 hours (**Fig. 16**).

If the hospital won't tolerate any such feeding of medicine or the parents won't accept it, just feed the infant only water during the first 20 to 30 hours until its first excrement. Only then start feeding the baby breast milk.

Mother's milk is the best choice for infant food, rich in nutrients to be readily absorbed. Since it is the natural course of life, breast-feeding also does a lot of good the mother's health, while milk powder may have been contaminated by chemicals that harm the digestive system. Commercially produced powdered food formulas are ill advised for infants as they will harm their digestive systems.

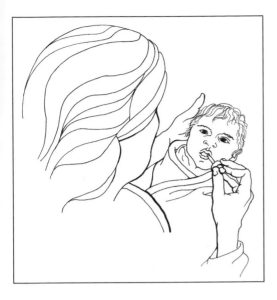

Fig. 16 Dripping *San Huang Tang* (Three Yellow Decoction) with dropper.

Infantile Jaundice

Newborn infants can develop jaundice either at birth or 1 week later. This disease can be treated with *niu huang* (dried cattle gallstones). Grind it with several drops of water into paste and feed the baby 1 g each time, 3 days a week, until jaundice disappears.

One Month after Birth

In order to refresh the blood of the infant, feed it with 3 g of *niu huang*, ground into a paste. Feed 1 g several portions each day, three times a week for 2 or 3 months.

From the First to the Sixth Month

It is of great importance to take good care of the newborn baby. During this period the child must be held in a horizontal position. If it is prematurely held in an upright position or thrown up into the air, this will put the baby in great danger. Sometimes the child has to sit up for a while, such as riding in a car. Such an occasion can be tolerated for only a short time. In this stage of life the internal organs of the baby are too delicate to suffer any displacement because of fragility of the elastic tissue that binds organs to the bony structure. Such mishandling will result in possible irregular circulation of blood and hindrance to the smooth running of *qi*.

All these activities will end up in germination of diseases retarding the natural growth of the child. These points are very important to ensure the healthy development of the baby after 4 or 5 years of age.

Infants should be fed with nothing hard to swallow, only milk before they are 20 months old. When the mother doesn't have enough milk for the child, gruel or porridge is full of nourishment. Infants are to be fed with food cooked at home only. Any prepared food bought from the market may contain chemicals and additives.

Infantile Nervous System Maladjustment

According to an old Chinese custom, infants were always wrapped up in a bundle called a "candle bundle." Infants below 6 months of age are liable to be alarmed. Noises or any other sorts of irritation might pose an irritant to them. When the infant is bundled up it will feel safer. Any sort of alarm might injure its nervous system.

Maladjustment of infantile nerves may come from several internal or external sources. During gestation if the mother is overwhelmed by some sort of emotional distress, it will in turn have an effect on the nerves of the infant. If the mother has a prolonged birth, or a Cesarean birth or a delivery with the help of instruments, all these will have a harmful impact on the nerves of the baby, thus weakening its physique. Until the baby is 3 years old, noises or a sudden fall to the ground will easily damage the nervous system.

Leon Hammer　In modern times the common practice of exposing infants and young children to loud noise (even rock concerts) is a significant source of shock to their nervous systems.

Nervous system maladjustment may have two possible manifestations. In one case, only the nervous system is maladjusted. In another case, the situation is complicated by a common cold. Maladjustment alone will make the child fidget, refuse to lie on the bed in peace, actively move its hands and feet, yet there is no fever. Children of 5 to 6 years of age may be fidgeting because of the maladjustment. If the maladjustment is also complicated by a common cold, the case will be aggravated. The child will not only have feverish spasms of fidgeting, but also even sleep with its mouth and eyes open. This fever is caused mainly by the maladjustment and fluctuates, usually rising in the afternoon. Even with a fever, the child doesn't show anything abnormal; it goes on sleeping and playing as usual.

A child troubled with nervous system maladjustment must have suffered some sort of alarm earlier in its infancy, such as a loud noise or a fall or even suffered from cold weather. Any or all of these might have irritated and affected its nervous system.

Formula for infantile nervous system maladjustment (without fever):

Pin Yin	Latin	English	Dosage
Shi chang pu	Acori Tatarinowii Rhizoma	Grass-leaved sweetflag rhizome, acorus	3 g
Chuan xiong	Chuanxiong Rhizoma	Chuanxiong root, Szechuan lovage root, cnidium	3 g
Jing jie	Schizonepeta Herba	Schizonepeta	3 g
Huang lian	Coptidis Rhizoma	Coptis rhizome	4.5 g
Fu shen	Poria Cocos Pararadicis Sclerotium	Poria fungus	9 g
Chao suan zao ren	Ziziphi Spinosae Semen	Fried zizyphus seeds, sour jujube seeds, zizyphus	12 g
Long chi	Fossilia Dentis Mastodi	Dragon teeth, fossilized teeth	18 g
Ci shi	Magnetitum	Magnetite	18 g
Yu jin	Curcumae Radix	Curcuma tuber	4.5 g
Zhi shi	Aurantii Immaturus Fructus	Immature bitter orange, unripe bitter orange, chih-shih	4.5 g
Deng xin cao	Medulla Junci Effusi	Rush pith, juncus	3 bundles

Leon Hammer
Face color and etiology:
- Constitutional etiology: the entire face will show a dark blue color, or the color can be confined just to the chin.
- Pregnancy (intrauterine): the blue color tends to be around the chin.
- At birth (congenital): the blue color is found around the mouth.
- After birth: from 6 months to 3 years the infant is most vulnerable to shock, which will have profound and long-lasting repercussions. The blue color tends to be found between the eyes and around the temples when the shock comes after birth.

Formula for infantile nervous system maladjustment (with fever):

Pin Yin	Latin	English	Dosage
Dan dou chi	Sojae Praeparatum Semen	Prepared soybean	9 g
Shi chang pu	Acori Tatarinowii Rhizoma	Grass-leaved sweetflag rhizome, acorus	3 g
Jing jie	Schizonepeta Herba	Schizonepeta	3 g
Fang feng	Saposhnikoviae Radix	Ledebouriella root, saposhnikoviae root, siler	3 g
Ge gen	Puerariae Radix	Kudzu root, pueraria	3 g
Shan zhi zi	Gardeniae Jasminoidis Fructus	Cape jasmine fruit, gardenia fruit	9 g
Lian qiao	Forsythiae Suspensae Fructus	Forsythia fruit	9 g
Long chi	Fossilia Dentis Mastodi	Dragon teeth, fossilized teeth	4.5 g
Ci shi	Magnetitum	Magnetite	18 g
Huang qin	Scutellariae Baicalensis Radix	Baical skullcap root, scutellaria, scute	3 g
Shen qu	Massa Medicata Fermentata	Medicated leaven (dough)	9 g
Zhi shi	Aurantii Immaturus Fructus	Immature bitter orange, unripe bitter orange, chih-shih	3 g
Deng xin cao	Medulla Junci Effusi	Rush pith, juncus	3 bundles

Administer infants of 2 to 12 months of age three small spoonfuls of the liquid every 2 to 3 hours. Infants older than 1 year can be fed with big spoons for more liquid.

Common Cold in a Child

A child may have caught a common cold with or without a low fever, but it shows signs of coughing, sneezing with a sore throat but not those signs of nervous system troubles.

Formula for a common cold:

Pin Yin	Latin	English	Dosage
Ge gen	Puerariae Radix	Kudzu root, pueraria	4.5 g
Jing jie	Schizonepeta Herba	Schizonepeta	3 g
Bai zhi	Angelicae Dahuricae Radix	Angelica root	3 g
Jie geng	Platycodi Radix	Root of balloonflower, platycodon root	3 g
Zhe bei mu	Fritillariae Thunbergii Bulbus	Zhejiang fritillaria, Thunberg fritillaria bulb, fritillaria	9 g
Mai ya	Hordei Germinatus Fructus	Barley sprout, malt	9 g
Cang er zi	Xanthii Sibirici Fructus	Cocklebur fruit, xanthium fruit	4.5 g

Digestive System Troubles

Even if the infant grows up breast-feeding, precautions should still be taken for it may still develop digestive system diseases. A comparatively effective way of diagnosis is to look at the radial aspect of the index finger where the large intestine channel is clearly embedded. If a thin blue line at the third joint is observed, then some phlegm is the problem. If the blue line goes up to the middle joint, there are

Diarrhea

Infantile diarrhea may arise from a common cold or troubles in the digestive system. Infants beyond 6 months can be treated with the massage method mentioned above. The following formula can also be used.

Formula for diarrhea:

Pin Yin	Latin	English	Dosage
Sheng jiang	Zingiberis Officinalis Recens Rhizoma	Fresh ginger rhizome	1 slice
Ping guo	Malum	Fresh apple	1 apple

Press the apple and ginger into a paste and feed the infant two to three times a day until diarrhea is relieved.

Infantile Hernia

Infantile hernia may arise from troubles in the digestive or nervous systems. Generally speaking, when the infant cries after feeding, there may be something wrong with the digestive system. If the child cries the whole night, this may be due to the cold disturbing its nervous system. This case may be accompanied by a fluctuating temperature. Different cases should be treated differently. The best policy for infants' meals is always to feed less food several times a day.

Formula for infantile hernia:

Pin Yin	Latin	English	Dosage
Xiao hui xiang	Foeniculi Fructus	Common fennel	5 g
Li zhi	Litchi Semen	Lychee pit	9 g
Ju he	Citri Reticulatae Semen	Tangerine seed	9 g
Rou gui fen	Cinnamomi Cassiae Cortex	Powdered inner bark of Saigon cinnamon	0.3 g

Allow the first three medicines to simmer for 10 minutes. Administer them without the residue. Roll the powder of cinnamon bark into little rice balls and have the child swallow. If there is some fluid inside the scrotum this is what doctors of Chinese medicine call "watery hernia." In such a case, boil 6 g che qian zi (plantago seeds) and bai zhu (white atractylodes rhizome) together with the other medicines.

Diaper Rash

Diaper rash is also called infantile red buttocks. Diaper rash occurs when dirty diapers are not changed often enough or when the diaper itself is made of some chemical textile material.

Formula for diaper rash:

Pin Yin	Latin	English	Dosage
Liu yi san	Talcum/Glycyrrhizae Radix	Six-to-one powder	6 parts talcum/ 1 part licorice
Bing pian	Borneolum Syntheticum	Borneol	20 % of total quantity

Grind ingredients together into a powder and apply to the troubled area. Do this two to three times a day.

Eczema

One month or more after its birth, the infant often develops fine, little, itchy, seeping blisters on its neck, cheeks or forehead. This is called infantile eczema. It is a sort of allergy. Newborns who haven't had timely cleaning of their digestive system with *San Huang Tang* liquid or haven't had good clean nourishment will tend to be have eczema. Eczema is a disease arising from the digestive system. Therefore it is suggested that the infant eat smaller portions of food more often each day.

Formula for eczema:

Pin Yin	Latin	English	Dosage
Di fu zi	Kochiae Fructus	Broom cypress, kochia fruit	4.5 g
Bai xian pi	Dictamni Dasycarpi Radicis Cortex	Cortex of Chinese dittany root, dictamnus root bark	3 g
Gan cao	Glycyrrhizae Radix	Licorice root	9 g
Gu ya	Oryzae Germinatus Fructus	Rice sprout	9 g
Mai ya	Hordei Germinatus Fructus	Barley sprout, malt	4.5 g
Xia ku cao	Prunellae Spica Vulgaris	Self-heal spike, prunella	4.5 g

The liquid is fed drop by drop for 1 to 2 weeks until the condition improves.

Night Sweats

To a doctor trained in TCM, night sweats in a child may come from constitutional deficiency or some trouble arising from the heart. Generally, when a sleeping child, although having a normal temperature on its head, sweats from it up to its neck, but not on the other parts of the body, this is night sweat. If the whole body sweats, including its head, at a high temperature, this is a normal result of the child having been covered with too much bedding.

Formula for night sweats:

Pin Yin	Latin	English	Dosage
Di fu zi	Kochiae Fructus	Broom cypress, kochia fruit	4.5 g
Bai xian pi	Dictamni Dasycarpi Radicis Cortex	Cortex of Chinese dittany root, dictamnus root bark	3 g
Gan cao	Glycyrrhizae Radix	Licorice root	9 g
Gu ya	Oryzae Germinatus Fructus	Rice sprout	9 g
Mai ya	Hordei Germinatus Fructus	Barley sprout, malt	4.5 g
Xia ku cao	Prunellae Spica Vulgaris	Self-heal spike, prunella	4.5 g

Fainting

A doctor trained in Western medicine may consider fainting a serious condition, but a doctor trained in Chinese medicine may not think so. From the viewpoint of Chinese medicine doctors, the cases can be delineated into three causes. Fainting may come from eating food, from phlegm, or from breath. If it is earnestly addressed in time, nothing serious will happen.

If the fainting comes from eating too much or too fast, it shows that the child is comparatively too weak to resist or is unable to swallow so much at a time, resulting in fainting. Or if it is too weak to digest so much food at one time, the undigested food turns to phlegm, seriously threatening the regular functioning of the pericardium. Or the child might have cried for so long that it gets short of breath and all of a sudden faints.

In this case dip a red-hot spoon into a cup of vinegar and promptly take it out of the cup. Then put the spoon close to the child's nose and let it smell it. The child will recover quickly. Needling CV-12 (*zhong wan*), GV-26 (*ren zhong*), and PC-6 (*nei guan*) will have the same effect.

In the case of a food faint open the child's mouth and administer ginger tea. At the same time massage the stomach area with ginger scallion juice. Needles should be placed at PC-6 (*nei guan*) and (*bi zhang*)*. The child will be revived shortly.

When the case of fainting is caused by phlegm, needle LU-11 (*shao shang*), GV-27 (*dui duan*), and CV-12 (*zhong wan*), and the child will return to consciousness.

If all these treatments fail to have any effect, take the child to a hospital immediately.

Cleaning Chemicals From the Body

For various reasons a woman may have taken chemically synthetic medicines during her pregnancy and in some cases she tends to take them as a habit.

In such a case, the fetus will unavoidably be affected. Only 6 months after its birth can we try to rid the infant of chemicals.

Formula to rid a child of chemicals:

Pin Yin	Latin	English	Dosage
Gan cao	Glycyrrhizae Radix	Licorice root	4.5 g
Jin yin hua	Lonicerae Flos	Honeysuckle flower, lonicera	6 g

External Bruise at Birth

If some instruments, such as forceps, were utilized to facilitate the birth, the infant may have suffered an external bruise that may be harmful to the circulation of blood in the head. The bruise will not show

its effect right away. However, in the process of its growth it will lead to such a wound. Therefore precautions must be taken against any possible harmful aftermath.

Formula to help prevent the aftermath of external injury:

Pin Yin	Latin	English	Dosage
Sang ji sheng	Taxilli Herba	Mulberry mistletoe stems, loranthus, taxillus, mistletoe	4.5 g
Dan shen	Salviae Miltiorrhiziae Radix	Salvia root	4.5 g
Fang feng	Saposhnikoviae Radix	Ledebouriella root, saposhnikoviae root, siler	3 g
Bai zhi	Angelicae Dahuricae Radix	Angelica root	4.5 g
Gan cao	Glycyrrhizae Radix	Licorice root	3 g

---

* It is possible that Dr. Shen was referring to the point *bi zhong*, an extra point located at the midpoint between the transverse creases of wrist and elbow, between radius and ulna, 1 cun proximal to PC-4 (*xi men*).

When the newborn baby shows some sort of nervousness or abnormal symptoms, add to the dosage one more medicine as follows:

Pin Yin	Latin	English	Dosage
San qi	Notoginseng Radix	Noto ginseng root, root of pseudo-ginseng	0.6 g

Heart Diseases

When an infant is found at birth to have some heart disease, such as trouble with the heart valves, generally a surgical operation is performed. If an operation is out of the question, the following formula is suggested:

Pin Yin	Latin	English	Dosage
Xi yang shen	Panacis Quinquefolii Radix	American ginseng root	3 g
Zi he che or tai pan	Placenta Hominis	Human placenta, placenta	3 g

American ginseng of the best quality must be chosen for this treatment. The boiled liquid is to be fed into the infant's mouth drop by drop, several drops a day; continue the process for several months to see if the infant's condition is any better.

Childhood

Great attention must be paid to the diet and sleep habits of children between the ages of 3 and 10 years. All-round nourishment is of primary importance for their diet. No partiality towards any kinds of food should be tolerated. They must be taught good habits of regularity in eating, sleeping, and getting up.

At 7 years of age children start school. Close observation reveals the fact that children are carrying ever heavier satchels on their backs, some weighing as much as 9 kg. This is certainly an abnormal phenomenon to be seriously studied by the whole of society. As the skeleton and internal organs of chil-

dren are far from being fully developed, the practice of carrying heavy loads will certainly inhibit their normal growth. Also observed among children is a difference in their physique. If heavy loads are placed on the shoulders of children of poor physique for a long time, it will make them still poorer, too poor to resist diseases. Investigations have shown that the health of children shows a declining tendency. When your children complain to you about their heavy satchel, we suggest that you buy two sets of books for them—one set for school, the other set for use at home. Let's sack the satchel!

Internal and External Bruises

Children tend to be lively and active. It is very possible for them to fall down or injure themselves somewhere on the body. When parents are told about an accident or a pain in their children, they must pay immediate attention. Whether or not there is any obvious external signs of a wound, they

should have a physician examine the child. Growing children, with their tender internal organs, are too delicate to resist any bumping or striking. Any such harm done to a child, in the eyes of a Chinese medicine doctor, will leave behind some sort of aftermath.

Yunnan Baiyao

For a Chinese medical doctor, *Yunnan Baiyao* is a powerfully effective medicine. Often adopted for

treating both internal and external wounds, it is available in any Chinese herbal medicine store. This

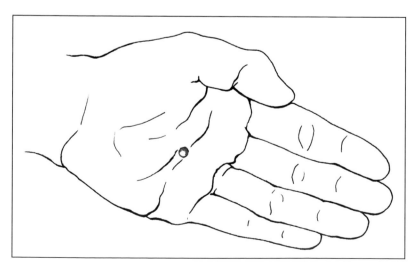

Fig. 19 Red pill, *Yunnan Baiyao.*

is a red-colored pill to be used only in a life-or-death emergency (**Fig. 19**).

In most cases, when someone is seriously injured, if their heart is still beating and their brain still working, this pill will restore them to health. Use half a pill daily for a child of 3 to 5 years of age and one pill daily for a child of 5 to 10 years of age.

Yunnan Baiyao was formerly called Hundred Herbal Powder and came into being with an interesting story. By the end of the 19th century there was a man named Qu in Szechuan Province in Western China who enjoyed a long life of more than 100 years. He was a herbal medicine physician interested in picking and collecting herbs in those remote, thickly forested, mountainous areas of the region. Once he came upon a snake. Although it was broken in two, the snake was still alive. The upper part of the snake, to Qu's great surprise, slithered its way as though looking for something. Curious, Qu followed at its heel to see what would happen to it. To his still greater surprise, the snake found a kind of grass and swallowed it. Upon this it returned to its lower part and a miraculous reunion occurred. The snake's wound perfectly healed, somehow, later. After that, Dr. Qu came to understand that nature gives even animals an instinct to cure their diseases. Thus he made up his mind to pay closer attention to other animals eating particular grasses, in order to ascertain their therapeutic effects. Once a monkey was found to have one of its legs broken. Qu diligently waited to see what would happen. A similar scene presented itself to him. The monkey also cured itself by swallowing a kind of grass. Dr. Qu made over 100 observations to learn the many herbs that were later concocted into that celebrated *Yunnan Baiyao*.

When China was suffering during the War of Resistance against Japan in 1937, the National Government of China intended to buy the recipe from Dr. Qu at a price of 100000 silver yuan, but failed. Dr. Qu, now a man of 75, being aware that there were millions upon millions of wounded, donated 100000 bottles of *Yunnan Baiyao* to the government, although he refused to sell his recipe.

When Dr. Qu died his son was still too young to know much about Chinese medicine. Only his daughter was big enough to serve her father as an assistant. According to an age-old tradition of China, personal property, including such a money-making recipe, was bequeathed only to sons, never to daughters. Regardless, Dr. Qu's daughter didn't know for sure the complete composition of the medicine. She later married a Yunnan merchant named Lu.

After her father's death, she produced the medicine without the complete recipe in the form of white, not red, pills and sold them. That is why *Yunnan Baiyao* has ever since been called Yunnan White Powder (YWP). It is sad to say that the present *Yunnan Baiyao* is concocted without all the original constituents, so it is not as effective as it once was.

In sports or games, it is very easy to have one's wrists or ankles injured. Even though the bones may not be broken, some *"jing mai"* or channels may have been hurt. Besides the YWP, the following recipe of medicines can be applied as an ointment on the injured wrists or ankles (see also "Dr. Shen's Formulas in Systems," p. 109):

Pin Yin	Latin	English	Dosage
Fen zhi zi	Gardeniae Jasminoidis Fructus	Powdered cape jasmine fruit, gardenia fruit	28 g
Mai fen	Tritici Fructus	Wheat flour	7 g
Ji dai qing	n. a.	Egg white	1
Gao liang jiu	n. a.	Vodka or Chinese rice wine	1 tsp

Make a paste out of the above four ingredients and apply it to area of injury and cover it with a piece of cellophane. Rest for 24 hours. When you remove the paste the skin will appear a blue color. This is a normal phenomenon of the curing effect. Repeat procedure until swelling is reduced. If the wound is rather serious, take contents from four to five capsules of the *Yunnan Baiyao*, grind them into fine powder and mix them into the paste for a more effective treatment.

Diarrhea in Children

Because children's digestive systems are often not yet fully developed, they are so weak as to end in indigestion and thus in diarrhea. They must be properly taken care of or they can further weaken their digestive capacity leaving them vulnerable to other diseases.

When their excrement doesn't coagulate into form, the following formula should be utilized to treat their diarrhea.

Formula for diarrhea in children:

Pin Yin	Latin	English	Dosage
Nuo mi	Oryzae Glutinosae Semen	Sweet rice	1 handful
Da zao	Zizyphi Jujubae Fructus	Chinese date, jujube	5–7 pieces

Boil three cups of water with sweet rice and red dates in the container for an hour-and-a-half until the dates have swollen. Give the gruel as breakfast or refreshments for the children until their stools become more firm and the excrement turns normal. If their excrement is very fluid, with much water, then add a piece of ginger to the rice and dates before boiling into gruel.

Leon Hammer Rice does not contain gluten, which is associated with celiac disease.

Constipation

There are three causes of constipation in children. Their weak physique, poor intestinal function, or poor digestive system as a whole.

Formula I for constipation:

Pin Yin	Latin	English	Dosage
Huo ma ren	Cannabis Sativae Semen	Hemp seed	6 g

Put the hemp seed into water and boil it. Drink one cup of the liquid before sleep every night until it is effective. If this is not effective, take the following formula II.

Formula II for constipation:

Pin Yin	Latin	English	Dosage
Huo ma ren	Cannabis Sativae Semen	Hemp seed	6 g
Yu li ren	Pruni Semen	Bush cherry pit	6 g

Boil the medicines in water and drink it as tea. If constipation persists it is due to *qi* deficiency in the physique.

Formula III for constipation:

Pin Yin	Latin	English	Dosage
Huo ma ren	Cannabis Sativae Semen	Hemp seed	6 g
Yu li ren	Pruni Semen	Bush cherry pit	6 g
Xi yang shen	Panacis Quinquefolii Radix	American ginseng root	3 g

Follow same preparation and dosage instructions.

Allergies

Children around 7 years of age tend to have allergies because of their weak physiques. Generally speaking, children have an underdeveloped immunity that can result in allergies. One precaution to take is to protect them from any harm done to their tender internal organs. For instance, never throw an infant into the air for fun. Even the slightest displacement of their internal organs can create an environment for allergies due to the fragility of the elastic tissue that binds organs to the fascia.

Formula for allergies:

Pin Yin	Latin	English	Dosage
Dang shen	Codonopsis Pilosulae Radix	Codonopsis root	4.5 g
Qiang huo	Notopterygii Rhizoma et Radix	Notopterygium root and rhizome, *chiang-huo*	4.5 g
Chuan xiong	Ligustici Chuanxiong Rhizoma	Szechuan lovage root, cnidium	4.5 g
Jing jie	Schizonepetae Herba	Schizonepeta	3 g
Lie geng	Platycodi Radix	Root of balloonflower, platycodon root	4.5 g
Zhe bei mu	Fritillariae Thunbergii Bulbus	Zhejiang fritillaria, Thunberg fritillaria bulb, fritillaria	9 g
Xing ren	Semen Armeniacae	Apricot kernel	9 g
Cang er zi	Xanthii Sibirici Fructus	Cocklebur fruit, xanthium fruit	6 g
Ge gen	Puerariae Radix	Kudzu root, pueraria	4.5 g
Shen qu	Massa Medicata Fermentata	Medicated leaven (dough)	9 g

The formula should be taken internally twice a day and at the same time the steam from the decoction should be inhaled.

Asthma

There are two causes of asthma in children. One scenario is that a child may have caught a cold that is accompanied by a cough. Without proper treatment, the child grows weaker and weaker, developing deficiency in the lungs and in the whole physique. Some slight exertion makes them pant with fatigue. In such a case, the child pants more and coughs less. Another case is where an external factor plays a major part in making the child pant. When a child gets a cold and coughs, his or her lungs suffer from the cold. Then it develops into bronchial asthma, which is generally treated by employing antibiotics. However, the very cause of the sickness, the "*han*" (coldness) is still trapped in the lungs. Whenever the temperature drops slightly, the susceptible child will get a cold right away and start panting again.

It is commonly the case that children with bronchial asthma have very feeble, deficient lungs and weak physiques. If they are active and at the same time undernourished, their cold will repeatedly recur, making them even weaker. Our advice is to pay serious attention to a common cold. Give the child timely treatment and enough rest to ensure full recovery.

One should not resort to Western synthetic medicines as the only cure, for they only suppress symptoms. The cold that is the cause still remains intact in the lungs, so the asthma will return whenever unfavorable conditions arise. Sufficient rest will restore the sick child to health and an improvement in overall health will certainly help rid the child of its panting. Some asthmatic children tend to be sensitive to some foods, so a careful examination of their diet is an essential part of treating the asthmatic child. For the two different cases of asthma, children can be treated in different ways.

Formula I for asthmatic children with symptoms of a common cold accompanied by a cough:

Pin Yin	Latin	English	Dosage
Mi ma huang	Ephedrae Herba	Honey-cooked ephedra stem	1.8 g
Su zi	Perillae Fructus	Perilla fruit	1.8 g
Qian hu	Peucedani Radix	Hogfennel root, peucedanum	3 g
Mi zhi zi wan	Asteris Radix	Honey-cooked purple aster, aster root	4.5 g
Zhe bei mu	Fritillariae Thunbergii Bulbus	Zhejiang fritillaria, Thunberg fritillaria bulb, fritillaria	12 g
Xing ren	Armeniacae Semen	Apricot kernel	12 g
Wu wei zi	Schisandrae Chinensis Fructus	Schisandra fruit	2.4 g
Ting li zi	Descurainae seu Lepidii Semen	Descurainia seeds, lepidium seeds	4.5 g
Bai jie zi	Sinapis Albae Semen	White mustard seed	6 g
Shan zha	Crataegi Fructus	hawthorn fruit, crataegus fruit	12 g

Formula II for asthmatic children with deficient lungs with less coughing:

Pin Yin	Latin	English	Dosage
Mi ma huang	Ephedrae Herba	Honey-cooked ephedra stem	1.8 g
Su zi	Perillae Fructus	Perilla fruit	1.8 g
Nan sha shen	Adenophorae seu Glehniae Radix	Adenophora root or glehnia root, ladybell root	6 g
Mi zhi zi wan	Asteris Radix	Honey-cooked purple aster, aster root	4.5 g
Zhe bei mu	Fritillariae Thunbergii Bulbus	Zhejiang fritillaria, Thunberg fritillaria bulb, fritillaria	12 g
Yu zhu	Polygonati Odorati Rhizoma	Solomon's seal rhizome, polygonatum	6 g
Wu wei zi	Schisandrae Chinensis Fructus	Schisandra fruit	2.4 g
Ting li zi	Descurainae seu Lepidii Semen	Descurainia seeds, lepidium seeds	4.5 g
Bai jie zi	Sinapis Albae Semen	White mustard seed	6 g
Shan zha	Crataegi Fructus	Hawthorn fruit, crataegus fruit	12 g

Asthmatic children can also be treated by cupping them two or three times a week to drive away the cold that has been imprisoned inside their lungs. The cupping jars are applied at UB-12, UB-13, and lung channel (**Figs. 20** and **21**).

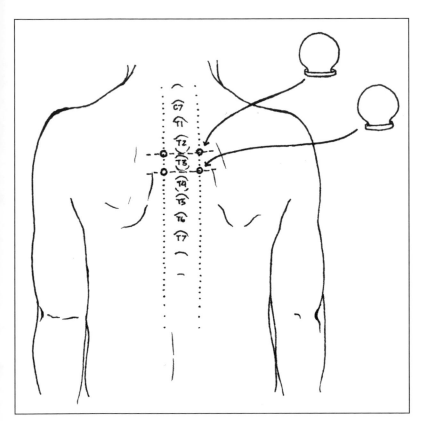

Fig. 20 Channel illustration of the cupping jars to treat asthma.

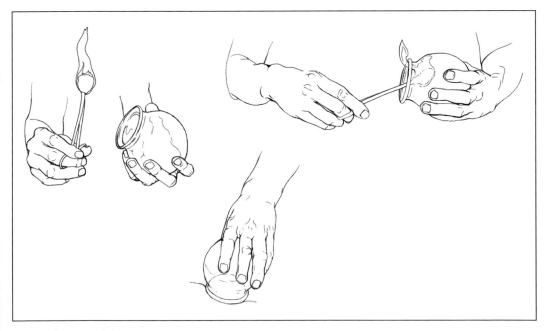

Fig. 21 Illustration of the cupping jars.

Measles and Chicken Pox

Measles

Measles and chicken pox are common diseases among children. Measles is associated with blood and water, pox with *qi*. Usually children who have been troubled with a common cold reveal patches of dark-reddish measles rash on their skin. In order to prevent or lessen the effect that will be exerted by measles, it is of great significance that a newborn infant should not be fed anything before its first excrement has been expelled (see above). This is an important measure taken to avoid the "heating" up of the blood that may possibly result in the appearance of measles. If the newborn baby is fed with milk immediately after its birth, it stands a greater risk of getting and/or suffering from a more serious case of measles. When our advice is followed by the parents, even if measles does appear, it is much less aggressive.

Generally, measles lasts a period of 1 week for children. For the first 3 days the child will have a low fever. Beginning on the third day, the measles will have subsided and the temperature will decrease. The fourth day will see the measles beat a retreat. The way to understand the degree of seriousness is to inspect the spots on the nose and chest on the third day. If they don't show red in color and the temperature is still high the measles hasn't yet played itself out. When the spots turn red, it is a sign that the measles has expressed itself and health is on the way.

During the week of suffering, the room should be kept dark with all the curtains drawn to safeguard the eyesight of the child from the irritation of light.

Formula for measles:

Pin Yin	Latin	English	Dosage
Dan dou chi	Sojae Praeparatum Semen	Prepared soybean	9 g
Chan tui	Periostracum Cicadae	Cicada moultings	2.4 g
Chao hei jing jie	Schizonepetae Herba	Fried, charred schizonepeta	4.5 g
Chao hei fang feng	Saposhnikoviae Radix	Fried, charred ledebouriella root, saposhnikoviae root, siler	4.5 g
Sang ye	Mori Folium	White mulberry leaf	4.5 g
Ge gen	Puerariae Radix	Kudzu root, pueraria	4.5 g
Zhe bei mu	Fritillariae Thunbergii Bulbus	Zhejiang fritillaria, Thunberg fritillaria bulb, fritillaria	9 g
Shan zhi zi	Gardeniae Jasminoides Fructus	Cape jasmine fruit, gardenia fruit	9 g
Shu huang qin	Scutellariae Baicalensis Radix	Prepared skullcap root, scutellaria, scute	4.5 g
Lian qiao	Forsythiae Suspensae Fructus	Forsythia fruit	9 g
Zhi ke	Citri Aurantii Fructus	Mature fruit of the bitter orange	4.5 g
Shen qu	Massa Medicata Fermentata	Medicated leaven (dough)	9 g
Fu ping	Lemnae seu Spirodelae Herba	Spirodela or duckweed	2.4 g

The medicines, boiled in water, are to be taken as tea for 3 to 4 days until the temperature falls and the measles on the nose, chest, and soles of the feet have turned red. That is to say, until all the measles have been expressed.

Chicken Pox

When children have chicken pox, they will not have a very high temperature. They must be fed a diet of liquid food. Even if their temperature has disappeared, for early recovery, it is suggested that they stay at home for 1 week or more. If they do not have sufficient rest and are fed carelessly, the function of their lungs will suffer. All this will lead to further weakening of the internal organs and indigestion.

As with measles, the optimum precaution against chicken pox is to feed newborn children only after their first excrement has been expelled (see above). Children with chicken pox must also avoid light.

Chicken pox makes them feel itchy and if they should scratch, scars will remain indelibly on their face or elsewhere, so put some gloves on their hands.

Formula for chicken pox:

Pin Yin	Latin	English	Dosage
Sheng jing jie	Schizonepetae Herba	Fresh schizonepeta	4.5 g
Sheng fang feng	Saposhnikoviae Radix	Fresh ledebouriella root, saposhnikoviae root, siler	4.5 g
Chan tui	Periostracum Cicadae	Cicada moultings	2.4 g
Jie geng	Platycodi Radix	Root of balloonflower, platycodon root	4.5 g
Fu ling	Poria Cocos Sclerotium	Sclerotium of tuckahoe, poria, China root, hoelen, Indian bread	9 g
Lian qiao	Forsythiae Suspensae Fructus	Forsythia fruit	9 g
Yi yi ren	Coicis Semen	Seed of Job's tears, coix seeds	12 g
Bai mao gen	Imperatae Cylindricae Rhizoma	Rhizome of woolly grass, imperata, white grass	9 g

Continue taking the formula until the itching is relieved.

Epidemic Parotitis or Mumps

When children come in contact with children who have mumps and one or both cheeks are feverish, you must be aware of their chance of getting infected too. Children with mumps must rest in bed and take fluid food.

Formula for epidemic mumps:

Pin Yin	Latin	English	Dosage
Jin yin hua	Lonicerae Flos	Honeysuckle flower, lonicera	9 g
Gan cao	Glycyrrhizae Radix	Licorice root	9 g

Epidemic mumps are also treated with ointment made in the following way:

Pin Yin	Latin	English	Dosage
Qing dai	Indigo Pulverata Levis	Processed da qing ye, woad leaf, istatis, indigo	as needed
Cu	Acetum	Vinegar	as needed

Mix ingredients with flour to make a plaster. Apply to swollen area.

Otitis Media

Otitis media among children often arises from a common cold, measles or something dirty getting into the ears. Children may experience fevers and the ear can ooze pus.

Formula for otitis media inflammation and its repeated recurrence:

Pin Yin	Latin	English	Dosage
Liu yi san	Talcum/Glycyrrhizae Radix	Six-to-one powder	6 parts talcum, 1 part licorice
Bing pian	Borneolum Syntheticum	Borneol	20 % of total quantity

Grind the medicines into powder. Use some absorbent cotton to sprinkle the ear with the power. This medicine is effective for both children and adults.

Nettle Rash, Urticaria

Children troubled by allergies also tend to have urticaria, patches of terribly itchy red rashes. They may also appear in their intestine, resulting in a running stomach. Treatment of rashes with Chinese medicine is very effective.

Formula I for nettle rash:

Pin Yin	Latin	English	Dosage
Lu lu tong	Liquidambaris Fructus	Sweetgum fruit, liquidambar fruit	30 g

Boil the medicine into fluid and take as a tea any time you like. It is very agreeable.

Formula II for nettle rash:

Pin Yin	Latin	English	Dosage
Chan tui	Periostracum Cicadae	Cicada moultings	9 g
Wu wei zi	Schisandrae Chinensis Fructus	Schisandra fruit	3 g
She tui	Serpentis Exuviae	Snake skin slough	9 g

Boil the medicines in water. Take one cup twice daily. Also effectively treats chronic nettle rash.

Tonsillitis

According to doctors trained in Western medicine, tonsillitis is easy to treat. A tonsillectomy is the routine treatment. In my Taiwan years I saw three patients die of tonsillectomies.

There are two classes of tonsillitis: acute and chronic. In an acute case, a child might have a cold that leads to sudden tonsillitis. That is a case arising from an external cause. In a chronic case, a child of poor physique who is feeble, yet very active, without adequate rest, develops tonsillitis gradually. Chronic conditions happen more frequently. Children with chronic conditions must be protected with sufficient rest, including time off from school.

Formula for acute tonsillitis:

Pin Yin	Latin	English	Dosage
Chao hei jing jie	Schizonepetae Herba	Fried, charred schizonepeta stem or bud	4.5 g
Fang feng	Saposhnikoviae Radix	Ledebouriella root, saposhnikoviae root, siler	4.5 g
Ma bo	Fructificatio Lasiosphaera seu Calvatia	Fruiting body of puff-ball	3 g
She gan	Belamcandae Rhizoma	Belamcanda rhizome	2.4 g
Gan cao	Glycyrrhizae Radix	Licorice root	3 g
Shan zhi zi	Gardeniae Jasminoidis Fructus	Cape jasmine fruit, gardenia fruit	9 g
Chao chi shao	Paeoniae Rubra Radix	Fried red peony root	6 g
Mu dan pi	Moutan Radicis Cortex	Tree peony root bark, moutan root bark	6 g
Shu huang qin	Scutellariae Baicalensis Radix	Prepared baical skullcap root, scutellaria, scute	4.5 g
Zhe bei mu	Fritillariae Thunbergii Bulbus	Zhejiang fritillaria, Thunberg fritillaria bulb, fritillaria	9 g
Lu gen	Phragmitis Communis Rhizoma	Reed rhizome	9 g

Formula for chronic tonsillitis:

Pin Yin	Latin	English	Dosage
Chao hei jing jie	Schizonepetae Herba	Fried, charred schizonepeta	4.5 g
Fang feng	Saposhnikoviae Radix	Ledebouriella root, saposhnikoviae root, siler	4.5 g
Shan zhi zi	Gardeniae Jasminoidis Fructus	Cape jasmine fruit, gardenia fruit	3 g
Xuan shen	Scrophulariae Radix	Ningpo figwort root, scrophularia	6 g
Chuan bei mu	Fritillariae Cirrhosae Bulbus	Szechuan fritillaria bulb, tendrilled fritillaria	9 g
Gan cao	Glycyrrhizae Radix	Licorice root	3 g
Zhe bei mu	Fritillariae Thunbergii Bulbus	Zhejiang fritillaria, Thunberg fritillaria bulb, fritillaria	9 g
Yu zhu	Polygonati Odorati Rhizoma	Solomon's seal rhizome, polygonatum	9 g
Xing ren	Armeniacae Semen	Apricot kernel	9 g
Bai he	Lilii Bulbus	Lily bulb	9 g

The above formula must be taken when the fever is absent and for quite a long time. At the same time the sick child must be allowed enough rest from activities. If the child gets a fever, switch to the formula for an acute case until fever is abated.

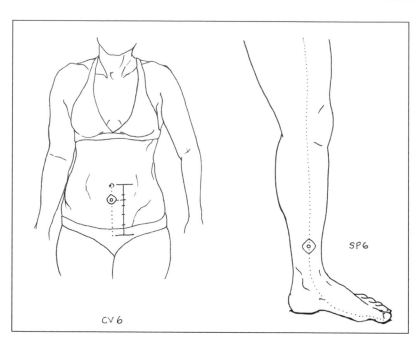

Fig. 22   *Chan su* plaster points.

Leon Hammer   The "brown sugar" as noted elsewhere is obtained in an oriental food store and is known as "red" sugar in block form. However, Dr. Shen said to me that the block "red" sugar was for excessive menstrual bleeding (menorrhagia) and white sugar was for pain (see above under "In Preparation for Conception").

The dosage for habitual period pain is as follows:

Pin Yin	Latin	English	Dosage
Yi mu cao	Leonuri Herba	Chinese motherwort, leonurus	9–15 g

Take 3 days before each period. When this dose doesn't have any effect, we use the following ointment, a medicated plaster method.

The medicated plaster is to be bought in the form of pills from a Chinese medicine store called "*chan su*" plaster (a toad cake, the dried venom of toads). Three days before the period place the plaster on CV-6 and SP-6 (**Fig. 22**).

Scanty Menstrual Flow

Formula for scanty menstrual flow due to blood deficiency:

Pin Yin	Latin	English	Dosage
Ji xiong pu	Gallus	Skinless chicken breast	2 pieces
Huang qi	Astragali Radix	Milk vetch root, astragalus root	15 g
Dang gui	Angelicae Sinensis Radix	Chinese Angelica root, *tang-kuei*	15 g
San qi	Notoginseng Radix	Noto ginseng root, root of pseudo-ginseng	6 g

Steam the medicine in a Chinese steam pot for 4 to 5 hours. Drink the liquid two to three times a week, before and after the period, to replenish the blood.

Menorrhagia

Sometimes a woman may lose too much blood during her period, sometimes going so far as to need to call for an ambulance to get first aid. This is usually mainly a matter of abnormal deficiency in the womb. For prevention in advance against ensuing cases, urgent measures must be taken to nourish the enfeebled woman and her womb. Those who have just started to show signs are treated differently from those women who have had the condition for several years.

Formula for recent manifestations of menorrhagia:

Pin Yin	Latin	English	Dosage
Dang gui	Angelicae Sinensis Radix	Chinese Angelica root, *tang-kuei*	9 g
Xi yang shen	Panacis Quinquefolii Radix	American ginseng root	9 g
Zi he che or tai pan	Placenta Hominis	Human placenta, placenta	12 g
Shan yao	Dioscoreae Oppositae Rhizoma	Chinese yam, dioscorea rhizome	12 g
Di yu	Sanguisorbae Radix	Sanguisorba, burnet-bloodwort root	12 g
Ou jie	Nelumbinis Nodus Rhizomatis	Node of lotus rhizome, lotus root node	12 g
Tu si zi	Cuscutae Chinensis Semen	Chinese dodder seeds, cuscuta	12 g
Duan mu li	Ostreae Concha	Calcined oyster shell	15 g
Da zao	Zizyphi Jujubae Fructus	Chinese date, jujube	7 dates
Dan shen	Salviae Miltiorrhiziae Radix	Salvia root	9 g

Boil the medicine in water and drink it as tea. Drink twice a day for 1 week before the period starts. Stop the day the period starts. Begin taking it again after the period.

Formula for a chronic case lasting several years:

Pin Yin	Latin	English	Dosage
Gao li shen	Ginseng Coreensis Radix	Korean ginseng	30 g
Xi yang shen	Panacis Quinquefolii Radix	American ginseng root	45 g
Lu rong	Cornu Cervi Parvum	Velvet of young deer antler, cervi	20 g
Ge jie	Gekko Gecko Linnaeus	Gecko	20 g
Zi he che or tai pan	Placenta Hominis	Human placenta, placenta	90 g

Grind the medicine into powder and divided it into 60 little portions or packets. Swallow one portion with water twice a day, once in the morning and once in the evening.

Irregularity of Menstrual Cycle

Leon Hammer Regarding menstrual patterns, during my time with Dr. Shen he taught that menses that occurred frequently, less than every 28 days, were associated with liver-kidney *yin* deficiency; delayed menses with kidney *yang* essence deficiency; missing months with liver *qi* stagnation; stopping and starting during a period with blood stagnation, in addition to what follows, which is sometimes at odds with the above.

Formula for frequent menses:

Pin Yin	Latin	English	Dosage
Dang gui	Angelicae Sinensis Radix	Chinese Angelica root, tang-kuei	6 g
Shu di huang	Rehmanniae Preparata Radix	Prepared Chinese foxglove root (cooked in red wine), cooked rehmannia rhizome	12 g
Bai zhu	Atractylodis Macrocephalae Rhizoma	White atractylodes rhizome	6 g
Fu ling	Poria Cocos Sclerotium	Sclerotium of tuckahoe, poria, China root, hoelen, Indian bread	9 g
Yuan zhi	Polygalae Radix	Chinese senega root, polygala root	6 g
Nu zhen zi	Ligustri Lucidi Fructus	Privet fruit, ligustrum	9 g
Tu si zi	Cuscutae Chinensis Semen	Chinese dodder seeds, cuscuta	12 g
Dan shen	Salviae Miltiorrhiziae Radix	Salvia root	6 g
Wu wei zi	Schisandrae Chinensis Fructus	Schisandra fruit	4.5 g
Bai shao	Paeoniae Alba Radix	White peony root	9 g
Fo shou	Citri Sarcodactylis Fructus	Finger citron fruit, Buddha's hand	6 g

Put the medicines in water and boil into tea; drink the tea twice a day until the periods are regular.

Leon Hammer During the time I spent with Dr. Shen and his immediate family as well as throughout China, I was impressed with the measures that were taken to protect women's *qi* and blood during their period, during pregnancy, and especially during the postprandial time both in terms of physical support, rest, and herbs. It was my impression that Chinese women of that time and before were spared the worst aspects of the menopause for this reason.

Hyperthyroidism

Hyperthyroidism is due to too much secretion from thyroid glands. The patient presents with a parched mouth and a dry throat, irritability, and a feeling of something burning hot inside. The tongue looks red and thinly coated with deficient but rapid pulses. Chinese medicine calls it, "deficiency in *yin* to induce vigorous fire." The patient also has swollen or enlarged thyroid glands. This condition could be seen as warm ambitions so suppressed that they rise in revolt into a sort of stagnant "fire" burning vehemently, thereby depleting the *yin* and harming both the liver and the kidneys. The Chinese medicine strategy is to nourish the *yin* to quell the deficient fire or to soften the stagnant rage to set up a compromise between *qi* and *yin*.

Formula for hyperthyroidism:

Pin Yin	Latin	English	Dosage
Sheng di huang	Rehmanniae Radix	Fresh Chinese foxglove root, rehmannia root	10 g
Sheng huang qi	Astragali Radix	Fresh milk vetch root, astragalus root	30 g
Dang gui	Angelicae Sinensis Radix	Chinese Angelica root, tang-kuei	10 g
Chao huang qin	Scutellariae Baicalensis Radix	Fried baical skullcap root, scutellaria, scute	10 g
Huang lian	Coptidis Rhizoma	Coptis rhizome	3 g

Pin Yin	Latin	English	Dosage
Huang bai	Phellodendri Cortex	Amur corktree bark, phellodendron bark	6 g
Sheng mu li	Concha Ostreae	Unprocessed oyster shell	30 g
Xuan shen	Scrophulariae Radix	Ningpo figwort root, scrophularia	15 g
Huang yao zi	Dioscoreae Bulbiferae Rhizoma	Airpotato yam rhizome	12 g
Jiang can	Bombyx Batryticatus	Silkworm, body of sick silkworm	10 g
Xia ku cao	Prunellae Spica Vulgaris	Self-heal spike, prunella	12 g

Boil the medicine with water. Take one dose daily, with 10 doses as one course of treatment, with some additions or some subtractions according to the condition.

Leon Hammer Hyperthyroidism, Graves disease, and mania, the psychological pattern closely resembling it, occur when the triple burner is unable to maintain a smooth transition in the nourishing (*sheng*) cycle between the water, wood, and fire. Perhaps related to repressed powerful and "hot" emotions, the wood begins to burn out of control (of the triple burner) and the fire goes to the heart beyond the ability of the water to control. The spirit housed in the heart becomes highly agitated in the form of mania and/or Graves disease (severe acute hyperthyroidism). This occurs when the heart attempts to retain the fire pathogen in a nonfatal yet vulnerable area of the body, in this instance, the thyroid. The thyroid is the organ that produces the normal metabolic heat that is one aspect of *qi*, and when out of control produces an excess of this metabolic heat. The water is depleted attempting to control the fire and gradually the wood is consumed and the fire banks into the condition we call depression. As long as the triple burner is unable to sustain a smooth transition between the phases, the pattern will begin again as soon as the wood recovers.

Hypothyroidism

Deficiency of thyroid gland function is due to the internal reduction of hormones in thyroid glands or from a thyroidectomy. Both are difficult tasks to tackle. Some improvement can be made, but not without side-effects.

This chronic condition manifests as sapped vitality and dire scarcity of blood and *qi* or internal organ deficiency. In Chinese medicine it falls into the category of consumptive diseases and is mainly a matter of *yang* deficiency in the spleen and kidneys. The nourishment of both the spleen and kidneys is the main treatment.

Formula for thyroid gland deficiency:

Pin Yin	Latin	English	Dosage
Xian mao	Rhizoma Curculifinis	Golden eye grass rhizome, curculigo	10 g
Yin yang huo	Epimedii Herba	Aerial parts of epimedium	15 g
Fu zi	Aconiti Lateralis Praeparata Radix	Aconite	6 g
Rou gui	Cinnamomi Cassiae Cortex	Inner bark of Saigon cinnamon	3 g
Dang shen	Codonopsis Pilosulae Radix	Codonopsis root	15 g
Huang qi	Astragali Radix	Milk vetch root, astragalus root	30 g
Lu jiao shuang	Cornu Cervi Degelatinatium	Leftover dregs after boiling deer antler glue	10 g
Shu di huang	Rehmanniae Preparata Radix	Prepared Chinese foxglove root (cooked in red wine), cooked rehmannia rhizome	15 g

Boil the medicine with water and drink one dose a day for 3 months. Long-term treatment produces better results.

Leon Hammer   Dr. Shen mentions three causes of gastric ulcer but does not mention the most common one in my clinical experience, both as a Western and Chinese medicine physician.

From early in my medical career and generally accepted by the medical community is the relationship between emotional stress and gastric-duodenal ulcers. When I was in medical college we admitted a 5-year-old child with a gastric ulcer who, in retrospect, was probably a victim of sexual abuse never confronted by medicine or society until recently.

The relationship between repressed emotions, liver *qi* stagnation, and stomach pathology is well known. The principal characteristic of liver *qi* is that it needs to move not only itself but also *qi* in many functions, especially the digestive tract, as we shall see later.

When liver *qi* moves from the contained to the repressed and the pressure to move overcomes the forces of resistance (the irrepressible force meets the immovable object), the *qi* can break loose and will move to the most vulnerable organ (liver "attacking" is a misconception). Almost always it carries with it the excess heat that has accumulated from failed attempts by the body to have metabolic heat move the *qi*.

The term "liver attacking" is unfortunate since the escaping liver *qi* is simply moving to the area of least resistance, the most vulnerable area or organ. There are internal pathological consequences as well as external, some of which are discussed below—liver blood stagnation, for example (the *qi* moves the blood), which can be the result of either *qi* stagnation due to excess or *qi* deficiency.

Blood Deficiency

Formula for blood deficiency (see also "Dr. Shen's Formulas in Systems," p. 94):

Pin Yin	Latin	English	Dosage
Huang qi	Astragali Radix	Milk vetch root, astragalus root	30 g
Dang gui	Angelicae Sinensis Radix	Chinese Angelica root, *tang-kuei*	15 g
Da zao	Zizyphi Jujubae Fructus	Chinese date, jujube	5 g
Ji xiong pu	Gallus	Skinless chicken breast	2 pieces

Put the medicines in a Yunnan steam pot and steam for 4 to 5 hours; eat one or two bowls of the soup a day, two to three times a week, to effectively promote the circulation of blood. If the case is serious consume each day. For gestational blood deficiency, add three kinds of livers to the soup.

Varicose Veins

Formula for varicose veins, see "Dr. Shen's Formulas in Systems," p. 34.

Common Cold in Adults

Common cold occurs when one meets abruptly warm or cold circumstances leading to coldness into the body. A little fever threatens our health to a great measure. If the patient takes no proper rest, leaving the cold still imprisoned in the body, other ailments will arise.

Formula for a common cold:

Pin Yin	Latin	English	Dosage
Jin yin hua	Lonicerae Flos	Honeysuckle flower, lonicera	15 g
Lian qiao	Forsythiae Suspensae Fructus	Forsythia fruit	15 g
Niu bang zi	Arctii Lappae Fructus	Great burdock fruit, arctium	10 g
Jing jie	Schizonepetae Herba	Schizonepeta	6 g
Fang feng	Saposhnikoviae Radix	Ledebouriella root, saposhnikoviae root, siler	6 g
Ge gen	Puerariae Radix	Kudzu root, pueraria	9 g
Bo he	Menthae Haplocalycis Herba	Field mint, mentha, peppermint leaves	6 g

Pin Yin	Latin	English	Dosage
Chan tui	Periostracum Cicadae	Cicada moultings	6 g
Jie geng	Platycodi Radix	Root of balloonflower, platycodon root	6 g
Sheng gan cao	Glycyrrhizae Radix	Fresh licorice root	6 g
Hei shan zhi zi	Gardeniae Jasminoidis Fructus	Charred cape jasmine fruit, gardenia fruit	10 g

Boil the medicine into tea and drink twice a day until condition improves.

Asthma

Asthma usually persists throughout a patient's life, with various causes leading to each stage. According to Chinese medicine, it is mainly deficiency of the heart, lungs, liver, kidneys, and spleen that leads to asthma. Generally speaking, it is the invasion of a penetrating coldness that has disarmed the body and remained latent within the body.

Overwork might also have exhausted the patient, thereby compromising their immunity. Any slight, careless cold will make the latent coldness surface again. The main strategy in treating asthma is to expel all the coldness. Cupping on UB-12 and UB-13 for 15 minutes three to four times a week can expel cold.

Formula for asthma:

Pin Yin	Latin	English	Dosage
Dong chong xia cao	Cordyceps Sinensis	Chinese caterpillar fungus	3 g
Chuan bei mu	Fritillariae Cirrhosae Bulbus	Szechuan fritillaria bulb, tendrilled, fritillaria	3 g
Feng mi	Mel Millis	Honey	1 g
Li	Pyri Fructus	Pear	1 pear

Stew the medicine in steam for 3 to 4 hours and drink the juice. Take the medicine before sleeping each night until asthma is relieved.

Formula for asthma with a cough:

Pin Yin	Latin	English	Dosage
Mi ma huang	Ephedrae Herba	Honey-cooked ephedra stem	1.8 g
Su zi	Perillae Fructus	Perilla fruit	4.5 g
Niu bang zi	Arctii Lappae Fructus	Great burdock fruit, arctium	6 g
Ting li zi	Descurainiae seu Lepidii Semen	Descurainia seeds, lepidium seeds	6 g
Mi zhi zi wan	Asteris Radix	Honey-cooked purple aster, aster root	9 g
Chuan bei mu	Fritillariae Cirrhosae Bulbus	Szechuan fritillaria bulb, tendrilled fritillaria	9 g
Bai jie zi	Sinapis Albae Semen	White mustard seed	9 g
Wu wei zi	Schisandrae Chinensis Fructus	Schisandra fruit	4.5 g
Xuan fu hua	Inulae Flos	Inula flower	6 g
Xing ren	Armeniacae Semen	Apricot kernel	9 g

If the patient has no more coldness inside, they can do very well without the cupping treatment and just take the above formula. They also have to pay more attention to taking rest to attain early recovery.

Sustained Fatigue

Sustained fatigue in Chinese medicine is called the "latent demon." Again, it is the coldness that has penetrated the physique after an illness. The pa-tient should rest and receive treatment at the very onset of a cold.

Formula for sustained fatigue:

Pin Yin	Latin	English	Dosage
Gui zhi	Ramulus Cinnamomi Cassiae	Cinnamon twig, cassia twig	2.4 g
Wei ge gen	Puerariae Radix	Roasted root of kudzu	9 g
Chao fang feng	Saposhnikoviae Radix	Fried ledebouriella root, saposhnikoviae root, siler	6 g
Zhi yuan zhi	Polygalae Radix	Prepared Chinese senega root, polygala root	6 g
Chao dang shen	Codonopsis Pilosulae Radix	Fried Codonopsis root	6 g
Chao huang qin	Scutellariae Baicalensis Radix	Fried baical skullcap root, scutellaria, scute	6 g
Zhi jiang can	Bombyx Batryticatus	Prepared silkworm, body of sick silkworm	9 g
Chuan bei mu	Fritillariae Cirrhosae Bulbus	Szechuan fritillaria bulb, tendrilled fritillaria	9 g
Shen qu	Massa Medicata Fermentata	Medicated leaven (dough)	12 g

Boil the medicines into tea and drink twice a day until condition improves.

Leon Hammer There are so many ways to exhaust *qi*, blood, *yin*, and *yang* as well as essence that Dr. Shen's concept as expressed here is somewhat limiting. I refer you to the introduction to this chapter for a discussion of "cold" invasion. Dr. Shen was well aware of the role of toxins and working beyond a person's energy as important factors in the etiology of chronic fatigue.

Migraine

Leon Hammer Discussed under "Headache" in "Dr. Shen's Formulas in Systems" regarding head trauma (see p. 116).

There are four causes of migraine. Either the nerves have been injured without receiving effective treatment; it is the sequela of a slight cerebral concus-sion; it is caused by anemia; or it is due to nervous tension. Migraines may persist from adolescence until old age.

Formula for those with latent injury:

Pin Yin	Latin	English	Dosage
Chao dang gui	Angelicae Sinensis Radix	Fried Chinese Angelica root, *tang-kuei*	6 g
Tian ma	Gastrodiae Rhizoma	Gastrodia rhizome	9 g
Chuan xiong	Chuanxiong Rhizoma	Chuanxiong root, Szechuan lovage root, cnidium	4.5 g
Bai zhi	Angelicae Dahuricae Radix	Angelica root	6 g

Pin Yin	Latin	English	Dosage
Sang ji sheng	Taxilli Herba	Mulberry mistletoe stems, loranthus, taxillus, mistletoe	12 g
Xiang fu	Cyperi Rotundi Rhizoma	Nutgrass rhizome, cypress	6 g
San qi	Notoginseng Radix	Noto ginseng root, root of pseudo-ginseng	3 g
Dan shen	Salviae Miltiorrhiziae Radix	Salvia root	6 g
Chao huang qin	Scutellariae Baicalensis Radix	Fried baical skullcap root, scutellaria, scute	6 g

In addition to the formula, the patient should take two pills a day of *Yunnan Baiyao* (Yunnan White Powder), for 7 days.

Formula for migraine due to anemia:

Pin Yin	Latin	English	Dosage
Chao dang gui	Angelicae Sinensis Radix	Chinese angelica root, *tang-kuei*	9 g
Shu di huang	Rehmanniae Preparata Radix	Prepared Chinese foxglove root (cooked in red wine), cooked rehmannia rhizome	12 g
Bai zhi	Angelicae Dahuricae Radix	Angelica root	6 g
Chuan xiong	Chuanxiong Rhizoma	Chuanxiong root, Szechuan lovage root, cnidium	6 g
Fu ling	Poria Cocos Sclerotium	Sclerotium of tuckahoe, poria, China root, hoelen, Indian bread	9 g
Zhi yuan zhi	Polygalae Radix	Prepared Chinese senega root, polygala root	6 g
Gou qi zi	Lycii Fructus	Chinese wolfberry, matrimony vine fruit, lycium fruit	12 g
Shan zhu yu	Corni Officinalis Fructus	Asiatic Cornelian cherry fruit, cornus	12 g
Man jing zi	Viticis Fructus	Vitex fruit	6 g
Chao huang qin	Scutellariae Baicalensis Radix	Fried baical skullcap root, scutellaria, scute	6 g

Boil the medicines into a tea and drink twice daily until conditions improve.

Vaginal Discharge

White mucus oozing out of the vagina, as if in the form of nasal mucus or sometimes dripping in a flow, is called vaginal discharge. Unrestrained diet or overwork that have hurt the spleen and the normal functioning of the internal organs lead to vaginal discharge. Sometimes the mucus looks yellowish, is sticky and smelly, sometimes reddish with blood, making the vagina itchy. When a woman takes a bath without clean water or towels, or has too much sex and is worn down by the so-called invasion of "damp toxin" she has to be treated in the following ways:

Formula for white vaginal discharge:

Pin Yin	Latin	English	Dosage
Bai zhu	Atractylodis Macrocephalae Rhizoma	White atractylodes rhizome	10 g
Chao shan yao	Dioscoreae Oppositae Rhizoma	Fried Chinese yam, dioscorea rhizome	15 g

nective tissue, where it stores excess damp (damp spleen).

Dr. Shen said that patients with edema should be advised to improve their improper ways of life, refrain from very spicy food, drinking wine, and eating too much salt and sugar. They should also abstain from sex in order to conserve their energies for recovery. When the patient can't follow these pieces of advice, even the best treatment will not help them. Again, "Chinese medicine is in the life."

Formula for facial edema:

Pin Yin	Latin	English	Dosage
Chao huang qi	Astragali Radix	Fried milk vetch root, fried astragalus root	12 g
Bai zhu	Atractylodis Macrocephalae Rhizoma	White atractylodes rhizome	9 g
Bai shao	Paeoniae Alba Radix	White peony root	9 g
Fu ling	Poria Cocos Sclerotium	Sclerotium of tuckahoe, poria, China root, hoelen, Indian bread	9 g
Yuan zhi	Polygalae Radix	Chinese senega root, polygala root	6 g
Wu wei zi	Schisandrae Chinensis Fructus	Schisandra fruit	4.5 g
Mu li	Ostreae Concha	Oyster shell	18 g
Mai men dong	Ophiopogonis Radix	Ophiopogon tuber	9 g
Chuan xiong	Chuanxiong Rhizoma	Chuanxiong root, Szechuan lovage root, cnidium	4.5 g
Chao jing jie	Schizonepetae Herba	Dry-fried schizonepeta	4.5 g
Chao hei fang feng	Saposhnikoviae Radix	Fried, charred ledebouriella root, saposhnikoviae root, siler	4.5 g
Huai niu xi or niu xi	Achyranthis Bidentatae Radix	Ox-knee root, achyranthes root from Huai	9 g

Formula for leg edema:

Pin Yin	Latin	English	Dosage
Dang shen	Codonopsis Pilosulae Radix	Codonopsis root	9 g
Bai zhu	Atractylodis Macrocephalae Rhizoma	White atractylodes rhizome	6 g
Shan yao	Dioscoreae Oppositae Rhizoma	Chinese yam, dioscorea rhizome	12 g
Fu ling	Poria Cocos Sclerotium	Sclerotium of tuckahoe, poria, China root, hoelen, Indian bread	9 g
Yuan zhi	Polygalae Radix	Chinese senega root, polygala root	6 g
Shan zhu yu	Corni Officinalis Fructus	Asiatic Cornelian cherry fruit, cornus	12 g
Qiang huo	Notopterygii Rhizoma et Radix	Notopterygium root and rhizome, chiang-huo	4.5 g
Yan hu suo	Corydalis Yanhusuo Rhizoma	Corydalis rhizome	9 g
Huai niu xi or niu xi	Achyranthis Bidentatae Radix	Ox-knee root, achyranthes root from Huai	12 g

Formula for leg edema due to water accumulation:

Pin Yin	Latin	English	Dosage
Xi xin	Asari Herba cum Radice	Chinese wild ginger, asarum	3 g
Du zhong	Eucommiae Cortex	Eucommia bark	12 g
Gou qi zi	Lycii Fructus	Chinese wolfberry, matrimony vine fruit, lycium fruit	12 g
Chi ling	Sclerotium Poriae Cocos Rubrae	Pink sclerotium of tuckahoe, china root, poria, hoelen	9 g
Shu di huang	Rehmanniae Preparata Radix	Prepared Chinese foxglove root (cooked in red wine), cooked rehmannia rhizome	12 g
Shu yi yi ren	Coicis Semen	Prepared seeds of Job's tears, coix seeds	12 g
Sheng yi yi ren	Coicis Semen	Fresh seeds of Job's tears, coix seeds	12 g
Ze xie	Alismatis Rhizoma	Water plantain rhizome, alisma rhizome	9 g
Rou cong rong	Cistanchis Herba	Cistanche, fleshy stem of the broomrape	9 g

Formula for edema in the whole body:

Pin Yin	Latin	English	Dosage
Bai zhu	Atractylodis Macrocephalae Rhizoma	White atractylodes rhizome	9 g
Bai shao	Paeoniae Alba Radix	White peony root	9 g
Qiang huo	Notopterygii Rhizoma et Radix	Notopterygium root and rhizome, chiang-huo	6 g
Fu ling	Poria Cocos Sclerotium	Sclerotium of tuckahoe, poria, China root, hoelen, Indian bread	9 g
Bi xie	Dioscoreae Hypoglancae Rhizoma	Fish-poison yam rhizome	4.5 g
Shan yao	Dioscoreae Oppositae Rhizoma	Chinese yam, dioscorea rhizome	12 g
Ze xie	Alismatis Rhizoma	Water plantain rhizome, alisma rhizome	9 g
Shi wei	Pyrrosiae Folium	Pyrrosia leaf	6 g
Yu mi xu	Stylus Zeae Mays	Cornsilk	12 g

Make an experiment. Take these formulas for a whole week. If no improvement has been made, go to see a doctor.

Diabetes

Formulas for diabetes, see "Dr. Shen's Formulas in Systems," p. 47–48.

Rheumatoid Arthritis

There are two causes leading to rheumatoid arthritis. Long exposure to extreme temperature changes results in the invasion of coldness into the patient's muscles and joints. The blood circulation becomes impaired, especially at the joints, where heat and pain are felt. If the blood is contaminated with chemicals, this can also cause inflammation and pain at the joints. For the first case, ingesting or bathing in Chinese medicine will do the patient good.

Insomnia

Formulas for insomnia, see "Dr. Shen's Formulas in Systems," p. 17–19.

Prostate Glands

Some men have troubles with their prostate glands, besides their innate physical weaknesses. Too much or too little sex can cause this. Make an analysis of the physical condition first, then counsel the patient to adapt their sexual activity to a normal degree, improving their way of life so as to arrive at a successful cure. When the disease is in full swing, the patient has to take Chinese medicines for an extended period of time.

Formula I for prostate glands:

Pin Yin	Latin	English	Dosage
Xuan shen	Scrophulariae Radix	Ningpo figwort root, scrophularia	9 g
Chi shao	Paeoniae Rubra Radix	Red peony root	9 g
Chao hei jing jie	Schizonepetae Herba	Fried, charred schizonepeta	4.5 g
Chao hei fang feng	Saposhnikoviae Radix	Fried, charred ledebouriella root, saposhnikoviae root, siler	4.5 g
Gan cao	Glycyrrhizae Radix	Licorice root	4.5 g
Mu dan pi	Moutan Radicis Cortex	Tree peony root bark, moutan root bark	6 g
Zhi mu	Anemarrhenae Asphodeloidis Rhizoma	Anemarrhena rhizome	9 g
Long gu	Fossilia Ossis Mastodi	Dragon bone, fossilized vertebrae and bones of the extremities (usually of mammals)	15 g
Sheng yi yi ren	Coicis Semen	Fresh seeds of Job's tears, coix seeds	12 g
Long dan cao	Gentianae Longdancao Radix	Chinese gentian root, gentiana	3 g

Boil the medicines into tea and drink twice a day for 2 or 3 months.

The typical trouble with prostate problems (benign prostatic hypertrophy) is that the patient finds it difficult to urinate or experiences urgency and frequency. This often occurs as a result of excessive sex. That is why men have to exercise moderation in their sexual activities in adulthood, and still more strictly in old age.

Formula II for prostate glands:

Pin Yin	Latin	English	Dosage
Dang shen	Codonopsis Pilosulae Radix	Codonopsis root	15 g
Huang qi	Astragali Radix	Milk vetch root, astragalus root	30 g
Fu ling	Poria Cocos Sclerotium	Sclerotium of tuckahoe, poria, China root, hoelen, Indian bread	15 g
Rou gui	Cinnamomi Cassiae Cortex	Inner bark of Saigon cinnamon	3 g
Wang bu liu xing	Vaccariae Segetalis Semen	Vaccaria seeds	10 g
Gan cao	Glycyrrhizae Radix	Licorice root	5 g
Che qian zi	Plantaginis Semen	Plantago seeds	12 g
Huai nui xi	Achyranthis Bidentatae Radix	Achyranthes root	10 g
Bi xie	Dioscoreae Rhizoma Hypoglaucae	Fish poison yam rhizome, tokoro	15 g

Boil the medicines into tea. If the case is prostrate cancer, the patient has to call on an expert doctor for treatment.

Impotence, Premature Ejaculation

There are three causes for these two conditions: overworking, a weak heart, and kidney *qi-yang* deficiency. The patient must readjust their way of life to include more rest and less sex.

Formula I for impotence and premature ejaculation due to overworking:

Pin Yin	Latin	English	Dosage
Huang qi	Astragali Radix	Milk vetch root, astragalus root	9 g
Dang gui	Angelicae Sinensis Radix	Chinese Angelica root, *tang-kuei*	9 g
Chuan xiong	Chuanxiong Rhizoma	Chuanxiong root, Szechuan lovage root, cnidium	4.5 g
Bai zhi	Angelicae Dahuricae Radix	Angelica root	4.5 g
Fu ling	Poria Cocos Sclerotium	Sclerotium of tuckahoe, poria, China root, hoelen, Indian bread	9 g
Yuan zhi	Polygalae Radix	Chinese senega root, polygala root	6 g
Suan zao ren	Ziziphi Spinosae Semen	Spiny zizyphus seeds, sour jujube seeds, zizyphus	12 g
Shan zhu yu	Corni Officinalis Fructus	Asiatic Cornelian cherry fruit, cornus	12 g
Long chi	Fossilia Dentis Mastodi	Dragon teeth, fossilized teeth	15 g

Boil the medicines into tea and drink twice a day until symptoms are relieved.

Formula II for impotence and premature ejaculation due to a weak heart:

Pin Yin	Latin	English	Dosage
Huang qi	Astragali Radix	Milk vetch root, astragalus root	12 g
Dang gui	Angelicae Sinensis Radix	Chinese Angelica root, *tang-kuei*	9 g
Bai shao	Paeoniae Alba Radix	White peony root	9 g
Bai zhu	Atractylodis Macrocephalae Rhizoma	White atractylodes rhizome	6 g
Mai men dong	Ophiopogonis Radix	Ophiopogon tuber	9 g
Yuan zhi	Polygalae Radix	Chinese senega root, polygala root	6 g
Shu di huang	Rehmanniae Preparata Radix	Prepared Chinese foxglove root (cooked in red wine), cooked rehmannia rhizome	9 g
Wu wei zi	Schisandrae Chinensis Fructus	Schisandra fruit	4.5 g
Mu li	Ostreae Concha	Oyster shell	15 g

Boil the medicine into tea and drink the tea twice a day until symptoms improve.

If the disease is caused mainly by deficiency in the kidneys, the patient should take medicines for the nourishment of the kidneys (we refer you to the discussion on preparation for conception and male infertility, p. 176).

Formula for early-stage breast cancer:

Pin Yin	Latin	English	Dosage
Chai hu	Bupleuri Radix	Hare's ear root, thorowax root, bupleurum	10 g
Dang gui	Angelicae Sinensis Radix	Chinese Angelica root, *tang-kuei*	10 g
Yu jin	Curcumae Radix	Curcuma tuber	10 g
Gua luo pi	Trichosanthis Pericarpium	Husk of trichosanthes fruit	30 g
Qing pi	Citri Reticulatae Pericarpium Viride	Unripe tangerine peel, green tangerine peel, blue citrus	6 g
San leng	Sparganii Stoloniferi Rhizoma	Bur-reed rhizoma, scirpus	10 g
E zhu	Curcumae Rhizoma	Zedoary rhizoma, zedoaria	10 g
Bai shao	Radix Paeoniae Alba	White peony root	10 g
Chi shao	Radix Paeoniae Rubra	Red peony root	10 g
Chuan bei mu	Fritillariae Cirrhosae Bulbus	Szechuan fritillaria bulb, tendrilled fritillaria	10 g
Bai ji li	Tribuli Terrestris Fructus	Caltrop fruit, puncture-vine fruit, tribulus	15 g

Boil the medicine into tea for daily drinking over an extended period of time.

Formula for later-stage breast cancer:

Pin Yin	Latin	English	Dosage
Nu zhen zi	Ligustri Lucidi Fructus	Privet fruit, ligustrum	30 g
Han lian cao	Ecliptae Prostratae Herba	Eclipta	10 g
Dang gui	Angelicae Sinensis Radix	Chinese Angelica root, *tang-kuei*	10 g
Xuan shen	Scrophulariae Radix	Ningpo figwort root, scrophularia	12 g
Shan zhu yu	Corni Officinalis Fructus	Asiatic Cornelian cherry fruit, cornus	10 g
Chuan bei mu	Fritillariae Cirrhosae Bulbus	Szechuan fritillaria bulb, tendrilled, fritillaria	10 g
Lu jiao shuang	Cornu Cervi Degelatinatium	Leftover dregs after boiling deer antler glue	15 g
Ji xue teng	Jixueteng Radix et Caulis	Spatholobus or milettia root and vine	30 g
Dan shen	Salviae Miltiorrhiziae Radix	Salvia root	15 g
Ban zhi lian	Scutellariae Barbatae Herba	Barbat skullcap, scutellaria	30 g
Si gua luo	Fasciculus Vascularis Luffae	Dried skeleton of vegetable sponge	10 g
Gua luo pi	Trichosanthis Pericarpium	Husk of trichosanthes fruit	30 g

Boil the medicines into tea for daily drinking with some addition or deduction of medicines to suit different cases.

Ovarian Cyst

An ovarian cyst was called in "*chang tan*" in ancient China. It arises from disharmony between the liver and kidneys and between the *ren* and the *chong*. The result of long-term suppression of *qi*, phlegm, and dampness collect on the collateral channels of the uterus and form lumps about the size of an egg at the early stages of ovarian cysts. They grow in size and the abdomen enlarges itself as if pregnant. These lumps feel soft and movable.

Formula for ovarian cysts:

Pin Yin	Latin	English	Dosage
Gui zhi	Ramulus Cinnamomi Cassiae	Cinnamon twig, cassia twig	6 g
Fu ling	Poria Cocos Sclerotium	Sclerotium of tuckahoe, poria, China root, hoelen, Indian bread	15 g
Mu dan pi	Moutan Radicis Cortex	Tree peony root bark, moutan root bark	10 g
Tao ren	Persicae Semen	Peach kernel, persica	10 g
Chi shao	Paeoniae Rubra Radix	Red peony root	10 g
Sheng yi yi ren	Coicis Semen	Fresh seeds of Job's tears, coix seeds	30 g
Wang bu liu xing	Vaccariae Segetalis Semen	Vaccaria seeds	10 g
Zhi shi	Aurantii Immaturus Fructus	Immature bitter orange, unripe bitter orange, chih-shih	10 g

Boil the medicines into tea and drink.

Uterine Tumor

Uterine tumors are not limited to only one etiology. There are three causes for their formation. It is made up either of blood or water or qi. These factors may intermingle in different compositions to be subdivided into still more forms. So the prerequisite for effective treatment is to first discern the etiology of the tumor.

When the tumor is made up of blood, the swellings in the uterus feel hard and remain constant in size. If the tumor is made up of water, some feel hard and others soft, while the size seems sometimes large and sometimes small. If the tumors are made up of qi, some are soft. Upon palpation they are sometimes large but disappear altogether at other times.

Formation of uterine tumors is the bitter aftermath of inappropriate ways of life. Tumors made up of blood have their root in deficiency of the womb (qi deficiency in the lower burner), which is too weak to expel all the menstrual blood freely so some is retained inside. If the patient's defective ways of life are not improved in time, clumps of blood will grow in size and number and become tumors.

Qi and water are gradually stockpiled in the womb due to deficient liver qi that is required to eliminate them along with blood, when appropriate. They will gradually grow into tumors. When the patient is stronger, her womb will expel the remnant stagnant blood or qi fluid. So the lumps are sometimes large and sometimes small.

Leon Hammer
Pulse:
• Pelvis lower body: choppy; slippery
• Proximal positions: choppy

Tongue:
Swollen with purple spots

The most important approach to treating uterine tumors is to overcome the defective ways of life and choose different formulas to suit different patients. See also "Dr. Shen's Formulas in Systems," p. 148–150.

Formula for uterine tumors arising from blood stagnation:

Pin Yin	Latin	English	Dosage
Dang gui	Angelicae Sinensis Radix	Chinese Angelica root, *tang-kuei*	6 g
Chuan xiong	Chuanxiong Rhizoma	Chuanxiong root, Szechuan lovage root, cnidium	6 g
Chi shao	Paeoniae Rubra Radix	Red peony root	9 g
Bai shao	Paeoniae Alba Radix	White peony root	6 g
Dan shen	Salviae Miltiorrhiziae Radix	Salvia root	6 g
Yi mu cao	Leonuri Herba	Chinese motherwort, leonurus	6 g
E zhu	Curcumae Rhizoma	Zedoary rhizoma, zedoaria	2.4 g
Xiang fu	Cyperi Rotundi Rhizoma	Nutgrass rhizome, cypress	4.5 g
Chuan lian zi	Meliae Toosendan Fructus	Szechuan pagoda tree fruit, Szechuan chinaberry, melia	9 g
Huai nui xi	Achyranthis Bidentatae Radix	Achyranthes root	9 g

Formula for uterine tumors arising from water accumulation:

Pin Yin	Latin	English	Dosage
Dang gui	Angelicae Sinensis Radix	Chinese Angelica root, *tang-kuei*	6 g
Cang zhu	Atractylodis Rhizoma	Black atractylodes rhizome	4.5 g
Bi xie	Dioscoreae Rhizoma Hypoglaucae	Fish poison yam rhizome, tokoro	4.5 g
Xiang fu	Cyperi Rotundi Rhizoma	Nutgrass rhizome, cypress	4.5 g
Chi fu ling	Poriae Cocos Rubrae Sclerotium	Red sclerotium of tuckahoe, china root, poria, hoelen	9 g
Lu lu tong	Liquidambaris Fructus	Sweetgum fruit, liquidambar fruit	12 g
Yan hu suo	Corydalis Yanhusuo Rhizoma	Corydalis rhizome	9 g
Yu jin	Curcumae Radix	Curcuma tuber	6 g
Ze xie	Alismatis Rhizoma	Water plantain rhizome, alisma rhizome	9 g
Sheng yi yi ren	Coicis Semen	Fresh seeds of Job's tears, coix seeds	12 g
Shu yi yi ren	Coicis Semen	Prepared seeds of Job's tears, coix seeds	12 g

Formula for uterine tumors arising from *qi stagnation*:

Pin Yin	Latin	English	Dosage
Dang gui	Angelicae Sinensis Radix	Chinese Angelica root, *tang-kuei*	6 g
Chuan xiong	Chuanxiong Rhizoma	Chuanxiong root, Szechuan lovage root, cnidium	6 g
Chai hu	Bupleuri Radix	Hare's ear root, thorowax root, bupleurum	3 g
Bai shao	Paeoniae Alba Radix	White peony root	9 g
Fu ling	Poria Cocos Sclerotium	Sclerotium of tuckahoe, poria, China root, hoelen, Indian bread	9 g
Yan hu suo	Corydalis Yanhusuo Rhizoma	Corydalis rhizome	9 g

Pin Yin	Latin	English	Dosage
E zhu	Curcumae Rhizoma	Zedoary rhizoma, zedoaria	3 g
Da fu pi	Arecae Catechu Pericarpium	Betel husk, areca peel	9 g
Huang qin	Scutellariae Baicalensis Radix	Baical skullcap root, scutellaria, scute	4.5 g
Huai nui xi	Achyranthis Bidentatae Radix	Achyranthes root	12 g

Boil the above medicines into tea and drink twice a day until the tumors disappear.

Glaucoma, Cataract

To effectively treat glaucoma and cataracts pay attention to harmonizing the functions of the internal organs and the hygiene of the eyes.

Formula for glaucoma or cataracts:

Pin Yin	Latin	English	Dosage
Huang qi	Astragali Radix	Milk vetch root, astragalus root	12 g
Gou qi zi	Lycii Fructus	Chinese wolfberry, matrimony vine fruit, lycium fruit	12 g
Bai shao	Paeoniae Alba Radix	White peony root	9 g
Gu jing cao	Eriocauli Flos	Pipewort scapus and inflorescence	9 g
Fu ling	Poria Cocos Sclerotium	Sclerotium of tuckahoe, poria, China root, hoelen, Indian bread	9 g
Sheng di huang	Rehmannia Radix	Fresh Chinese foxglove root, fresh rehmannia root	12 g
Yu jin	Curcumae Radix	Curcuma tuber	9 g
Mu zei	Equiseti Hiemalis Herba	Equisetum, scouring rush, shave grass, Dutch rushes, rough horsetail	9 g
Tu si zi	Cuscutae Chinensis Semen	Chinese dodder seeds, cuscuta	12 g
Da qing ye	Daqingye Folium	Woad leaf, isatis, indigo	9 g
Lu e mei	Pruni Mume Flos	Plum blossom	3 g

Boil the medicines into tea and drink twice a day until the symptoms disappear.

Leon Hammer Cataracts and glaucoma are etiologically separate so I do not know how one formula could address both. The cataracts are associated with a drying process due to *yin* deficiency and the glaucoma with excess heat in the eyes (upper burner) with accumulating fluid brought to reduce the heat.

Deafness in Old Age

According to Chinese medical theory, kidneys have their outward manifestation in the ears, so listening proficiency reflects the physical ability of the kidneys. During old age, the kidneys' ability is on the wane, with the ears' acuity likewise retarding, the degree depending on individual kidney *qi*. The patient has to limit sexual activities and always be optimistic, as well as taking herbs to nourish the kidneys.

Formula for old-age deafness:

Pin Yin	Latin	English	Dosage
Shu di huang	Rehmanniae Preparata Radix	Prepared Chinese foxglove root (cooked in red wine), cooked rehmannia rhizome	12 g
Dang gui	Angelicae Sinensis Radix	Chinese Angelica root, tang-kuei	9 g
Tu si zi	Cuscutae Chinensis Semen	Chinese dodder seeds, cuscuta	12 g
Shan zhu yu	Corni Officinalis Fructus	Asiatic Cornelian cherry fruit, cornus	12 g
Rou cong rong	Cistanchis Herba	Cistanche, fleshy stem of the broomrape	9 g
Bu gu zhi	Psoraleae Corylifoliae Fructus	Psoralea fruit	9 g
Wu wei zi	Schisandrae Chinensis Fructus	Schisandra fruit	6 g
Long chi	Fossilia Dentis Mastodi	Dragon teeth, fossilized teeth	15 g
Shi chang pu	Acori Tatarinowii Rhizoma	Grass-leaved sweetflag rhizome, acorus	3 g
Yuan zhi	Polygalae Radix	Chinese senega root, polygala root	6 g
Dan shen	Salviae Miltiorrhiziae Radix	Salvia root	9 g

Boil the medicines into tea and drink twice a day for an extended period of time.

Dull-witted Old Age, Dementia

Well into old age, brain cells for memory decrease and some patients can always recollect stories of their youth but are very forgetful of the events of the day. This can be likened to the hardware of a computer with limited memory capacity for new data.

The following formula is effective for senility and those who have Parkinson disease can also possibly benefit:

Pin Yin	Latin	English	Dosage
Huang qi	Astragali Radix	Milk vetch root, astragalus root	12 g
Ren shen	Ginseng Radix	Ginseng root	6 g
Dang gui	Angelicae Sinensis Radix	Chinese Angelica root, tang-kuei	9 g
Sheng di huang	Rehmannia Radix	Fresh Chinese foxglove root, fresh rehmannia root	12 g
Bai zhi	Angelicae Dahuricae Radix	Angelica root	6 g
Chuan xiong	Chuanxiong Rhizoma	Chuanxiong root, Szechuan lovage root, cnidium	6 g
Shi chang pu	Acori Tatarinowii Rhizoma	Grass-leaved sweetflag rhizome, acorus	3 g
Xiang fu	Cyperi Rotundi Rhizoma	Nutgrass rhizome, cypress	4.5 g
Long chi	Fossilia Dentis Mastodi	Dragon teeth, fossilized teeth	15 g
Ding xiang	Caryophylli Flos	Clove flower bud	4.5 g
Mei gui hua	Rosae Rugosae Flos	Young flower of Chinese rose	4.5 g

Boil the herbal medicines into tea and drink twice a day as a long practice.

Old Age Health Care, Chinese Medicated Jelly Herbs

All organ functions wane over 50 years of age and especially over 60 years. People find that if they have had nervous tension throughout their life, severe neurological and psychological problems will be more likely to manifest as one ages. If the patient has paid little attention to adjusting their diet, they will suffer from illnesses arising from the stomach and intestines, which impair digestion and absorption. This will, in turn, weaken other organs.

Fortunately in Chinese medicine there is an abundance of health care resources for the aged. Included in the measures advocated are doing physical exercises (*tai chi* and *qi gong*), keeping one's heart happy (meditation), leading a moderate way of life in terms of diet and sex, supplemented with Chinese herbal treatment.

Smoking is only detrimental to human health and has no benefits. According to some old Chinese pharmacopoeia, our forefathers warned us against smoking long ago. According to Western medicine, smoking leads to cancer and heart diseases so we must avoid smoking. Drinking a little wine helps activate the channels of the body and sharpen the appetite. However, a long habit of excessive drinking certainly endangers health.

Tea does us more good than harm. It helps refresh the drinker in their meditation, quickens their efficiency at work, stimulates their saliva for better digestion, reduces inflammation, and facilitates urination and excretion of toxins. Therefore, by drinking tea we strengthen our body condition, our heart and prevent obesity. Drinking tea is an age-old agreeable tradition.

Using Jelly Herbs

The best practice for the preservation of good health in old age is to employ medicated "jelly" specifically concocted for a particular person's daily nourishment. This has been practiced in China for thousands of years. The "jelly" creates harmony among the organs and supplements what is missing as well as discards the long-accumulated unwholesome retained toxic pathogens, after taking every aspect of the patient's specific condition into long-range consideration.

The usual procedure to make the medicated syrup is as follows:

1. A well-experienced Chinese medical doctor must first diagnose the patient's specific physical condition and illness on which to base a formula of some 20 to 30 medicinal herbs.
2. Buy all of the medicines prescribed.
3. Soak all of the medicines in water, with a sufficient margin of 15 cm above them, for 12 hours so that all the effective ingredients will be dissolved in the solution.
4. Boil the solution in a porcelain or pottery pot (never in a vessel made of iron) on a low heat until all the herbs swell sufficiently. Then continue on a high heat so that the solution boils vigorously. Now simmer on a low heat for 2 to 5 hours. Filter. Pour another portion of water into the pot—enough to cover all the medicines—and boil the medicines again to get the filtrate.

Repeat the process two more times. Then pour all the filtrate together and let it set for some time. Filter the filtrate if there is fine residue in it.

5. Concentration. Pour all the filtrate in the pot and boil it on a high heat while skimming off the supernate, if any, from the surface. When the filtrate grows more and more concentrated, carry on boiling it on a slow heat. Stir it from time to time to prevent carbonization. Drop some of the concentrate on a piece of paper; if there is no more water seeping through the paper, the concentration is ready.
6. Continue to boil the concentrate on a still lower heat, add sugar, rock sugar, or honey about one-quarter of the weight of the medicine, add E-gelatin or other kinds of gelatin (best in the form of powder for a better solution); dissolve the gelatin in yellow wine, an indigenous product of Shaoxin, Zhejiang Province, while still stirring, until all has been dissolved. Now see whether it has been concentrated sufficiently. If the paste will drop from a spoon, then experience tells us it is sufficiently concentrated.
7. Let it cool down and put it in the jar or some other vessel made of glass for storage.

If the "jelly" herbs are meant only for nourishment, the most opportune season for their ingestion is in the 8 to 90 days after the winter solstice. If they are meant for treatment of some illness, the patient will take the "jelly" herbs whenever their condition requires it as a long-term practice. The patient is asked to take one or two teaspoons of the "jelly" both in the morning and evening on an empty stomach and wash it down with some hot water.

During the period of treatment the patient is advised not to drink tea or to eat turnip/radish, which are said to counteract the effect of the medicines. During the period, if the patient gets a cold and develops a fever, or they are troubled with indigestion and diarrhea, they are advised to stop the medicine until recovered.

Apoplexy (Stroke)

There are several causes of apoplexy. The patient has a long-term suppressed discontent or even anguish, so strong as to even make the *qi* at the heart and liver coagulate. The muffled *qi* will in turn be transformed into "fire"; and the fire will refine *qi* into phlegm as the final consummation of the disease. The patient may also be a gourmet or glutton (see below).

Leon Hammer   The pathogenesis of coagulation that we call "phlegm-fire misting the orifices" is as follows. Metabolic heat is required to move chronic liver *qi* stagnation, a condition in which the liver contains strong negative emotions, which if acted upon could cause grave social consequences. If it fails to overcome the stagnation, excess heat accumulates. While the body brings fluid to balance the heat, if that fails the excess heat grows into liver fire. Eventually it will escape the liver to the most vulnerable organ, which is often the heart, where heart and kidney *yin* will again try to cool the fire.

When the fluid and the heat come together in the heart the result is phlegm that "mists" the orifices and is one pathological scenario leading to one kind of stroke. The damp from the spleen *qi*'s difficulty in "digesting" fluid will also complicate the phlegm condition in the heart. The scenario described above can also begin with *qi* stagnation that begins in the heart when shock causes heart *qi* stagnation (flat, inflated, muffled qualities at the LDP).

Gourmet or glutton:

The problem is compounded when a glutton spends a lifetime eating too much fatty food. An enormous amount of thermal energy is produced and over time this results in the formation of phlegm and fire. With the reduction of *qi* in middle and old age, the ability to metabolize phlegm and fire diminishes and it accrues to the phlegm-fire in the heart.

Stroke:

The following discussion regarding stroke is entirely Dr. Shen's with an unknown editor.

From a Chinese medicine perspective, this will end in a tempest of liver *yang* that disturbs the upper clear calmness. In addition to their overworking, if the patient is much afflicted by their anguish and gives vent to their feelings by eating and drinking too much, then an interior cyclone of *yang* "*qi*" is formed and can suddenly dash upward ("wind"), resulting in apoplexy. That is why in Chinese medicine we call this disease, "stricken by the tempest." We always put precautions and prevention before treatment, especially in the potential case of apoplexy. Advise the patient to mend their defective way of life, carefully readjust dietary habits, refrain from sexual activity, and put turbulent emotions under control.

When the channels are struck by "wind" it is collateral channel apoplexy. The patient will suffer from deviation of the mouth and awry eyes. The skin may be numb and the limbs less dexterous, although the condition hasn't advanced to hemiplegia, aphasia, or collapse. The channels must be relieved of the wind that has clogged them up. The treatment is better supplemented with acupuncture and moxibustion treatment.

Leon Hammer   Once again, metabolic heat is required to relieve chronic liver *qi* stagnation. If it fails to overcome the stagnation, excess heat accumulates. The liver mobilizes its *yin* to balance the excess heat and over time, possibly years, the *yin* is depleted. Eventually the depleted *yin* cannot hold onto *yang*, "*yin* and *yang* separate" and *yang*, without the centrifugal force of the *yin*, becomes out of control and dysfunctional. In our time, liver *qi-yang* deficiency is even more prevalent than liver *yin* deficiency and more involved with the "separation of *yin* and *yang*."

Once separated, *yang*, the lighter warm energy, rises, becoming the condition "liver *yang* rising," whose consequences are well known as being disruptive to the function of whatever vulnerable organ area it reaches. This is a deficient condition, a severe *yin* and/or *qi-yang*-deficient condition resulting in the "separation of *yin* and *yang*." It is *not an excess condition* simply because the symptoms, intermittent high-pitched tinnitus, throbbing headache, and so on may have excess characteristics. The remedy is to nourish *yin* or *yang* or both. Do not drain as if the condition were excess heat.

Formula for treating the attacked channels:

Pin Yin	Latin	English	Dosage
Sheng di huang	Rehmanniae Radix	Fresh Chinese foxglove root, fresh rehmannia root	15 g
Dang gui	Angelicae Sinensis Radix	Chinese Angelica root, *tang-kuei*	10 g
Bai shao	Paeoniae Alba Radix	White peony root	10 g
Gui zhi	Ramulus Cinnamomi Cassiae	Cinnamon twig, cassia twig	6 g
Du huo	Angelicae Pubescentis Radix	Pubescent Angelica root	8 g
Qin jiao	Gentianae Qinjiao Radix	Gentiana macrophylla root, *chin-chiu*	8 g
Sang zhi	Ramulus Mori Albae	Mulberry twig, morus twig	30 g
Huai niu xi or niu xi	Achyranthis Bidentatae Radix	Ox-knee root, achyranthes root from Huai	10 g
Fang feng	Saposhnikoviae Radix	Ledebouriella root, saposhnikoviae root, siler	10 g

Boil the medicines into tea and drink. May be taken long term.

Zhong fu or hollow visceral apoplexy is another type of being "stricken by the tempest." It is manifested as sudden attacks of aphasia. Though the patient is still alert in their mind, they suffer from sudden aphasia and hemiplegia with deviation or trembling of their tongue. They suffer from constipation, but have no control over urination and, when not constipated, bowel movements are out of their control. Treat by nourishing the *yin* and restraining the *yang*, which will check the liver and calm the "tempest."

Formula for *zhong fu* apoplexy:

Pin Yin	Latin	English	Dosage
Ling yang jiao	Cornu Antelopsis	Antelope horn powder	1 g
Tian ma	Gastrodiae Rhizoma	Gastrodia rhizome	10 g
Jiang can	Bombyx Batryticatus	Silkworm, body of sick silkworm	10 g
Dan nan xing	Arisaematis Praeparatum Rhizoma cum Felle Bovis	Arisaema pulvis, Jack in the pulpit rhizome with cow bile	4 g
Gou teng	Ramulus cum Uncis Uncariae	Stems and thorns of the gambir vine, uncaria	15 g

Pin Yin	Latin	English	Dosage
Huai niu xi or niu xi	Achyranthis Bidentatae Radix	Ox-knee root, achyranthes root from Huai	12 g
Bai shao	Paeoniae Alba Radix	White peony root	10 g
Mai men dong	Ophiopogonis Radix	Ophiopogon tuber	10 g
Sheng di huang	Rehmanniae Radix	Fresh Chinese foxglove root, fresh rehmannia root	12 g

Boil the medicines into tea.

If the patient still has some after-effects of aphasia and hemiplegia, this is a sequela. It is primarily due to *qi* deficiency and blood stasis. Nourish the *yang* to tonify the *qi* and dissolve the coagulated blood. If the patient still has aphasia, add *yuan zhi* (polygala root) and *shi chang pu* (grass-leaved sweetflag rhizome).

Zhong zhuang, "visceral apoplexy," is typically manifested in the following ways: sudden attacks of fainting, lockjaw, and clenched fists, loud snoring and the sound of phlegm in the throat. The tongue is red with a curdy coating. The pulses are thin, slippery, and rapid. It is certainly a difficult problem. One must pry the mouth open to introduce a medicinal decoction. Try *Zhi Bao Dan* (Greatest Treasure Special Pill) or *An Gong Niu Huang Wan* (Calm the Palace Pill with Cattle Gallstone) for resuscitation and to calm down the wind as well as the following formula.

Formula for the closing up of *zhong zhuang*:

Pin Yin	Latin	English	Dosage
Niu huang	Calculus Bovis	Cattle gallstone, bezoar	2 g
Hu po	Succinum	Amber powder	5 g
Huang lian	Coptidis Rhizoma	Coptis rhizome	3 g
Dan shen	Salviae Miltiorrhiziae Radix	Salvia root	10 g
Yuan zhi	Polygalae Radix	Chinese senega root, polygala root	5 g
Shi chang pu	Acori Tatarinowii Rhizoma	Grass-leaved sweetflag rhizome, acorus	6 g
Ju hong	Pars Rubra Epicarpii Citri Erythrocarpae	Red part of Tangerine peel	3 g
Dan nan xing	Arisaematis Praeparatum Rhizoma cum Felle Bovis	Arisaema pulvis, Jack in the pulpit rhizome with cow bile	3 g
Mai men dong	Ophiopogonis Radix	Ophiopogon tuber	6 g
Dan zhu ye	Lopatheri Gracilis Herba	Lophatherum stem and leaves	10 g

Boil the medicines into tea.

If a patient has a sudden collapse due to deficiency, is in a comatose state, with shallow breathing, fecal and urinary incontinence, cold limbs with sweating, low and slight pulses, this is a very serious life-threatening condition treated with the following formula.

Formula for treating a sudden collapse of apoplexy patients as a trial:

Pin Yin	Latin	English	Dosage
Shu di huang	Rehmanniae Preparata Radix	Prepared Chinese foxglove root (cooked in red wine), cooked rehmannia rhizome	20 g
Fu zi	Aconiti Lateralis Praeparata Radix	Aconite	10 g
Ren shen	Ginseng Radix	Ginseng root	6 g
Gou qi zi	Lycii Fructus	Chinese wolfberry, matrimony vine fruit, lycium fruit	10 g
Fu shen	Poria Cocos Pararadicis Sclerotium	Poria fungus	10 g
Yuan zhi	Polygalae Radix	Chinese senega root, polygala root	6 g
Gan jiang	Zingiberis Rhizoma	Dried ginger	3 g

Boil the medicines into tea and drink from time to time. If the case is very serious, the patient must be given emergency treatment or undergo a medical operation, if necessary.

Cervical Vertebra Nerve Ache

A life of office work, sitting at a desk with little chance to move the head and neck or an attack of external dampness or traumatic injury can all be possible causes of this condition. From the point of view of Chinese medicine, this disease originates from stagnation of blood in channels, which result in their deficiency such that the evil wind-and-dampness prevails. There is degeneration of the cervical vertebrae.

This condition extends its effect in making the upper limbs numb and the shoulders ache. The patient will experience a severe unilateral headache. When they try to turn their head, they tend to feel dizzy, or faint and nauseous. The proper treatment lies in the revitalization of the blood to extinguish the wind; when the blood flows freely, the wind will vanish of its own accord.

Formula for cervical vertebra nerves ache:

Pin Yin	Latin	English	Dosage
Dang gui	Angelicae Sinensis Radix	Chinese Angelica root, tang-kuei	15 g
Chi shao	Paeoniae Rubra Radix	Red peony root	12 g
Qin jiao	Gentianae Qinjiao Radix	Gentiana macrophylla root, chin-chiu	10 g
Tian ma	Gastrodiae Rhizoma	Gastrodia rhizome	10 g
Gou teng	Ramulus cum Uncis Uncariae	Stems and thorns of the gambir vine, uncaria	15 g
Jiang can	Bombyx Batryticatus	Silkworm, body of sick silkworm	10 g
Bai ji li	Tribuli Terrestris Fructus	Caltrop fruit, puncture-vine fruit, tribulus	15 g
Wu gong[a]	Scolopendra Subspinipes	Centipede, scolopendra	2 pieces
Gui zhi	Ramulus Cinnamomi Cassiae	Cinnamon twig, cassia twig	8 g
Ge gen	Puerariae Radix	Kudzu root, pueraria	15 g
Di long	Lumbricus	Earthworm, lumbricus	10 g

[a] Toxic
Boil the medicines into tea.

Inflammation at Shoulder Joints, Arthritis

This condition appears when there is a combination of etiologies including overall *qi* and blood deficiency that cannot expel external wind-cold-damp and recover from trauma. In the beginning there is a dull pain, aching only upon movement. These symptoms are aggravated with time as the condition extends to the soft tissue around the shoulders, causing unbearable pain and functional hindrances.

Treat the disease by relaxing the tendons to revitalize the blood and warm the tendons to dispel the cold.

Formula for shoulder-joint arthritis:

Pin Yin	Latin	English	Dosage
Qiang huo	Notopterygii Rhizoma et Radix	Notopterygium root and rhizome, chiang-huo	10 g
Du huo	Angelicae Pubescentis Radix	Pubescent Angelica root	10 g
Fang feng	Saposhnikoviae Radix	Ledebouriella root, saposhnikoviae root, siler	9 g
Dang gui	Angelicae Sinensis Radix	Chinese Angelica root, tang-kuei	12 g
Xu duan	Dipsaci Asperi Radix	Japanese teasel root, dipsacus	12 g
Wu jia pi	Acanthopanacis Gracilistyli Radicis Cortex	Acanthopanax root bark	10 g
Xi xin	Asari Herba cum Radice	Chinese wild ginger, asarum	5 g
Hong hua	Carthami Tinctorii Flos	Safflower flower, carthamus	6 g
Qing pi	Citri Reticulatae Pericarpium Viride	Unripe tangerine peel, green tangerine peel, blue citrus	6 g

Boil the medicines into tea:
- If the pain changes from place to place, add two pieces of *wu gong* and 10 g of *di long* (earthworm).
- If the channels are aching as if they were pricked by needles, add 20 g of *ji xue teng* (spatholobus or milettia root and vine), 10 g of *chuan shan jia* (anteater scales [pangolin—deemed obsolete because of its endangered status]).
- In the case of old patients, add 30 g of *huang qi* (milk vetch root).

Schizophrenia

Formula for derangement (see also "Dr. Shen's Formulas in Systems," p. 133):

Pin Yin	Latin	English	Dosage
Sheng zhi shi	Immaturus Citri Aurantii Fructus	Fresh immature bitter orange	10 g
Zhu ru	Bambussae in Taeniis Caulis	Bamboo shavings	10 g
Zhi ban xia	Pinelliae Preparatum Rhizoma	Dried processed pinellia rhizome	6 g
Chen pi	Citri Reticulatae Pericarpium	Tangerine peel	6 g
Fu ling	Poria Cocos Sclerotium	Sclerotium of tuckahoe, poria, China root, hoelen, Indian bread	12 g
Sheng gan cao	Glycyrrhizae Radix	Fresh licorice root	6 g

Pin Yin	Latin	English	Dosage
Yuan zhi	Polygalae Radix	Chinese senega root, polygala root	6 g
Shi chang pu	Acori Tatarinowii Rhizoma	Grass-leaved sweetflag rhizome, acorus	10 g
Yu jin	Curcumae Radix	Curcuma tuber	15 g
Tian zhi huang	Concretio Silicea Bambusae Textillis	Tabasheer or siliceous secretions of bamboo	10 g

Boil the medicines into tea.

Hepatitis

Allopathic medicine identifies hepatitis as an infectious disease caused by the hepatitis virus. In Chinese medicine hepatitis is called "yellow hepatitis" and understood as an "external pathogenic evil dampness with ominous heat and toxin." It is differentiated as follows.

Yellow Hepatitis

If the patient has more heat toxin than damp, his or her whole body appears jaundiced. The patient feels hot and thirsty, the urine turns red and stools pale white. The main treatment principle is to relieve heat (by means of antipyretic measures) and clear the toxin.

Leon Hammer
Pulse:
• Rate: rapid

• Left middle positions (LMP): tense, flooding excess, robust pounding, the latter especially at the organic and organic-blood and organic-substance depths

Formula for yellow hepatitis:

Pin Yin	Latin	English	Dosage
Yin chen hao	Artemisiae Yinchenhao Herba	Yinchenhao shoots and leaves, capillaries, oriental wormwood	30 g
Zhi zi	Gardeniae Jasminoidis Fructus	Cape jasmine fruit, gardenia fruit	10 g
Da huang	Rhei Rhizoma et Radix	Rhubarb root and rhizome	10 g
Huang bai	Phellodendri Cortex	Amur corktree bark, phellodendron bark	10 g
Ban lan gen	Isatidis seu Baphicacanthis Radix	Woad root, isatis root	15 g
Gan cao	Glycyrrhizae Radix	Licorice root	6 g
Hu zhang	Polygoni Cuspidati Radix et Rhizoma	Bushy knotweed root and rhizome	15 g
Bai jiang cao	Herba cum Radice Patriniae	Patrina, thiaspi	30 g

Boil the medicines into tea.

If the patient has more dampness than any other heat, his or her entire body will have a dull yellow cast. There is fatigue, a heavy head, and a stuffy chest with a white curdy tongue. The main treatment is to remove the dampness and to relieve the heat.

Leon Hammer One needs to understand that *qi* stagnation and excess heat are still the underlying issues and that the damp appears only as the organism's way of cooling the heat.

Pulse:
• Rate: rapid but slower than with pure heat toxin
• LMP: more slippery and leisurely with less flooding excess and robust pounding.

Formula for hepatitis with more dampness:

Pin Yin	Latin	English	Dosage
Yin chen hao	Artemisiae Yinchenhao Herba	Yinchenhao shoots and leaves, capillaries, oriental wormwood	15 g
Fu ling	Poria Cocos Sclerotium	Sclerotium of tuckahoe, poria, China root, hoelen, Indian bread	15 g
Zhu ling	Sclerotium Polypori Umbellati	Polyporus sclerotium	10 g
Hua shi	Talcum	Talcum	15 g
Ze xie	Alismatis Rhizoma	Water plantain rhizome, alisma rhizome	10 g
Hu zhang	Polygoni Cuspidati Radix et Rhizoma	Bushy knotweed root and rhizome	15 g
Bai jiang cao	Patriniae Herba cum Radice	Patrina, thiaspi	15 g
Yu jin	Curcumae Radix	Curcuma tuber	15 g
Huang bai	Phellodendri Cortex	Amur corktree bark, phellodendron bark	8 g
Da zao	Zizyphi Jujubae Fructus	Chinese date, jujube	10 dates

Boil the medicine into tea.

Hepatitis without Jaundice

Pain felt at the ribs with a stuffinotess or fullness in the abdomen. The patient does not want to eat, especially fatty food. This is hepatitis in its true sense and the patient is in a more precarious situation than those with jaundicing hepatitis. The patient is advised to receive medical treatment as early as possible and rest. For its treatment, one must clear the liver and strengthen the spleen, cool blood, and relieve toxins.

Leon Hammer It is not clear to me as to why Dr. Shen considered the patient with "true hepatitis" to have a more dangerous condition than one with jaundice, which in Western medicine is considered more serious.

Formula for hepatitis without symptomatic jaundice:

Pin Yin	Latin	English	Dosage
Chai hu	Bupleuri Radix	Hare's ear root, thorowax root, bupleurum	8 g
Chuan xiong	Chuanxiong Rhizoma	Chuanxiong root, Szechuan lovage root, cnidium	6 g
Zhi shi	Aurantii Immaturus Fructus	Immature bitter orange, unripe bitter orange, chih-shih	10 g
Mu dan pi	Moutan Radicis Cortex	Tree peony root bark, moutan root bark	12 g
Hu zhang	Polygoni Cuspidati Radix et Rhizoma	Bushy knotweed root and rhizome	15 g
Sheng gan cao	Glycyrrhizae Radix	Fresh licorice root	6 g
Zi cao	Arnebiae seu Lithospermi Radix	Groomwell root, lithospermum, arnebia	10 g
Huang lian	Coptidis Rhizoma	Coptis rhizome	34 g
Mu xiang	Saussureae Lappae Radix or Aucklandia Lappae Radix	Costus root, saussurea, aucklandia	5 g

Boil the medicines into tea.

Chronic Hepatitis

Chronic hepatitis often takes place when the treatment of acute hepatitis is delayed or when the treatments have been inadequate in completely re-

Leon Hammer   Chronic hepatitis occurs when the body is unable to eliminate the hepatitis virus and diverts it to a less immediately dangerous location as a retained pathogen.
Except as observed as a retained pathogen deep in the organic-blood and organic-substance depths with robust pounding, slippery, and choppy qualities often on the entire pulse, the exact retained location is not clear to me.

moving the heat toxins. The infection persists, further undermining the patient's health.

Perhaps it is retained in the relatively safer gallbladder, which in many of these patients shows *qi* stagnation (muffled), micro-bleeding (choppy), excess heat (robust pounding), damp (slippery) and sometimes accumulation of gases from bacteria and deteriorating walls (inflated).

Formula for chronic hepatitis:

Pin Yin	Latin	English	Dosage
Chai hu	Bupleuri Radix	Hare's ear root, thorowax root, bupleurum	6 g
Dang gui	Angelicae Sinensis Radix	Chinese Angelica root, *tang-kuei*	10 g
Bai zhu	Rhizoma Atractylodis Macrocephalae	White atractylodes rhizome	10 g
Bai shao	Paeoniae Alba Radix	White peony root	10 g
Fu ling	Poria Cocos Sclerotium	Sclerotium of tuckahoe, poria, China root, hoelen, Indian bread	15 g
Dan shen	Salviae Miltiorrhiziae Radix	Salvia root	15 g
Hu zhang	Polygoni Cuspidati Radix et Rhizoma	Bushy knotweed root and rhizome	15 g
Gan cao	Glycyrrhizae Radix	Licorice root	6 g
Tai zi shen	Pseudostellariae Heterophyllaceae Radix	Pseudotellaria root	30 g
Mai ya	Hordei Germinatus Fructus	Barley sprout, malt	15 g

Gallstones

The formation of gallstones is related to repressed emotions and a diet rich in fat and spices. The former creates excess heat and damp in the liver as explained elsewhere in this book, and the latter places a heavy burden on the liver and gallbladder. To digest increased amounts of fat and hot spices add to the heat in the liver. Also consider that living in a damp environment will exacerbate the damp aspect of the damp-heat.

When a patient suffers from damp-heat in the liver and gallbladder, the right ribs ache and the pain gradually develops in the back. The abdomen feels bloated and the mouth bitter. The patient will have dry stools and an intermittent fever. Jaundice can be seen in the eyes and whole body. Of course, this is a serious medical condition that should be addressed immediately to remove the *qi* stagnation in the liver and clear the damp-heat condition in both the liver and the gallbladder.

Formula for gallstones arising from dampness and heat:

Pin Yin	Latin	English	Dosage
Chai hu	Bupleuri Radix	Hare's ear root, thorowax root, bupleurum	10 g
Huang qin	Scutellariae Baicalensis Radix	Baical skullcap root, scutellaria, scute	10 g
Sheng da huang	Rhei Rhizoma et Radix	Fresh rhubarb root and rhizome	9 g
Yu jin	Curcumae Radix	Curcuma tuber	15 g
Zhi shi	Aurantii Immaturus Fructus	Immature bitter orange, unripe bitter orange, chih-shih	9 g
Yin chen hao	Artemisiae Yinchenhao Herba	Yinchenhao shoots and leaves, capillaries	15 g
Mu xiang	Radix Saussureae Lappae or Radix Aucklandia Lappae	Costus root, saussurea, aucklandia	8 g
Bai shao	Paeoniae Alba Radix	White peony root	10 g
Hu zhang	Polygoni Cuspidati Radix et Rhizoma	Bushy knotweed root and rhizome	15 g

Boil the medicines into tea.

Leon Hammer   The gallbladder serves to relieve excess heat from the liver through the bile that it stores and releases to digest fats in the intestines. Again, wherever excess heat accumulates the body supplies fluid to balance the heat and we arrive at a damp-heat condition that over time becomes phlegm, which increasingly becomes harder, turning into gallstones.

The process begins with repression of emotions, such as frustration and associated anger, that we call liver qi stagnation. Another source of this stagnation is the inability to arrive for long periods of time at crucial life decisions such as separating from a part-ner or changing an unsatisfactory but essential job. The metabolic heat that is brought to move the stagnation builds up and is removed by the bile through the bile ducts to the gallbladder. The other sources of heat are from spicy heat-producing foods.

Pulse:
- LMP: tense, slippery with robust pounding
- Gallbladder: tense-tight; slippery; choppy (here a sign of inflammation); inflated

Tongue:
Red body with a yellow coat

Urine:
Deep yellow

Urethra Stone

Formation of a urethra stone refers to the particles or grains formed in the kidneys, urethra, bladder or ureter of the urinary system. They are called stone *lin* or bloody *lin* in Chinese medicine.

These stones are the consummation of liver *qi* deficiency together with lower *jiao* damp-heat. The lower *jiao* denotes the overall activities within the realm of, or shared by, the kidneys, bladder, and small and large intestines.

Treatment is mainly focused on expelling or dissolving these particles of/from the system by means of the medicines in the following formula, with some appropriate modifications according to different cases.

Treatment is as follows:

Pin Yin	Latin	English	Dosage
Jin qian cao	Lysimachiae Herba	Lysimachia	30 g
Hai jin sha	Lygodii Japonici Spora	Japanese fern spores, lygodium	15 g
Dong kui zi	Abutili seu Malvae Semen	Musk mallow seeds, abutilon seeds	10 g

Pin Yin	Latin	English	Dosage
Che qian zi	Plantaginis Semen	Plantago seeds	10 g
Hua shi	Talcum	Talcum	20 g
Shi wei	Pyrrosiae Folium	Pyrrosia leaf	15 g
Sheng di huang	Rehmanniae Radix	Fresh Chinese foxglove root, fresh rehmannia root	15 g
Chuan niu xi	Cyathulae Officinalis Radix	Ox-knee root from Szechuan	10 g

Boil the medicines into tea.

If the patient has abdominal pain, add:

Pin Yin	Latin	English	Dosage
Bai shao	Paeoniae Alba Radix	White peony root	12 g
Gan cao	Glycyrrhizae Radix	Licorice root	12 g
Yan hu suo	Corydalis Yanhusuo Rhizoma	Corydalis rhizome	3–9 g

If the stone particles do not respond to the above formula, add:

Pin Yin	Latin	English	Dosage
Hu po	Succinum	Amber powder	6 g

Use 6 g of amber powder for each dose, two doses a day, to be taken when the stomach is empty.

Lupus Erythematosus

Lupus erythematosus arises from an imbalance in "systems" relations (nervous, circulatory, digestive, and organ systems) (Hammer, 2005).

The main symptoms are fever, an internal burning sensation, sore joints, and butterfly-like spots on the face. Hereditary kidney *yin* deficiency is the root cause of the disease. Unfortunately, viruses or chemicals in the person's blood make things worse. At the same time, the condition will be exacerbated by external heat if the person works under the sun for long periods of time.

Consider the following three differential diagnoses and treatments:

With Toxic Heat

Symptomatic features are high temperature with a fiery red face; all muscles and joints are suffering from painful agitation. The patient is often lost in delirious wild talking or bleeding, becoming so thirsty as to ask for cold drinks.

Treat by clearing toxic heat and cool the blood to protect the *yin*.

Leon Hammer   Whereas the conventional etiology of the high temperatures is *yin* deficiency there is little evidence from my experience or from others that *yin*-nourishing herbs are effective.

It is my impression that there is a "separation of *yin* and *yang*" and a "*qi* wild" condition in which the *yang* has separated from the *yin* and is rising out of control and responsible for the uncontrollable heat. The *yin*, being separated from the *yang*, is no longer available to cool the heat and is itself quickly exhausted. However, the fire that is out of control is *yang*. This view needs to be tested clinically since I have seen few patients with this condition.

There is possibly a hereditary disposition. However, the exhaustion of *yin* and/or *yang* involved could also be from infection or toxic chemicals. It can be found upon the face of young women's cheeks or nose in the form of red butterflies. It may also be seen on the scalp, ears, or lips.

Tongue:
- Red to magenta with a yellow coating to no coating
- Thin and dry

Inside lower eyelids:
Vessels very red

Formula for lupus erythematosus with toxic heat:

Pin Yin	Latin	English	Dosage
Sheng di huang	Rehmanniae Radix	Fresh Chinese foxglove root, fresh rehmannia root	30 g
Chi shao	Paeoniae Rubra Radix	Red peony root	10 g
Xuan shen	Scrophulariae Radix	Ningpo figwort root, scrophularia	10 g
Jin yin hua	Lonicerae Flos	Honeysuckle flower, lonicera	15 g
Lian qiao	Forsythiae Suspensae Fructus	Forsythia fruit	15 g
Shi gao	Gypsum Fibrosum	Gypsum	30 g
Zhi mu	Anemarrhenae Asphodeloidis Rhizoma	Anemarrhena rhizome	10 g
Mu dan pi	Moutan Radicis Cortex	Tree peony root bark, moutan root bark	10 g
Mai men dong	Ophiopogonis Radix	Ophiopogon tuber	10 g

Boil into tea. Take with 6 g of powdered buffalo horn (*shui niu jiao*).

With *Qi* and *Yin* Deficiency

This condition is slightly different from the foregoing case in that there is a persistent low fever and hot sensations on the palms and soles of the feet. The patient is perturbed as if exhausted and there are night sweats. The face looks swollen red with painful joints and soles of the feet.

Leon Hammer

Night sweats:

Again the *yin* and *yang* are separated and the *yang* is escaping, experienced as hot flashes, and the *yin* will follow through hot sweats since the *yin* always wants to be with the *yang*. During the day the sun inhibits the *yang* from leaving so this occurs principally in the night unless the protective *qi* (*wei*) is too weak to restrain the *yang* from leaving during the day.

Pulse:
- With *qi* deficiency: yielding to feeble and slow
- With *yin* deficiency: thin, tight, rapid
- With "separation of *yin* and *yang*": empty quality or changing qualities in a single position and with "*qi* wild" in many positions

Tongue:
- *Qi* deficiency: pale wet body and thin white coating
- *Yin* deficiency: thin, dry, darker red body and less coating

Inside of lower eyelid:
- *Qi* deficiency: vessels are less bright
- *Yin* deficiency: vessels have lost their distinctness and cross over one another

---

Treat by nourishing the *yin* and invigorating *qi*, activating the blood and clearing the channels.

Formula for lupus erythematosus with both *qi* and *yin* deficiency:

Pin Yin	Latin	English	Dosage
Sha hen	Adenophorae seu Glehniae Radix	Adenophora root or glehnia root	10 g
Shi hu	Dendrobii Herba	Dendrobium	10 g
Yu zhu	Polygonati Odorati Rhizoma	Solomon's seal rhizome, polygonatum	10 g
Huang qi	Astragali Radix	Milk vetch root, astragalus root	15 g
Dang shen	Codonopsis Pilosulae Radix	Codonopsis root	10 g
Dan shen	Salviae Miltiorrhiziae Radix	Salvia root	10 g
Ji xue teng	Jixueteng Radix et Caulis	Spatholobus or milettia root and vine	15 g
Huang lian	Coptidis Rhizoma	Coptis rhizome	3 g
Qing hao	Artemisiae Annuae Herba	Wormwood, *ching-hao*	10 g
Bai wei	Cynanchi Baiwei Radix	Swallowwort root	10 g

Boil the medicines into tea.

With Spleen and Kidney *Yang* Deficiency

The symptoms in this case include a pale and slightly swollen warm face and cool swollen hands and feet. There is fatigue, painful joints and soles, sore sides and knees, a thirsty mouth and dry throat, a pale, fatty, tender tongue with a scanty coat and the pulse is deep and feeble. Mild invigoration of the spleen and kidneys and facilitation of the *yang* to correct the water metabolism will treat this disease.

Formula for lupus with deficiency of both the spleen and kidney *yang*:

Pin Yin	Latin	English	Dosage
Sheng huang qi	Astragali Radix	Fresh milk vetch root, astragalus root	30 g
Sheng dang shen	Codonopsis Pilosulae Radix	Fresh codonopsis root	15 g
Bai zhu	Actractylodis Macrocephalae Rhizoma	White atractylodes rhizome	10 g
Fu ling	Poria Cocos Sclerotium	Sclerotium of tuckahoe, poria, China root, hoelen, Indian bread	30 g
Shan yao	Dioscoreae Oppositae Rhizoma	Chinese yam, dioscorea rhizome	15 g
Tu si zi	Cuscutae Chinensis Semen	Chinese dodder seeds, cuscuta	10 g
Nu zhen zi	Ligustri Lucidi Fructus	Privet fruit, ligustrum	10 g
Gou qi zi	Lycii Fructus	Chinese wolfberry, matrimony vine fruit, lycium fruit	10 g
Che qian zi	Plantaginis Semen	Plantago seeds	10 g
Dan shen	Salviae Miltiorrhiziae Radix	Salvia root	12 g
Ji xue teng	Jixueteng Radix et Caulis	Spatholobus or milettia root and vine	15 g
Zao xiu	Paridis Rhizoma	Paris rhizome	10 g

Boil the medicines into tea.

Leon Hammer
Spleen and Kidney-*yang* Deficiency:
Pulse:
• RMP and SPEP:
  – Reduced substance
  – Diffuse
  – Feeble/absent or empty
• Proximal positions:
  – Deep
  – Reduced substance
  – Diffuse

  – Feeble/absent
  – Empty

Again, my own tentative concept of the later-stage "burning-up" of lupus is not of a pure *yin*-deficient condition that does not respond to conventional *yin*-nourishing herbs but rather a "separation of *yin* and *yang*" due to a severe deficiency of both and an aimlessly wandering *yang* that is out of control, masquerading as devastating heat and responding better to reuniting *yin* and *yang* as well as nourishing both (Hammer, 1998).

Psoriasis

In Chinese medicine this is called pine-bark tinea. It is caused by an attack of a scorching ill wind blowing upon the patient. This pathogenic heat has wasted so much of their blood that the skin has been deprived of nourishment. There are two measures taken for treatment of psoriasis.

In acute cases the blood contains chemical toxins or some invading bacteria. The patient's skin often looks bright red, covered with drops or coins made of silvery fine scales. If one should try to peel them off, they will bleed. The patient feels anxiously thirsty. The tongue is red with a yellow coat and the pulses are tense and rapid. Dissipation of the heat and detoxification of the blood are the main measures taken.

Leon Hammer I do not find consistent signs with this condition. At earlier stages there is usually a great deal of heat in the blood and blood stagnation with what we call blood "heat" or "thick" at and above the blood depth. However, in other patients there seems to be more blood deficiency or a generally thin pulse and may correspond to Dr Shen's second example below.

Formula I for psoriasis:

Pin Yin	Latin	English	Dosage
Sheng di huang	Rehmanniae Radix	Fresh Chinese foxglove root, fresh rehmannia root	30 g
Chi shao	Paeoniae Rubra Radix	Red peony root	10 g
Mu dan pi	Moutan Radicis Cortex	Tree peony root bark, moutan root bark	10 g
Tu fu ling	Smilacis Glabrae Rhizoma	Glabrous greenbrier rhizome, smilax	30 g
Sheng huai hua mi	Sophorae Japonicae Flos	Fresh pagoda tree flower (bud), sophora flower	30 g
Bai xian pi	Dictamni Dasycarpi Radicis Cortex	Cortex of Chinese dittany root, dictamnus root bark	30 g
Da qing ye	Daqingye Folium	Woad leaf, isatis, indigo	12 g
Zao xiu	Paridis Rhizoma	Paris rhizome	10 g
Wu xiao she	Zaocys Dhumnades	Garter snake	10 g

Boil the medicines into tea.

When the condition presents with blood deficiency and dryness arising out of the "wind," this often shows that the disease is in its static stage or is on the ebb. The patient's skin appears a pale color, upon which coin-like patterns or spots are seen under a thin layer of scaly substances. The tongue is pale with a clear coat. The pulse is tense and thin.

Leon Hammer The use of the expression "is arising out of the 'wind'" is unclear to me here since the term "wind" seems to be used in Chinese medicine when there is a changeable somewhat uncontrolled condition that does not seem to be applicable with this type of psoriasis. I can comprehend the "wind" arising from the dryness but not causing it.

It is necessary to nourish blood and moisten dryness to eliminate the wind and stop itching.

Formula II for psoriasis:

Pin Yin	Latin	English	Dosage
Sheng di huang	Rehmanniae Radix	Fresh Chinese foxglove root, fresh rehmannia root	30 g
Dang gui	Angelicae Sinensis Radix	Chinese Angelica root, tang-kuei	10 g
He shou wu	Polygoni Multiflori Radix	Fleece-flower root, polygonum hosuwu	15 g
Dan shen	Salviae Miltiorrhiziae Radix	Salvia root	15 g
Xuan shen	Scrophulariae Radix	Ningpo figwort root, scrophularia	10 g
Ku shen	Sophorae Flavescentis Radix	Sophora root	10 g
Bai xian pi	Dictamni Dasycarpi Radicis Cortex	Cortex of Chinese dittany root, dictamnus root bark	15 g
Wu xiao she	Zaocys Dhumnades	Garter snake	10 g

Boil the medicines into tea.

The patient is also advised to put as many poplar leaves into the water as the pot can hold and boil them. Filter the solution and keep the filtrate, which is to be concentrated into a black sticky substance together with 30% Vaseline. Apply this concentrated poplar plaster to the skin.

Formula III for psoriasis (see also "Dr. Shen's Formulas in Systems," p. 41):

Pin Yin	Latin	English	Dosage
Di fu zi	Kochiae Fructus	Broom cypress, kochia fruit	12 g
Gan cao	Glycyrrhizae Radix	Licorice root	6 g
Huang bai	Phellodendri Cortex	Amur corktree bark, phellodendron bark	9 g
Bai xian pi	Dictamni Dasycarpi Radicis Cortex	Cortex of Chinese dittany root, dictamnus root bark	12 g
Bi xie	Discoreae Hypoglaucae Rhizoma	Fish poison yam rhizome, tokoro	6 g
Xia ku cao	Prunellae Spica Vulgaris	Self-heal spike, prunella	6 g
Fang feng	Saposhnikoviae Radix	Ledebouriella root, saposhnikoviae root, siler	6 g
Zhi shi	Aurantii Immaturus Fructus	Immature bitter orange, unripe bitter orange, chih-shih	4.5 g
Chi shao	Paeoniae Rubra Radix	Red peony root	9 g

Itching as a Disease in Old Age

Itching in old age is a disease covering the whole body and there are no obvious causes. Just as one of the old Chinese medical classics has put it: "Though without ringworm, the patient feels an itching all over the body."

The cause of the disease may be that the already enfeebled body condition suffers from an external wind pathogenic factor, which penetrates into the skin and stagnates the blood and *qi*, enough to cause itching but at first not enough to cause pain.

Nourishing the blood and moistening the dryness will stop the itching.

Formula for old-age itching:

Pin Yin	Latin	English	Dosage
Sheng di huang	Rehmanniae Radix	Fresh Chinese foxglove root, fresh rehmannia root	15 g
He shou wu	Polygoni Multiflori Radix	Fleece-flower root, polygonum hosuwu	10 g
Bai shao	Paeoniae Alba Radix	White peony root	10 g
Dang gui	Angelicae Sinensis Radix	Chinese Angelica root, *tang-kuei*	10 g
Bai ji li	Tribuli Terrestris Fructus	Caltrop fruit, puncture-vine fruit, tribulus	10 g
Mu dan pi	Moutan Radicis Cortex	Tree peony root bark, moutan root bark	10 g
Jing jie	Schizonepetae Herba	Schizonepeta	6 g
Fang feng	Saposhnikoviae Radix	Ledebouriella root, saposhnikoviae root, siler	6 g
Chan tuii	Periostracum Cicadae	Cicada moultings	6 g
Jiang can	Bombyx Batryticatus	Silkworm, body of sick silkworm	10 g
Ku shen	Sophorae Flavescentis Radix	Sophora root	10 g
Gan cao	Glycyrrhizae Radix	Licorice root	6 g

Boil the medicine into tea.

Leon Hammer The stagnation due to deficiency can lead to interference with peripheral circulation of *qi* and blood and the nourishment of the skin, and cause dryness of superficial nerves, and the body's call for help in the form of the symptom of itching. From the inside, the precipitous decline of *yang* essence with age and the concomitant increase in blood stagnation in the vessels, whose movement it would ordinarily advance, will contribute as much or more to this loss of nourishment to the superficial circulation and nerves.

Herpes Zoster (Shingles)

In ancient China zoster was called snake-like ulcer. In Chinese medicine it is considered the result of liver fire rashly moving upward while moistened heat moves inward, causing an abrupt emergence of rash upon the skin. It is first felt painfully on the face and/or on only one side of the ribs. These rashes group themselves into big or small glittering clusters, or into scaly substances, as if they were sparkling stars, with the red skin as their background in normal conditions. The patient finds the rashes painful and burning hot for 2 weeks.

Leon Hammer Herpes zoster in the aged is a condition moving from rash and itching as with the former formula to severe debilitating pain, usually for a very long time and difficult to relieve. Herpes zoster that forms a complete belt around the abdomen, as with Dr. Shen's "snake-like ulcer," is associated with cancer of no specificity and is a serious sign of impending decline and death.

Formula for zoster:

Pin Yin	Latin	English	Dosage
Long dan cao	Gentianae Longdancao Radix	Chinese gentian root, gentiana	6 g
Chai hu	Bupleuri Radix	Hare's ear root, thorowax root, bupleurum	6 g
Huang qin	Scutellariae Baicalensis Radix	Baical skullcap root, scutellaria, scute	6 g
Ban lan gen	Isatidis seu Baphicacanthis Radix	Woad root, isatis root	15 g
Yan hu suo	Corydalis Yanhusuo Rhizoma	Corydalis rhizome	15 g
Sheng gan cao	Glycyrrhizae Radix	Fresh licorice root	6 g
Qing pi	Citri Reticulatae Pericarpium	Unripe tangerine peel, green tangerine peel, blue citrus	6 g
Mu dan pi	Moutan Radicis Cortex	Tree peony root bark, moutan root bark	10 g

Boil the medicines into tea.

Apply *Ru Yi Huang Jing San* (Wish Fulfilling Golden Yellow Poultice) dissolved in rice vinegar on the troubled skin.

Alopecia Areata (Losing of Hair in Patches)

Deficiency in kidney *yin* accompanied by blood deficiency and dryness results in loss of hair on the head in patches, especially when the case is triggered by the patient's nervous tension. The patient is often found taken by a surprise by big or small hairless patches on his or her head, which neither itch, nor are reddish or scaly. Sometimes some individual patches may develop into a bald head, which we in China call "devil's barber tricks."

Leon Hammer   Dr. Shen taught that women tended to lose hair in the front of their head due to blood deficiency and that men lose their hair at the back due to kidney essence deficiency.

Formula for alopecia areata:

Pin Yin	Latin	English	Dosage
He shou wu	Polygoni Multiflori Radix	Fleece-flower root, polygonum hosuwu	15 g
Dang gui	Angelicae Sinensis Radix	Chinese Angelica root, *tang kuei*	15 g
Sheng di huang	Rehmanniae Radix	Fresh Chinese foxglove root, fresh rehmannia root	15 g
Hei dou	Semen Glycines Hispidae	Prepared black soybean	30 g
Sang shen	Mori Albae Fructus	White mulberry, morus fruit	12 g
Tian ma	Gastrodiae Rhizoma	Gastrodia rhizome	6 g
Chuan xiong	Chuanxiong Rhizoma	Chuanxiong root, Szechuan lovage root, cnidium	6 g
Bai shao	Paeoniae Alba Radix	White peony root	12 g

Boil the medicines into tea.

The medicine for external use: put 35 g of *ce bai ye* (Platycladi Cacumen, oriental arborvitae leaves into 100 mL of 75% alcohol and let them remain immersed in it for 7 days. Dip a swab into the liquid and apply it to the patches.

Appendix 1: Additions to Dr. Shen's Life Cycle Formulas

Formulas for Specific Conditions

Maladjustment of Heart Nerves

This maladjustment is termed by Chinese medicine as palpitation with fright. The patient has been greatly frightened, suffering from frequent heart palpitations. Even a slight bit of irritating news provokes palpitations in this patient. The left pulses are small and stringy, and the number of their pulses are felt unevenly. The treatment must be done without distressing them with new worries. Keep the patient in a pleasant mood by using sedating herbs that calm, thereby invigorating *qi* and enriching the heart.

Formula for maladjustment of heart nerves:

Pin Yin	Latin	English	Dosage
Wu wei zi	Schisandrae Chinensis Fructus	Schisandra fruit	6 g
Fu ling	Poria Cocos Sclerotium	Sclerotium of tuckahoe, poria, China root, hoelen, Indian bread	10 g
Sheng di huang	Rehmanniae Radix	Fresh Chinese foxglove root, fresh rehmannia root	10 g
Tian men dong	Asparagi Radix	Asparagus root	10 g
Yuan zhi	Polygalae Radix	Chinese senega root, polygala root	6 g
Suan zao ren	Ziziphi Spinosae Semen	Spiny zizyphus seeds, sour jujube seeds, zizyphus	15 g
Long chi	Fossilia Dentis Mastodi	Dragon teeth, fossilized teeth	15 g
Dan shen	Salviae Miltiorrhiziae Radix	Salvia root	10 g
Shi chang pu	Acori Tatarinowii Rhizoma	Grass-leaved sweetflag rhizome, acorus	3 g
Chuan xiong	Chuanxiong Rhizoma	Chuanxiong root, Szechuan lovage root, cnidium	5 g
Bai shao	Paeoniae Alba Radix	White peony root	6 g

Boil the medicines into tea and drink twice a daily. Continue until condition improves.

Neuralgia Among the Ribs on Both Sides

This is a common disease occurring only on one side or bilaterally. The pain is indistinctly felt among the ribs as a needling sensation aggravated by deep breathing. It comes from suppressed emotions aggravated by anger that injure the liver *qi*. It can also be caused by external injury such as carrying a heavy load on the shoulders, which has an adverse effect upon the ribs. In Chinese medicine, a troubled liver channel, which is distributed bilaterally, weakens the nervous system and circulatory systems, thereby hindering the free circulation of *qi* and blood. Treatment strategy should be to clear and regulate liver *qi* to activate the channels and thus kill the pain.

Formula to relieve pain among the ribs:

Pin Yin	Latin	English	Dosage
Chai hu	Bupleuri Radix	Hare's ear root, thorowax root, bupleurum	3 g
Zhi shi	Aurantii Immaturus Fructus	Immature bitter orange, unripe bitter orange, chih-shih	9 g
Xiang fu	Cyperi Rotundi Rhizoma	Nutgrass rhizome, cyperus	9 g
Qian cao gen	Rubiae Radix	Rubia root	9 g
Xuan fu hua	Inulae Flos	Inula flower	9 g
Qing pi	Citri Reticulatae Pericarpium Viride	Unripe tangerine peel, green tangerine peel, blue citrus	6 g
Chuan lian zi	Meliae Toosendan Fructus	Szechuan pagoda tree fruit, Szechuan chinaberry, melia	9 g
Yan hu suo	Corydalis Yanhusuo Rhizoma	Corydalis rhizome	12 g

Boil the medicines into tea and drink twice daily.

Numbness

There are usually two cases of numbness. The less serious one is when the patient feels neither itching nor aching, but rather feels as if worms were crawling just beneath the skin somewhere in their body. The more serious case is when some part of the body, especially the limbs, feel numb or paralyzed. The patient may find their fingers or toes insensitive to touch. More frequently the two occur at the same time. The numbness can also affect the face.

This condition is often found in patients who abruptly cease engaging in intense physical activity, which interrupts the usual circulation in the body and places stress on the adaptation mechanism. This change in tempo from allegro to almost a full stop, from fortissimo to pianissimo, from activity to inertia creates a lethargic revolt in the *qi* and blood, resulting in numbness. A contributing factor can be overindulgence in sex, which saps vitality and wastes blood. The best treatment is to nourish *qi* and blood and clear the channels to increase circulation.

Formula for numbness:

Pin Yin	Latin	English	Dosage
Sheng huang qi	Astragali Radix	Fresh milk vetch root, astragalus root	30 g
Sheng dang shen	Codonopsis Pilosulae Radix	Fresh codonopsis root	15 g
Chao dang gui	Angelicae Sinensis Radix	Fried Chinese angelica root, tang-kuei	10 g
Chao chuan xiong	Chuanxiong Rhizoma	Fried Chuanxiong root, Szechuan lovage root, cnidium	10 g
Dan shen	Salviae Miltiorrhiziae Radix	Salvia root	10 g
Hong hua	Carthami Tinctorii Flos	Safflower flower, carthamus	10 g
Tao ren	Persicae Semen	Peach kernel, persica	10 g
Ji xue teng	Jixueteng Radix et Caulis	Spatholobus or milettia root and vine	15 g

Boil the medicines into tea and drink twice a day until symptoms improve.

Another case of numbness is observed when the patient feels numbness in half of the face, with either the mouth or eyes askew. This can be due to poor circulation of *qi* and blood or to phlegm and wind interrupting the normal circulation of *qi* and blood. If this is the case, then acupuncture is also advised.

Formula to cure facial numbness:

Pin Yin	Latin	English	Dosage
Zhi bai fu zi	Typhonii seu Radix Aconiti Rhizoma	Honey-fried typhonium root	6 g
Jiang can	Bombyx Batryticatus	Silkworm, body of sick silkworm	9 g
Quan xie	Buthus Martensi	Scorpion	6 g
Wu gong[a]	Scolopendra Subspinipes	Centipede, scolopendra	2 pieces
Bai zhi	Angelicae Dahuricae Radix	Angelica root	9 g
Fang feng	Saposhnikoviae Radix	Ledebouriella root, saposhnikoviae root, siler	5 g
Gou teng	Ramulus cum Uncis Uncariae	Stems and thorns of the gambir vine, uncaria	12 g
Dang gui	Angelicae Sinensis Radix	Chinese angelica root, *tang-kuei*	10 g
Chuan xiong	Chuanxiong Rhizoma	Chuanxiong root, Szechuan lovage root, cnidium	10 g

[a] Toxic

Boil the medicines in water into tea and drink twice a day; continue the application until the symptoms are relieved.

Paralysis

Paralysis, in the essence of the Chinese character, means nothing but a blockage, something like a traffic jam. It is the foul combination of wind, coldness, dampness, and heat that has penetrated deep into the flesh. The limbs are sore and aching, hindering bodily activities. Generally speaking, it includes what Western doctors call rheumatism, rheumatoid arthritis, sciatica, and so on.

The primary expression of paralysis is a sensation of pain in some part of the body. It is due to the clogging up of *qi* and blood of the circulatory system that causes such a pain. The main treatment strategy is to clear up the passageways. According to our forefathers, it is recommended to first treat the blood before treating a rheumarthritis pain. When the blood has free passage, the pain of course gives way. This is especially true when treating a recurrent case. Elimination of the foul combination must go hand in hand with nourishment of the *qi* and blood to clear the passageways for circulation.

Formula for nourishing *qi* and blood and dispelling paralysis:

Pin Yin	Latin	English	Dosage
Sheng huang qi	Astragali Radix	Fresh milk vetch root, astragalus root	30 g
Gui zhi	Ramulus Cinnamomi Cassiae	Cinnamon, cassia	6 g
Bai shao	Paeoniae Alba Radix	White peony root	9 g
Chao dang gui	Angelicae Sinensis Radix	Fried Chinese angelica root, *tang-kuei*	15 g
Zhi gan cao	Glycyrrhizae Radix	Honey-fried licorice root	6 g
Sheng jiang	Zingiberis Officinalis Rhizoma	Fresh ginger rhizome	3 g

Pin Yin	Latin	English	Dosage
Chao fang feng	Saposhnikoviae Radix	Fried ledebouriella root, saposhnikoviae root, siler	5 g
Hong hua	Carthami Tinctorii Flos	Safflower flower, carthamus	9 g
Ji xue teng	Jixueteng Radix et Caulis	Spatholobus or milettia root and vine	15 g
Wei ling xian	Clematidis Radix	Chinese clematis root	12 g

Boil the medicines in water into tea and drink twice a day until condition is improved.

Prone to Sudden Rage

To be prone to sudden rage or the tendency to fall into sudden indignation is seen when the patient experiences suppressed agony concerning the lack of fulfillment of their long-cherished aspirations. This makes the liver stagnant and its revolting *qi* upturns to give vent in the form of rage. The patient's two sides swell, and they tend to exhale long sighs.

The reasonable way to cure such a disease is to clear the liver *qi* by cultivating a harmonious mood and with proper nourishment.

Formula for sudden rage:

Pin Yin	Latin	English	Dosage
Chai hu	Bupleuri Radix	Hare's ear root, thorowax root, bupleurum	5 g
Bai shao	Paeoniae Alba Radix	White peony root	10 g
Zhi ke	Aurantii Fructus	Mature fruit of the bitter orange	10 g
Mu dan pi	Moutan Radicis Cortex	Tree peony root bark, moutan root bark	10 g
Sheng gan cao	Glycyrrhizae Radix	Fresh licorice root	6 g
Xiang fu	Cyperi Rotundi Rhizoma	Nutgrass rhizome, cyperus	10 g
Chuan xiong	Chuanxiong Rhizoma	Chuanxiong root, Szechuan lovage root, cnidium	5 g
Bai ji li	Tribuli Terrestris Fructus	Caltrop fruit, puncture-vine fruit, tribulus	15 g
Mei gui hua	Rosae Rugosae Flos	Young flower of Chinese rose	6 g

Boil the medicine into tea and drink.

Prone to Inappropriate Laughter

In this case the heart fire is burning too briskly and the mind is not strong enough to contain an outpouring of laughter even when nothing particular has occurred to provoke that response. Instead the fire is set free and throws the mind into confusion. The patient is unable restrain themselves from laughing and merry-making. There are sores on the tongue and inside the mouth. The mouth waters and the tongue point is red hot. The heart fire must be dissipated before health can be restored.

Formula to dissipate excess heart fire:

Pin Yin	Latin	English	Dosage
Huang lian	Coptidis Rhizoma	Coptis rhizome	3 g
Huang qin	Scutellariae Baicalensis Radix	Baical skullcap root, scutellaria, scute	6 g
Huang bai	Phellodendri Cortex	Amur corktree bark, phellodendron bark	6 g
Zhi da huang	Rhei Radix et Rhizoma	Honey-cooked rhubarb root and rhizome	6 g
Sheng gan cao	Glycyrrhizae Radix	Fresh licorice root	6 g

Boil the medicine in water into tea and drink.

Qi-deficiency Constipation

When the patient is found distressed in low spirits and physically worn out, panting, with their tongue dilute in color and the coating white, and their pulses weak, then this is a case of qi-deficiency constipation.

Formula for qi-deficiency constipation:

Pin Yin	Latin	English	Dosage
Mi zhi huang qi	Astragali Radix	Honey-processed milk vetch root, astragalus root	30 g
Huo ma ren	Cannabis Sativae Semen	Hemp seed	10 g
Yu li ren	Pruni Semen	Bush cherry pit	10 g
Chen pi	Citri Reticulatae Pericarpium	Tangerine peel	6 g
Bai mi	Mel Millis	Light-colored honey	1 tsp

Boil the medicines in water into tea. Add a spoonful of honey and drink twice a day. Continue the practice as long as you like.

Sweating

Sweating signals the discord between qi and blood, which impairs the opening and closing of the pores. The perspiration can present in two forms, either as spontaneous or night sweats. Patients who have spontaneous sweating both day and night, especially upon exertion, are found to have very weak pulses and thin white tongue coats. Patients who sweat at night when sleeping and stop sweating upon waking up, have small stringy pulses and a very dilute coating upon the tongue. Those who sweat during the day, must be treated by invigorating the qi and strengthening the exterior, while patients with night sweats should be treated by invigorating the yin and clearing the fire, as well as nourishing the blood and heart.

Formula for those who sweat when awake:

Pin Yin	Latin	English	Dosage
Sheng huang qi	Astragali Radix	Fresh milk vetch root, astragalus root	15 g
Chao bai zhu	Atractylodis Macrocephalae Rhizoma	Fried white atractylodes rhizome	9 g
Chao fang feng	Saposhnikoviae Radix	Fried ledebouriella root, saposhnikoviae root, siler	4 g

Pin Yin	Latin	English	Dosage
Bai shao	Paeoniae Alba Radix	White peony root	9 g
Chao dang gui	Angelicae Sinensis Radix	Fried Chinese angelica root, tang-kuei	9 g
Duan mu li	Ostreae Concha	Calcined oyster shell	20 g
Sheng jiang	Zingiberis Officinalis Rhizoma	Fresh ginger rhizome	3 slices
Da zao	Zizyphi Jujubae Fructus	Chinese red date, jujube	6 pieces
Bi tao gan	Prunus Persica Fructus	Immature peach seed	15 g

Boil the medicines into tea and drink twice a day. Continue until symptoms improve.

Formula for those who sweat at night:

Pin Yin	Latin	English	Dosage
Dang gui	Angelicae Sinensis Radix	Chinese angelica root, tang-kuei	10 g
Sheng di huang	Rehmanniae Radix	Chinese foxglove root, fresh rehmannia root	15 g
Wu wei zi	Schisandrae Chinensis Fructus	Schisandra fruit	6 g
Suan zao ren	Ziziphi Spinosae Semen	Spiny zizyphus seeds, sour jujube seeds, zizyphus	12 g
Duan mu li	Ostreae Concha	Calcined oyster shell	20 g
Bai zi ren	Platycladi Semen	Biota seed	10 g
Chao huang bai	Phellodendri Cortex	Fried amur corktree bark, phellodendron bark	6 g
Nuo dao gen xu	Oryzae Glutinosae Radix	Glutinous rice root	30 g

Boil the medicines into tea and drink twice a day.

Tendency to Get Alarmed

In this chronic case the male patient experiences continued fright due to excessive sexual intercourse, which leads to a low sperm count and loss of vitality. The patient may feel sore and soft on the sides of his trunk and in his knees. In the bewilderment and dejection the patient sweats and is unable to control the lower gates, resulting in urinary incontinence and seminal emission. The pulses, particularly the kidneys, are felt to be deficient.

Treatment must be done by invigorating the kidneys and nourishing the whole body.

Formula to dispel fright:

Pin Yin	Latin	English	Dosage
Shu di huang	Rehmanniae Preparata Radix	Prepared Chinese foxglove root (cooked in red wine), cooked rehmannia rhizome	15 g
Shan yao	Dioscoreae Oppositae Rhizoma	Chinese yam, dioscorea rhizome	15 g
Shan zhu yu	Corni Officinalis Fructus	Asiatic Cornelian cherry fruit, cornus	12 g
Fu ling	Poria Cocos Sclerotium	Sclerotium of tuckahoe, poria, China root, hoelen, Indian bread	10 g
Mu dan pi	Moutan Radicis Cortex	Tree peony root bark, moutan root bark	10 g

Pin Yin	Latin	English	Dosage
Yuan zhi	Polygalae Radix	Chinese senega root, polygala root	6 g
Gou qi zi	Lycii Fructus	Chinese wolfberry, matrimony vine fruit, lyceum fruit	12 g
Lu jiao shuang	Cornu Cervi Degelatinatium	Leftover dregs after boiling deer antler glue	10 g

Boil the medicines in water into tea and drink it.

Tendency to be Sad

In this case the patient is always lost in grief and weeps uncontrollably without cause. This kind of chronic brooding injures the heart and mind and sends the other organs into confusion. Other symptoms may include insomnia and sweating and a lack of independent thought. This patient must be mentally enlightened with optimism as well as the following formula.

Formula for treating a patient in great grief:

Pin Yin	Latin	English	Dosage
Sheng mai ya	Hordei Germinatus Fructus	Fresh barley sprout, malt	30 g
Sheng gan cao	Glycyrrhizae Radix	Fresh licorice root	6 g
Da zao	Zizyphi Jujubae Fructus	Chinese date, jujube	12 g
Bai shao	Paeoniae Alba Radix	White peony root	10 g
Fu shen	Poria Cocos Pararadicis Sclerotium	Poria fungus	10 g
Suan zao ren	Ziziphi Spinosae Semen	Spiny zizyphus seeds, sour jujube seeds, zizyphus	10 g
Long chi	Fossilia Dentis Mastodi	Dragon teeth, fossilized teeth	15 g
Wu wei zi	Schisandrae Chinensis Fructus	Schisandra fruit	6 g
Yuan zhi	Polygalae Radix	Chinese senega root, polygala root	6 g

Boil the medicines in water into tea and drink.

Trembling

This usually refers to the quivering of a part of the body, such as the shaking of the head or the trembling of the hands. This is a symptom especially seen in the aged, more frequently occurring in men. The disease arises mainly from overwork, which has squandered the vitality so much that the nervous system becomes out of balance and a deficiency wind invades. In order to take precautions one must always lead an optimistic life, never being molested by melancholia or wrath. The patient should be advised to lessen sexual intercourse and eat more vegetables and less fatty foodstuffs. It is rather difficult to cure such a disease. However, one may still try the following formula to calm down the marauding wind.

Formula for trembling:

Pin Yin	Latin	English	Dosage
Sheng di huang	Rehmanniae Radix	Fresh Chinese foxglove root, fresh rehmannia root	15 g
Shu di huang	Rehmanniae Preparata Rhizoma	Prepared Chinese foxglove root (cooked in red wine), cooked rehmannia rhizome	15 g
Shan zhu yu	Corni Officinalis Fructus	Asiatic Cornelian cherry fruit, cornus	12 g
Gou teng	Ramulus cum Uncis Uncariae	Stems and thorns of the gambir vine, uncaria	15 g
Bai ji li	Tribuli Terrestris Fructus	Caltrop fruit, puncture-vine fruit, tribulus	15 g
Mu li	Ostreae Concha	Oyster shell	30 g
Jing jie	Schizonepetae Herba	Schizonepeta	5 g
Bai shao	Paeoniae Alba Radix	White peony root	10 g
Long chi	Fossilia Dentis Mastodi	Dragon teeth, fossilized teeth	30 g
Ci shi	Magnetitum	Magnetite	30 g
Chuan xiong	Chuanxiong Rhizoma	Chuanxiong root, Szechuan lovage root, cnidium	6 g
Ji zi huang	Gallus	Egg yolk	1 piece

Boil the medicines in water into tea. Stir in the egg yolk and drink. The residue is to be boiled again into tea. Take one dose daily until symptoms improve.

Formulas for Specific Organs

Heart Blood Deficiency

Heart blood deficiency can be a result of chronic loss of blood from bleeding hemorrhoids, excessive menstruation, or from transmission of too much blood. In other cases, it can be due to over-exhaustion from too much work and poor diet so that the patient presents with dizziness, an abnormal heart beat, weakness of the limbs, and a pale face. The tongue is pale white and the pulses feel weak, small, and rapid.

The treatment must focus on the nourishment of heart blood along with guarding against further loss of blood. At the same time, good rest and quality nourishment should be employed to ensure early recovery and good health.

Formula for the nourishment of heart blood:

Pin Yin	Latin	English	Dosage
Dang shen	Codonopsis Pilosulae Radix	Codonopsis root	15 g
Huang qi	Astragali Radix	Milk vetch root, astragalus root	15 g
Bai zhu	Atractylodis Macrocephalae Rhizoma	White atractylodes rhizome	10 g
Shu di huang	Rehmanniae Preparata Rhizoma	Prepared Chinese foxglove root (cooked in red wine), cooked rehmannia rhizome	10 g
Dang gui	Angelicae Sinensis Radix	Chinese angelica root, tang-kuei	10 g
Suan zao ren	Ziziphl Spinosae Semen	Spiny zizyphus seeds, sour jujube seeds, zizyphus	10 g
E jiao	Corii Colla Asini	Donkey hide gelatin	10 g
Yuan zhi	Polygalae Radix	Chinese senega root, polygala root	6 g
Guang mu xiang	Saussureae Lappae Radix or Aucklandia Lappae Radix	Costus root, saussurea, aucklandia from Guangdong Province	6 g
Zhi gan cao	Glycyrrhizae Radix	Honey-fried licorice root	6 g

Boil the medicines into tea and drink twice a day. Continuation of this practice will benefit the patient.

Heart Qi Deficiency

This is the result of long-term hard work in a very low spirit, so much so that the internal organs, especially the heart, are greatly affected or even weighed down. The patient has palpitations, panting from exhaustion, sweating upon slight activity, a pale face, and feeble pulses. Their treatment must include relaxation of their mind and body to obtain a good rest. Special emphasis must be on nourishment of their qi and heart and maintaining a pleasant mood.

Formula for the nourishment of heart *qi*:

Pin Yin	Latin	English	Dosage
Dang shen	Codonopsis Pilosulae Radix	Codonopsis root	15 g
Huang qi	Astragali Radix	Milk vetch root, astragalus root	15 g
Dang gui	Angelicae Sinensis Radix	Chinese angelica root, *tang-kuei*	10 g
Chuan xiong	Chuanxiong Rhizoma	Chuanxiong root, Szechuan lovage root, cnidium	6 g
Zhi gan cao	Glycyrrhizae Radix	Honey-fried licorice root	6 g
Suan zao ren	Ziziphi Spinosae Semen	Spiny zizyphus seeds, sour jujube seeds, zizyphus	10 g
Bai zi ren	Platycladi Semen	Biota seed	10 g
Yuan zhi	Polygalae Radix	Chinese senega root, polygala root	6 g
Wu wei zi	Schisandrae Chinensis Fructus	Schisandra fruit	6 g
Fu ling	Poria Cocos Sclerotium	Sclerotium of tuckahoe, poria, China root, hoelen, Indian bread	9–15 g

Boil the medicines in water into tea and drink twice a day.

Kidney *Yin* Deficiency

In Chinese medicine, the kidneys are considered to be of congenital significance among all the internal organs. If a patient has been worn down with old age or chronic disease, postpartum weakness, excessive sex or masturbation, kidney *yin* deficiency is the result.

When a patient has kidney *yin* deficiency, the signs are: depletion of physique, dizziness, a kind of tinnitus that sounds like a murmuring stream gurgling nearby and diminished hearing. The patient feels sore and soft on the sides and their feet feel exhausted. There are frequent nocturnal emissions and frequent thirst. The tongue is red and the pulses are small and rapid. Inside the lower eyelid the blood vessels no longer run in straight separate lines, but cross over into each other (**Fig. 24a,b**).

Nourish the kidneys and invigorate the *yin* to treat this condition. Rest is advised, supplemented with adequate physical exercises. Sexual intercourse is forbidden.

Formula for the nourishment of the kidneys and invigoration of *yin*:

Pin Yin	Latin	English	Dosage
Sheng di huang	Rehmanniae Radix	Fresh Chinese foxglove root, fresh rehmannia root	15 g
Shu di huang	Rehmanniae Preparata Rhizoma	Prepared Chinese foxglove root (cooked in red wine), cooked rehmannia rhizome	15 g
Shan zhu yu	Corni Officinalis Fructus	Asiatic Cornelian cherry fruit, cornus	12 g
Shan yao	Dioscoreae Oppositae Rhizoma	Chinese yam, dioscorea rhizome	12 g
Fu ling	Poria Cocos Sclerotium	Sclerotium of tuckahoe, poria, China root, hoelen, Indian bread	10 g
Gou qi zi	Lycii Fructus	Chinese wolfberry, matrimony vine fruit, lyceum fruit	9 g
Huai niu xi or niu xi	Achyranthis Bidentatae Radix	Ox-knee root, achyranthes root from Huai	9 g

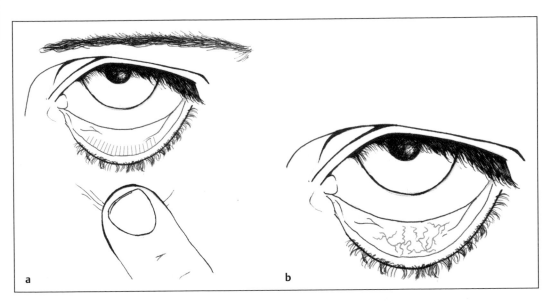

Fig. 24a,b
a Normal: arteries appear as uniform, thin, red, straight lines.
b *Yin* deficiency: artery lines appear squiggly and random, connecting together.

Pin Yin	Latin	Engllsh	Dosage
Tu si zi	Cuscutae Chinensis Semen	Chinese dodder seeds, cuscuta	10 g
Gui ban	Plastrum Testudinis	Tortoise shell	15 g
Sheng yi yi ren	Coicis Semen	Fresh seeds of Job's tears, fresh coix seeds	12 g

Boil the medicines into tea and drink twice a day. Long-term ingestion is beneficial.

Kidney *Yang* Deficiency

A patient suffering from kidney *yang* deficiency feels their hands and feet chilled and looks pale, physically exhausted, and spiritually dejected. There is possible dizziness, tinnitus, aching sides, nocturnal emission, and impotence. There can be either urinary difficulty or incontinence and cock's crow diarrhea or running bowels. Other possible signs are edema all over the body, shortness of breath, and panting.

Formula to mildly nourish the kidney *yang*:

Pin Yin	Latin	English	Dosage
Fu zi	Aconiti Lateralis Praeparata Radix	Aconite	10 g
Rou gui	Cinnamomi Cassiae Cortex	Inner bark of Saigon cinnamon	3 g
Shu di huang	Rehmanniae Preparata Rhizoma	Prepared Chinese foxglove root (cooked in wine), cooked rehmannia rhizome	15 g
Shan yao	Dioscoreae Oppositae Rhizoma	Chinese yam, dioscorea rhizome	15 g
Shan zhu yu	Corni Officinalis Fructus	Asiatic Cornelian cherry fruit, cornus	12 g

Pin Yin	Latin	English	Dosage
Sheng yi yi ren	Coicis Semen	Fresh seeds of Job's tears, fresh coix seeds	30 g
Fu ling	Poria Cocos Sclerotium	Sclerotium of tuckahoe, poria, China root, hoelen, Indian bread	20 g
Chao ze xie	Alismatis Rhizoma	Water plantain rhizome, alisma rhizome	10 g
Huai niu xi or niu xi	Achyranthis Bidentatae Radix	Ox-knee root, achyranthes root from Huai	10 g
Bai zhu	Atractylodis Macrocephalae Rhizoma	White atractylodes rhizome	6 g
Cang zhu	Atractylodis Rhizoma	Black atractylodes rhizome	6 g

Boil the medicines into tea and drink twice a day. This formula can be taken long term.

We have given a brief introduction to the symptoms and treatment of the deficiency of internal organs. They are so closely interrelated as an entity that clinical investigation/analysis should be made according to concrete conditions before the doctor comes to any conclusion or decision. For instance, in the case of heart disease, there can be deficiency in both heart *qi* and blood, or deficiency in both heart and spleen. In the case of liver diseases there can be deficiency both in the liver and in the kidneys. Spleen diseases may involve lungs and spleen *qi* deficiency or spleen or kidney *yin* deficiency, and so on. That is to say, the internal organs are so closely interrelated and interactive with each other that we have to use our discretion and display flexibility according to concrete conditions before we can be sure of our of treatment.

Liver *Yin* Deficiency

According to Chinese medicine theory, the liver is equipped with a versatile capacity for the regulation and restoration of the physical strength of the body. It is also a storage tank of blood to help facilitate the smooth transmission of *qi* and blood throughout the body and help the digestive system. When overwork and a lack of rest have become chronic the patient becomes depressed and irritable and the digestive and absorbing function of the system will suffer. In other cases, the patient may have been born with an innate blood defect, such as a chemical or viral toxicity or a genetic anomaly that leaves the circulatory system in need of sufficient blood. In some cases, the blood is harmful enough to deteriorate the function of the liver, so that the circulating blood fails to meet the urgent demands of the whole body. That is why the patient feels terribly exhausted and always dizzy as if going to fall due to their feeble limbs. The patient feels their sides aching slightly and presents with a red tongue without coating. The pulses on the left arm are small and stringy. This is called liver *yin* deficiency or liver blood deficiency.

Formula for the nourishment of liver blood:

Pin Yin	Latin	English	Dosage
Dang gui	Angelicae Sinensis Radix	Chinese angelica root, *tang-kuei*	15 g
Sheng di huang	Rehmanniae Radix	Chinese foxglove root, fresh rehmannia root	15 g
Bai shao	Paeoniae Alba Radix	White peony root	10 g
Chuan xiong	Chuanxiong Rhizoma	Chuanxiong root, Szechuan lovage root, cnidium	6 g

Pin Yin	Latin	English	Dosage
Gou qi zi	Lycii Fructus	Chinese wolfberry, matrimony vine fruit, lyceum fruit	10 g
Nu zhen zi	Ligustri Lucidi Fructus	Privet fruit, ligustrum	10 g
Wu wei zi	Schisandrae Chinensis Fructus	Schisandra fruit	6 g

Boil the medicines into tea and drink twice a day. Long-term ingestion will benefit the patient.

Liver *qi* deficiency is a rather rare case, so it is not dealt with here.

Lung *Qi* Deficiency

According to Chinese medicine, the lungs work not only as an organ of breathing, but are also involved in the distribution of water. Known as the "tender organ," they are easily hurt by outside influences. Lung *qi* deficiency always comes as a result of a chronic condition or habit, such as a teacher or a singer who, because of the overuse of the voice, enfeebles their breath *qi*. Dysfunction in other organ systems can adversely affect the lungs, as well.

The patient with lung *qi* deficiency may experience panting, a low speaking voice, cough, diluted phlegm, spontaneous sweating, aversion to wind or a tendency to catch colds. The tongue has a white coat and the *cun* pulse of the right arm feels deficient, deep, and small.

The treatment must be focused on invigoration of the lung *qi*. Counsel the patient to create an agreeable environment, neither too warm nor too cold. The diet must be well adapted to their health and regular routine. Neither smoking nor drinking are allowed and very little sexual intercourse should be engaged in.

Formula for the nourishment of lung *qi*:

Pin Yin	Latin	English	Dosage
Dang shen	Codonopsis Pilosulae Radix	Codonopsis root	15 g
Bai zhu	Atractylodis Macrocephalae Rhizoma	White atractylodes rhizome	10 g
Fu ling	Poria Cocos Sclerotium	Sclerotium of tuckahoe, poria, China root, hoelen, Indian bread	10 g
Wu wei zi	Schisandrae Chinensis Fructus	Schisandra fruit	6 g
E jiao	Corii Colla Asini	Donkey hide gelatin	10 g
Sang bai pi	Mori Cortex	Mulberry root bark, morus bark	9 g
Chuan bei mu	Fritillariae Cirrhosae Bulbus	Szechuan fritillaria bulb, tendrilled, fritillaria	6 g
Xing ren	Armeniacae Semen	Apricot kernel	9 g
Gan cao	Glycyrrhizae Radix	Licorice root	6 g

Boil the medicines into tea and drink twice a day. This formula can be taken long term.

Lung *Yin* Deficiency

Lung *yin* deficiency results from the loss of so much saliva that the lungs have insufficient moisture to support their normal workings. So the patient has a dry cough without phlegm or with phlegm that is dry and sticky. There may be a cough with phlegm stained with blood or blood clots. As a rule, when *yin* is in a state of insufficiency, then *yang* will flourish. When evening fades out like a shadow into night, the patient will sweat and become fidgety and sleepless. Very small yet rapid pulses are felt and the tongue has little coating.

The treatment must be focused on moistening the lung *yin*, as in the treatment of lung *qi* deficiency, and make the patient magnanimously light-hearted, without being troubled by daily worries.

Formula for the moistening of lung *yin*:

Pin Yin	Latin	English	Dosage
Sheng di huang	Rehmanniae Radix	Fresh Chinese foxglove root, fresh rehmannia root	15 g
Mai men dong	Ophiopogonis Radix	Ophiopogon tuber	15 g
Xuan shen	Scrophulariae Radix	Ningpo figwort root, scrophularia	9 g
Chuan bei mu	Fritillariae Cirrhosae Bulbus	Szechuan fritillaria bulb, tendrilled, fritillaria	6 g
Bai shao	Paeoniae Alba Radix	White peony root	9 g
Gan cao	Glycyrrhizae Radix	Licorice root	6 g
Jie geng	Platycodi Radix	Root of balloonflower, platycodon root	6 g
Sha shen[a]	Adenophorae seu Glehniae Radix	Adenophora root or glehnia root	9 g
Bei sha shen[a]	Glehniae Littoralis Radix	Coastal glehnia root	9 g
Di gu pi	Lycii Radicis Cortex	Cortex of wolfberry root, lyceum bark	9 g
Bie jia	Carapax Amydae Sinensis	Chinese soft-shelled turtle shell	12 g

[a] Harvested in spring, autumn.
Boil the medicines into tea and drink twice a day. Long-term administration of this formula is helpful.

Spleen *Qi* Deficiency

The main function of the spleen is to help transport and dissolve the mixture of the grain and water. Many factors may have an unfavorable impact upon its normal functioning. When the patient is heavily burdened with deep thinking or has been greatly exhausted by heavy labor and an irregular habit of eating, this will greatly inhibit the normal function of spleen and stomach. If such a way of life has been practiced a long time, the patient will have a pale face, weak limbs, and talk intermittently with panting. If the patient has running bowels through eating a simple, moderate diet, the tongue coating is white and the right arm pulses are deficient, small, and weak. These are typical signs of spleen *qi* deficiency, also called "*zhong jiao*" deficiency. For treatment, strengthen and invigorate the spleen *qi* of the patient.

Formula for strengthening the spleen *qi*:

Pin Yin	Latin	English	Dosage
Dang shen	Codonopsis Pilosulae Radix	Codonopsis root	15 g
Chao bai zhu	Atractylodis Macrocephalae Rhizoma	Fried white atractylodes rhizome	10 g
Fu ling	Poria Cocos Sclerotium	Sclerotium of tuckahoe, poria, China root, hoelen, Indian bread	10 g
Zhi gan cao	Glycyrrhizae Radix	Honey-fried licorice root	6 g

Pin Yin	Latin	English	Dosage
Sheng jiang	Zingiberis Officinalis Rhizoma	Fresh ginger rhizome	3 g
Da zao	Zizyphi Jujubae Fructus	Chinese date, jujube	10 g
Chen pi	Citri Reticulatae Pericarpium	Tangerine peel	6 g

Boil the medicines into tea and drink twice a day.

In addition to the symptoms described above, if the patient suffers from edema all over the body, feels cold, prefers hot drinks, has very pale urine, and the pulses on the right arm feel small and deep, this is spleen *yang* deficiency. The treatment strategy should be to warm up the *yang* in order to excrete the dampness.

Formula for strengthening the spleen *yang* and excreting the dampness:

Pin Yin	Latin	English	Dosage
Zhi fu zi	Aconiti Lateralis Praeparata Radix	Processed aconite	8 g
Chao bai zhu	Atractylodis Macrocephalae Rhizoma	Fried white atractylodes rhizome	10 g
Fu ling	Poria Cocos Sclerotium	Sclerotium of tuckahoe, poria, China root, hoelen, Indian bread	30 g
Wei jiang	Zingiberis Officinalis Recens Rhizoma	Baked ginger	3 g
Zhi gan cao	Glycyrrhizae Radix	Honey-fried licorice root	6 g
Cao guo	Fructus Amomi Tsao-Ko	Tsaoko amomum fruit	3 g
Huang qi	Astragali Radix	Milk vetch root, astragalus root	15 g
Da fu pi	Arecae Catechu Pericarpium	Betel husk, areca peel	9 g
Chi xiao dou	Phaseoli Calcarati Semen	Aduki bean	30 g

Boil the medicines into tea and drink twice a day. Continue until the edema resolves.

Spleen *Yin* Deficiency

In this case the patient is very depleted. Signs and symptoms include weak hands and feet, poor appetite, stuffy bowels, constipation, dry mouth, and tongue. The tongue is scarlet and the pulses on the right arm are small and rapid. This is a case of spleen *yin* deficiency. The treatment strategy is to nourish the spleen *yin* and at the same time the patient should rest well, abstain from smoking, consuming wine or any food that is pungent, spicy, or deep-fried in oil.

Formula for the nourishment of spleen *yin*:

Pin Yin	Latin	English	Dosage
Nan sha shen	Adenophorae seu Glehniae Radix	Adenophora root or glehnia root, ladybell root	10 g
Mai men dong	Ophiopogonis Radix	Ophiopogon tuber	10 g
Shan yao	Dioscoreae Oppositae Rhizoma	Chinese yam, dioscorea rhizome	10 g

Pin Yin	Latin	English	Dosage
Fu ling	Poria Cocos Sclerotium	Sclerotium of tuckahoe, poria, China root, hoelen, Indian bread	10 g
Shi hu	Dendrobii Herba	Dendrobium	10 g
Bai shao	Paeoniae Alba Radix	White peony root	10 g
Bai bian dou	Lablab Semen Album	White hyacinth bean	10 g
Chao gu ya	Oryzae Germinatus Fructus	Fried rice sprout	20 g
Zhi gan cao	Glycyrrhizae Radix	Honey-fried licorice root	6 g

Boil the medicines into tea and drink twice a day.

Appendix 2: Pulse Legend

CP	Complementary position	
DP	Diaphragm position	Informs us about the condition of *qi* stagnation in the chest-diaphragm area measured by degree of inflation felt at that position. Left diaphragm: If significantly inflated we have reason to believe that the person is repressing tender feelings and substituting angry ones as a form of protecting their vulnerable heart feelings. If the situation is severe the right diaphragm will also be inflated at the same time to the same degree. Right diaphragm: When this side is inflated the reason is usually lifting beyond a person's 'energy.' Bilateral inflation: Trauma is another etiology for which the history is usually available.
EP	Esophageal position	
FI	First impressions	
LB	Lower burner	
L,R-DP	Distal positions	
L,R-MP	Middle positions	
L,R-PP	Proximal positions	
LS	Left side	
MB	Middle burner	
MV	Mitral valve	
NP	Neurological positions	
PLB	Pelvic lower body	
PP	Principal positions	
RS	Right side	
SI	Small intestine	This position informs us of the functional condition of the physical small intestines; excess heat, inflammation, stagnation of *qi*, food, damp, and strength.
SLP	Special lung positions	These bilateral positions inform us of the functional condition of the anatomical lung on the opposite side of the body beyond the regular lung position (right distal). It gives us a more in-depth picture of the past history of the lung as well as the present.
SPEP	Stomach-pylorus extension	
UB	Upper burner	
~	Transient	The pulse quality occurs occasional-intermittent.

References

Bibliography to Introduction

AOM. Pioneers & Leaders: A Commemorative Book of Challenge and Courage, Volume 1 1982–2007. A collaborative work of the American Association of Acupuncture and Oriental Medicine (AAAOM), the National Certification Commission for Acupuncture and Oriental Medicine (NCCAOM), the Council of Colleges for Acupuncture and Oriental Medicine (CCAOM), and the Accreditation Commission for Acupuncture and Oriental Medicine (ACCAOM); 2007

Hammer LI. Chinese Pulse Diagnosis: A Contemporary Approach. Seattle: Eastland Press; 2001

Hammer LI. Dragon Rises Red Bird Flies. Seattle: Eastland Press; 2005

Maciocia G, et al. In memoriam, Dr. John Shen. J Chin Med 2001;67:22

References to Dr. Shen's Formulas in Systems

Bensky D, Clavey S. Stöger S. Chinese Herbal Medicine Materia Medica. 3rd ed. Seattle: Eastland Press; 2004.

Fruehauf H. Qianyang Dan: A key formula of the Sichuan fire spirit school. An in-depth interview with Heiner Fruehauf. www. Classicalchinesemedicine.org; 2009

Hammer LI. Dragon Rises, Red Bird Flies. New York: Station Hill Press; 1990

Hammer LI. Towards a unified theory of chronic disease: with regard to the separation of yin and yang and "the qi is wild." Oriental Medicine 1998;6;2&3:15

Hammer LI. Chinese Pulse Diagnosis: A Contemporary Approach. Seattle: Eastland Press; 2001

Hammer LI. Dragon Rises Red Bird Flies. Revised ed. Seattle: Eastland Press; 2005

Hammer LI. The concept of "blocks": structure. The American Acupuncturist 2006;38:25

Hammer LI. Awareness in Chinese medicine. The American Acupuncturist 2007;41

Hammer LI. The liver in Chinese medicine. Medical Acupuncture 2009;21;3:173–178

Hammer LI. Case study—stopping long-term strenuous exercise suddenly: an epidemic treated with Chinese herbal medicine. Chinese Medicine Times 2011a;6:1

Hammer LI. The relationship between the kidney and heart in Chinese medicine, part one. Chinese Medicine Times, 2011b;6:3

Jacob J. The Acupuncturist's Clinical Handbook. New York: Integrative Wellness; 1996

Jio Shu-De. Ten Lectures on the Use of Formulas from the Personal Experience of Jiao Shu-De. Edited by Nigel Wiseman. New Mexico: Paradigm Publications; 2005

Maciocia G. The Foundations of Chinese Medicine. New York: Churchill Livingstone; 1989

Maciocia G. Obstetrics and Gynecology in Chinese Medicine. 8th ed. New York: Churchill Livingstone; 1997

MEDLINE, Unified Medical Language System (UMLS): http://ghr.nlm.nih.gov/glossary=meconium.

Mitchel C, Ye F, Wiseman N. Shang Han Lun on Cold Damage. New Mexico: Paradigm Publications; 1999

Scheid V, Bensky D, Ellis A, Barolet R. Chinese Herbal Medicine: Formulas and Strategies. 2nd ed. Seattle: Eastland Press; 2009

References to Dr. Shen's Life-cycle Formulas

Hammer LI. The Chinese medical model in thyroid disease. American Journal of Acupuncture1982;10(1): 1–17

Hammer LI. Towards a unified theory of chronic disease: with regard to the separation of yin and yang and "the qi is wild." Oriental Medicine 1998;6;2&3:15

Hammer LI. Chinese Pulse Diagnosis: A Contemporary Approach. Seattle: Eastland Press; 2001

Hammer LI, Heffron R, Leavy K. Inflammation in atherosclerosis. Medical Acupuncture 2003;15:2

Hammer LI. Dragon Rises Red Bird Flies. Seattle: Eastland Press; 2005

Hammer LI, Rosen R. The pulse, the electronic age and radiation: early detection. The American Acupuncturist 2009; 49

Hammer LI. A discussion of terrain, stress, root and vulnerability. Chinese Medicine Times 2010a;5:1

Hammer LI. Science east and west. Medical Acupuncture 2010b;22:2

Hammer LI. Case study—stopping long-term strenuous exercise suddenly: an epidemic treated with Chinese herbal medicine. Chinese Medicine Times 2011;6:1

Indexes

General Index

Pin Yin Pharmaceutical Index

F

Fang feng Saposhnikoviae Radix 2, 4, 39, 40, 41, 43, 45, 89, 90, 106, 107, 112, 113, 119, 123, 129, 131, 143, 155, 156, 165, 166, 167, 168, 189, 194, 205, 224, 234, 247, 250, 259, 265

Fen zhi zi Gardeniae jasminoidis Fructus 108, 197, 251

Feng mi Mel Millis 44, 206, 225

Fo shou Citri Sarcodactylis Fructus 6, 56, 63, 102, 212, 230, 239

Fu hai shi Costaziae Os 163

Fu ling Poria Cocos Sclerotium 9, 12, 14, 16, 23, 24, 48, 49, 54, 57, 58, 59, 62, 63, 64, 72, 76, 80, 86, 101, 103, 120, 121, 125, 126, 132, 141, 145, 147, 149, 172, 173, 174, 184, 203, 211, 212, 214, 222, 227, 228, 231, 232, 233, 236, 237, 241, 242, 243, 250, 252, 253, 257, 263, 268, 272, 274, 275, 276, 277, 278

Fu pen zi Rubi Fructus 66, 174

Fu ping Lemnae seu Spirodelae Herba 202

Fu shen Poria Cocos Pararadicis Sclerotium 7, 8, 9, 11, 13, 19, 33, 51, 119, 128, 180, 188, 230, 238, 249, 269

Fu xiao mai or *xiao mai* Tritici Levis Fructus 33

Fu zi Aconiti Lateralis Praeparata Radix 15, 32, 146, 213, 249, 273

G

Gan cao Glycyrrhizae Radix 2, 33, 37, 38, 39, 40, 41, 42, 43, 44, 45, 48, 78, 94, 96, 97, 105, 126, 134, 141, 151, 152, 167, 168, 193, 194, 203, 205, 215, 216, 222, 234, 236, 251, 253, 255, 259, 260, 275, 276

Gan jiang Zingiberis Rhizoma 59, 60, 69, 71, 79, 83, 84, 146, 172, 178, 210, 221, 249

Gan ju hua Chrysanthemi Flos 216

Gao li shen Ginseng Coreensis Radix 15, 20, 61, 87, 181, 209

Gao liang jiang Alpiniae Officinari Rhizoma 31, 144, 221

Gao liang jiu 108, 197

Ge gen Puerariae Radix 37, 90, 106, 107, 112, 125, 127, 129, 131, 134, 155, 156, 165, 166, 189, 199, 202, 224, 234, 249

Ge jie Gekko Gecko Linnaeus 10, 87, 158, 209

Gou ji Cibotii Rhizoma 109, 110, 123, 146

Gou qi zi Lycii Fructus 46, 102, 109, 115, 128, 137, 152, 179, 182, 217, 227, 233, 243, 249, 257, 269, 272, 275

Gou teng Ramulus cum Uncis Uncariae 134, 179, 247, 249, 265, 270

Gu jing cao Eriocauli Flos 151, 152, 243

Gu ya Oryzae Germinatus Fructus 25, 54, 63, 64, 78, 85, 92, 177, 185, 193

Gua lou pi Trichosanthis Pericarpium 11, 13, 14, 20, 22, 35, 55, 56, 60, 90, 125, 127, 130, 138, 139, 184, 217, 222, 223, 230, 234, 240

Guang mu xiang Saussureae Lappae Radix or Aucklandia Lappae Radix 121, 271

Gui ban Plastrum Testudinis 273

Gui zhi Ramulus Cinnamomi Cassiae 105, 107, 131, 156, 157, 226, 234, 241, 247, 249, 265

H

Hai jin sha Lygodii Japonici Spora 254

Hai piao xiao Sepiae Endoconcha 140, 144

Hai zao Sargassum 137, 140

Han fang ji Stephaniae Tetrandrae Radix 34, 107

Han lian cao Ecliptae Prostratae Herba 41, 139, 240

He huan pi Albiziae Cortex 33

He shou wu Polygoni Multiflori Radix 33, 103, 147, 259, 260, 261

He ye Nelumbinis Folium 92

Hei dou Semen Glycines Hispidae 261

Hei fang feng Saposhnikoviae Radix 3

Hei shan zhi zi Gardeniae jasminoidis Fructus 2, 39, 43, 72, 133, 167, 172, 216, 225

Hei zhi ma Sesami Nigrum Semen 157

Hong hua Carthami Tinctorii Flos 34, 68, 73, 80, 83, 84, 97, 106, 111, 113, 120, 122, 129, 173, 178, 211, 234, 250, 264, 266

Hong tang Saccharum 207

Hou po Magnoliae Officinalis Cortex 60, 68, 84, 130, 145, 178, 222

Hu po, Succinum 34, 35, 248, 255

Hu tao ren Juglandis Regiae Semen 157

Hu zhang Polygoni Cuspidati Radix et Rhizoma 2, 251, 252, 253, 254

Hua shi Talcum 252, 255

Huai hua Sophorae Flos 139

Huai jiao Sophorae Fructus 139

Huai niu xi Achyranthis Bidentatae Radix 16, 68, 69, 79, 80, 87, 120, 128, 136, 139, 148, 149, 210, 211, 232, 236, 238, 242, 243, 247, 248, 272, 274

Huang bai Phellodendri Cortex 41, 42, 136, 144, 154, 168, 186, 213, 216, 228, 251, 252, 259, 267

Huang dou Glycine 185

Huang lian Coptidis Rhizoma 7, 9, 23, 34, 59, 60, 64, 133, 141, 146, 154, 186, 188, 212, 221, 230, 248, 252, 257, 267

Huang qi Astragali Radix 23, 24, 61, 74, 83, 90, 93, 126, 128, 173, 176, 181, 183, 184, 213, 224, 236, 237, 238, 243, 244, 257, 271, 272, 277

Huang qin Scutallariae Baicalensis Radix 3, 9, 12, 14, 22, 39, 41, 43, 48, 54, 60, 62, 64, 79, 84, 104, 149, 167, 178, 183, 189, 230, 239, 243, 254, 261, 267

Huang yao zi Dioscoreae Bulbiferae Rhizoma 140, 144, 213

Huo ma ren Cannabis Sativae Semen 198, 267

Huo xiang Agastaches seu Pogostemi Herba 48

P

Pang da hai Sterculiae Lychnophorae Semen 45
Pao jiang Rhizoma Zingiberis Officinalis 220
Pei lan Eupatorii Herba 92
Pi pa ye Eriobotryae Folium 140, 143, 164
Ping guo Malum 192
Pu gong ying Taraxaci Herba 137

Q

Qian cao gen Rubiae Radix 264
Qian hu Peucedani Radix 200
Qian shi Euryales Ferocis Semen 146, 218
Qiang huo Notopterygii Rhizoma et Radix 4, 36, 37, 83, 84, 89, 106, 107, 110, 111, 112, 113, 114, 122, 129, 134, 143, 146, 155, 165, 166, 178, 179, 199, 232, 233, 234, 250
Qin jiao Gentianae Qinjiao Radix 247, 249
Qin pi Fraxini Cortex 220
Qing dai Indigo Pulverata Levis 203
Qing feng teng Sinomenii Caulis 215
Qing hao Artemisiae Annuae Herba 48, 125, 257
Qing pi Citri Reticulatae Viridae Pericarpium 60, 137, 138, 221, 240, 250, 261, 264
Quan gua lou Trichosanthis Fructus 137
Quan xie Buthus Martensi 134, 265

R

Ren dong teng Lonicerae Caulis 215
Ren shen Ginseng Radix 15, 32, 49, 77, 87, 126, 238, 244, 249
Rou cong rong Cistanches Herba 66, 88, 128, 157, 233, 244
Rou gui Cinnamomi Cassiae Cortex 18, 19, 32, 57, 69, 71, 113, 146, 172, 192, 210, 213, 221, 236, 273
Rou wu mei Pruni Mume Fructus 220
Ru xiang Gummi Olibanumi 113, 129, 130, 234

S

Sa zao Zizyphi Jujubae Fructus 184
San leng Sparganii Stoloniferi Rhizoma 138, 240
San qi Notoginseng Radix 31, 88, 109, 110, 111, 114, 116, 119, 122, 184, 195, 208, 223, 227, 234
San yu cao 31
Sang bai pi Mori Cortex 43, 275
Sang ji sheng Taxilli Herba 4, 20, 22, 23, 25, 35, 36, 57, 68, 107, 111, 112, 114, 116, 120, 143, 179, 194, 227
Sang shen Mori Albae Fructus 261
Sang ye Folium Mori 43, 202
Sang zhi Ramulus Mori Albae 4, 25, 107, 112, 123, 247
Sha ren Amomi Fructus 6, 54, 59, 144, 146, 220, 221
Sha shen Adenophorae seu Glehniae Radix 257, 276
Sha yuan zi Astragali Complanati Semen 140
Shan dou gen Menispermi Rhizoma/ Sophorae Tonkinensis Radix 96, 136
Shan yao Dioscoreae Oppositae Rhizoma 24, 31, 46, 54, 57, 62, 76, 83, 103, 115, 121, 126, 128, 145, 146, 157, 173, 178, 182, 183, 184, 209, 232, 233, 238, 257, 268, 272, 273, 277
Shan zha Crataegi Fructus 60, 145, 183, 200
Shan zhi zi Gardeniae jasminoidis Fructus 189, 202, 205, 221, 228, 234
Shan zhu yu Corni Officinalis Fructus 47, 57, 58, 62, 103, 118, 128, 139, 157, 182, 227, 232, 237, 240, 244, 268, 270, 272, 273
She chuang zi Cnidii Fructus 66, 174, 228
She gan Belamcandae Rhizoma 44, 167, 205
She tui Serpentis Exuviae 204
Shen jin cao Lycopodii Herba 113
Shen qu Massa Medicata Fermentata 40, 48, 59, 60, 90, 145, 168, 184, 189, 199, 202, 222, 226
Sheng bai zhu Atractylodis Macrocephalae Rhizoma 174

Sheng cang zhu Atractylodis Rhizoma 215
Sheng da huang Rehi Rhizoma et Radix 254
Sheng dang shen Codonopsis Pilosulae Radix 257, 264
Sheng di huang Rehmannia Radix 38, 44, 45, 46, 47, 55, 61, 68, 72, 84, 94, 96, 97, 109, 133, 146, 151, 172, 179, 211, 212, 215, 243, 244, 247, 248, 255, 256, 258, 260, 261, 263, 268, 270, 272, 274, 276
Sheng fang feng Saphoshnikoviae Radix 203
Sheng gan cao Glycyrrhizae Radix 92, 100, 121, 132, 133, 153, 174, 215, 221, 225, 228, 250, 252, 261, 266, 267, 269
Sheng huai hua mi Sophorae Japonicae Flos 258
Sheng huang qi Astragali Radix 34, 47, 212, 257, 264, 265, 267
Sheng jiang pian Rhizoma Zingiberis Officinalis 265
Sheng jiang Zingiberis Officinalis Recens Rhizoma 40, 85, 174, 177, 185, 190, 192, 207, 268, 277
Sheng jing jie Schizonepetae Herba 203
Sheng ma Cimicifugae Rhizoma 181, 182
Sheng mai ya Hordei Germinatus Fructus 269
Sheng mi ren Oryza Sativa 215
Sheng mu li Concha Ostreae 213
Sheng shan yao Dioscoreae Oppositae Rhizoma 47
Sheng yi yi ren Coicis Semen 38, 92, 149, 215, 228, 233, 236, 241, 242, 273, 274
Sheng zhi shi Fructus Immaturus Citri Aurantii 132, 250
Shi chang pu Acori Tatarinowii Rhizoma 3, 7, 8, 9, 11, 12, 13, 23, 24, 32, 33, 51, 68, 124, 127, 128, 130, 132, 184, 188, 189, 217, 230, 244, 248, 251, 263
Shi fen 235
Shi gao Gypsum Fibrosum 215, 256
Shi hu Dendrobii Herba 54, 55, 62, 63, 64, 223, 257, 278
Shi jun zi Quisqualis Fructus 216

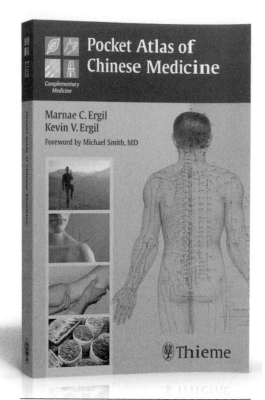

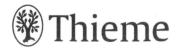

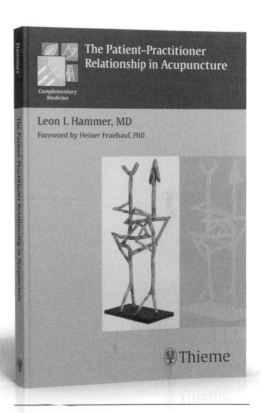
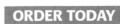

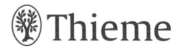